The Duke University
Medical Center
Book of Arthritis

Also in the Duke University Medical Center Series:

**THE DUKE UNIVERSITY MEDICAL CENTER
BOOK OF DIET AND FITNESS**

The Duke University Medical Center Book of Arthritis

David S. Pisetsky, M.D., Ph.D.
with Susan Flamholtz Trien

FAWCETT COLUMBINE

NEW YORK

A Fawcett Columbine Book
Published by Ballantine Books

Copyright © 1992 by the Duke University Medical Center and Engel & Engel, Inc.

All rights reserved under International and Pan-American Copyright
Conventions. Published in the United States by Ballantine Books,
a division of Random House, Inc., New York, and simultaneously
in Canada by Random House of Canada Limited, Toronto.

Library of Congress Catalog Card Number: 94-94637

ISBN: 0-449-90887-9

Cover design by Judy Herbstman

Manufactured in the United States of America

First Ballantine Books Trade Paperback Edition: April 1995

10 9 8 7 6 5 4 3 2 1

Contents

Acknowledgments

This book represents a highpoint in my association with an outstanding group of physicians, nurses, and other health professionals at the Duke University Medical Center and its affiliate, the Durham VA Hospital. These institutions have been my academic home, and I want to especially acknowledge at Duke Dr. Ralph Snyderman, Chancellor of Health Affairs, Dr. Joseph Greenfield, Chairman of the Department of Medicine, and Dr. Barton Haynes, Chief of the Division of Rheumatology and Immunology. Together, they have maintained the strong medical tradition at Duke and have provided an environment where excellence in patient care, teaching, and research are so valued. Dr. Snyderman, my first division chief, brought me to the faculty at Duke in 1978 and has ever since been a friend, guide, and role model.

Many colleagues, friends, and neighbors have read chapters of this book at various stages of development. Their comments and insights were very valuable in assuring relevance and accuracy and are greatly appreciated. Dr. Stephen Lang, my good neighbor in Durham and surgeon at Duke, reviewed the chapter on orthopedics and provided many useful suggestions. While Duke is an amalgam of individuals with their own approaches to patient care, I have tried to distill a set of principles that could fairly be called the Duke approach. Some of the opinions expressed in the book necessarily reflect my own clinical experience and philosophy, although its overall content is representative of a shared perspective.

Over the years, I have been a physician to a large number of patients whose struggles with arthritis are truly the foundation of this book. By sharing with me their life stories, concerns, and feelings, these very fine people have taught me much about arthritis and what it means to be a patient. Their good humor, despite pain and adversity, and appreciation of my efforts as their doctor have been a source of inspiration in my writing and one of my greatest satisfactions as a physician.

Finally, I would like to thank my family, who have been so supportive during the writing of this book. My parents, Lillian and Joseph, have encouraged me in all my life's endeavors and have always wanted me to be a good doctor in its highest sense. There is a special pleasure for me in writing a book on arthritis since my father, also a doctor, loves medical books and can now have a volume in his collection with our family name. My children, Emily and Michael, have had to endure dad's scribbling in notebooks and proofreading when we should have been playing. They are great children and I want to thank them for completely ignoring my requests for peace and quiet; without their interruptions and joyful mischief, writing this book would have been much less fun. Finally, I want to thank my wife Ingrid. Her grace and equanimity make everything in our lives much better and were unfailing during my time as author. This book is therefore dedicated to my family, with love and appreciation.

—*David S. Pisetsky, M.D., Ph.D.*

I would like to thank the Arthritis Foundation of Genesee Valley for graciously inviting me to attend arthritis support group meetings and the Monroe County Medical Society for granting me complete access to their videotape library. A special thanks to my family—David, Stacey, and Adam—who are always there to lend support; and to my literary agent Lynn Seligman.

—*Susan Flamholtz Trien*

The Duke University Medical Center Book of Arthritis

Introduction

This book is an outgrowth of my long-standing professional interest in arthritis and immunology. I am Professor of Medicine at Duke University and also see arthritis patients regularly at the nearby Durham Veterans Administration Hospital, where I am chief of the rheumatology division. In addition, I am actively involved in arthritis research and teach medical students, house staff, and fellows. This marriage of laboratory research, patient care, and teaching has given me valuable insights on arthritis from several perspectives.

I first came to Duke University Medical Center in 1978, when I was fortunate enough to be asked to join the faculty. Duke is considered to have one of the most distinguished rheumatology divisions in the country, and it has a strong commitment to research.

My tenure at Duke has been professionally rewarding, but through the years I've become concerned with the lack of understanding about arthritis among patients and their families. Some of the most alarming and discouraging misconceptions are the prevailing notions that there's nothing to be done for arthritis; that everybody gets it; and that you just have to grin and bear it. Perhaps these misconceptions have taken hold because rheumatology, the study of arthritic diseases, is a relatively new medical specialty. When I came to Durham, North Carolina, more than a decade ago, there were very few rheumatologists in the entire state; now there are probably fifty to a hundred specialists. Though there are now thousands of rheumatologists nationwide, a large part of the country still doesn't have access to this type of specialty care.

One of my goals in writing this book is to let everyone know that there *are* things to be done for arthritis. I'd like you to be aware that early medical intervention *can* affect the course of your disease significantly, and that there are many good treatments available, no matter what form of arthritis you may have.

I've devoted my professional life to patient care and arthritis research. I see *The Duke University Medical Center Book of Arthritis* as an opportunity to share with you some of the more important and intriguing aspects of current research. I have tried to make some of the complex concepts and terminology more accessible so that you can be better informed about the latest developments in the field.

This book also gives me the opportunity to increase public awareness of arthritis. Arthritis affects nearly forty million people in the United States. Though it is not usually a life-threatening disease, it can be a lifelong problem. I feel that, as a nation, we should begin to recognize that arthritis can be a potentially serious medical problem and that we need to learn all we can about it so that it can be diagnosed and treated early on.

In the writing of this book, I've tried to address readers as I do my patients. Health professionals at Duke believe it is important to practice what could be called an old-fashioned approach to medicine. We like to spend time talking to patients so we can get to know them better and can make sure they understand their condition and the possible treatment options. We try to treat our patients intelligently and, when appropriate, encourage them to participate in medical decisions.

Having you understand your condition is an important part of your therapy. You're more likely to take your medicine and adhere to your treatment regimen; you also feel more in control of your life and have the sense that you and your doctor are partners in planning your care.

Sometimes doctors—including me—get too busy to give as lengthy an explanation of your illness and treatment options as we might wish. This book gives me the opportunity to give you the explanations I'd ideally like to provide each patient and to walk you through treatment decisions at a more leisurely pace. I'll discuss, for example, why your physician may choose to order a detailed workup for certain types of arthritis and simpler workups for others; or how physicians make treatment choices by weighing the possible benefits of a drug against the potential risks of taking it. I hope this book will be reassuring to you as a patient and help you see that doctors are indeed very concerned about their patients' welfare, though they may not always have the time to express these concerns to you.

The book is divided into four major parts. Part One, "What's Happening to Me?", acquaints you with the basic facts and dispels some of the misconceptions surrounding arthritis. You'll learn what goes wrong in the arthritic joint, which specialists to consult if you think you have arthritis, and what specific types of tests doctors use to diagnose various forms of arthritis.

Part Two, "What Kind of Arthritis Do I Have?", provides you with in-depth descriptions of the major forms of arthritis. You may wish to focus on those particular chapters that apply to your condition.

While each chapter reviews treatment options, I'll discuss these individual treatments in great detail in Part Three, "Treating Arthritis." This section includes all the elements of The Duke Basic Arthritis Program offered to patients at the Duke University Medical Center. This Basic Program, while not unique to Duke, is one of the best, most comprehensive programs in the nation. Duke uses a multidisciplinary team approach to arthritis that involves rheumatologists, nurses, physicians' assistants, physical therapists, occupational therapists, dietitians, social workers, psychologists, and other appropriate medical specialists, including orthopedic surgeons. Together we try to see each patient in terms of his lifestyle and develop treatments tailored to his individual needs. Major components of the Duke plan are covered in separate chapters and include: medication, physical therapy, occupational therapy, diet, and psychological techniques. I've also included a chapter on surgery and many helpful, practical suggestions to help you accomplish your daily activities more comfortably.

The book concludes with Part Four, "What's in the Future?", an overview of trends in research and new and future treatments for arthritis. Rheumatology is a dynamic, rapidly changing field, and this section should give you a good sense of the breakthroughs we hope to see in the years ahead.

I've learned a great deal from my patients over the years. I like them and try to do right by them, and they've been important in shaping my thinking as a doctor and my approach to clinical problems. My patients in turn have revealed to me the issues that concern them most as patients. If you or someone you know has arthritis, you probably share many of those questions and concerns. I hope that after reading this book you will have a better understanding of arthritis and will feel reassured that there's a great deal you can do to make living with arthritis easier and more rewarding.

PART ONE

What's Happening To Me?

1

What Is Arthritis?

Theresa, a seventy-two-year-old retired schoolteacher, gets a great deal of pleasure from doing needlepoint and belongs to a weekly sewing club. This past year she found that her fingers sometimes became stiff and painful. On some days the pain and stiffness were bad enough to prevent her from embroidering. Theresa was understandably annoyed at this development. She was beginning to worry that next summer she might not be able to do gardening, another of her favorite hobbies.

Joan, a thirty-two-year-old public relations executive, carries a sports bag to work and jogs during her lunch hours. Several months ago, she noticed some pain and swelling in her ankles, knees, and feet. She also noticed that she felt stiff in the morning when she woke up, and that she felt tired most afternoons. She tried to stick to her active lifestyle, but the pain grew so bad that she was forced to modify her busy work schedule and to give up jogging.

Victor, a forty-six-year-old computer software analyst, travels a great deal, visiting corporate clients throughout the country. One night while on the road he took a client out for a couple of drinks and a big dinner. He returned to his hotel and went to bed feeling fine, but then awoke at 3:00 A.M. with a red, swollen, and painful big toe. The pain was so bad that he was forced to cancel all his business appointments the next day and return home.

Glen, a nineteen-year-old college athlete, had to drop out of basketball after his lower back began to ache. He tried bed rest, but the pain continued to grow worse. In addition, Glen's right knee became swollen, red, and tender. Glen knows that his father and uncle both have arthritis, but he thinks he's much too young to be getting the disease.

These four people have distinctly different symptoms. Yet each of these patients eventually came to Duke University for a medical evaluation and was diagnosed as having arthritis.

What exactly is arthritis? Many people use the term as if all kinds of arthritis were one disease. In fact, this is probably the most common misconception about arthritis. When a patient says, "I think I have arthritis," he may not be aware that arthritis encompasses not just one, but actually more than a hundred different diseases, each with its own distinctive set of causes, symptoms, and treatments.

According to the Arthritis Foundation, approximately 37 million people in the United States have some form of the hundred or so diseases we call arthritis. This translates to one out of seven people, or one in three families. Chances are good that most of us have friends, relatives, or acquaintances who have been diagnosed with an arthritic condition.

Despite the prevalence of arthritis, the general public isn't as well informed about the subject as it could be. Many medical consumers know the indications of a heart attack or skin cancer, but how many can say the same for arthritis?

According to one recent study, most people said they relied mainly on the mass media for their information on arthritis. In fact, many people learn about arthritis through TV commercials for over-the-counter pain relievers. A typical ad may feature an older woman with a pained expression complaining of her aching fingers. After swallowing a few pills for "those minor aches and pains of arthritis," she's smiling, pain-free, and able to slice the cake at her grandson's birthday party. Such commercials are potentially misleading. They imply that arthritis is a minor annoyance that can be self-diagnosed and self-treated. This discourages patients from seeing their doctors early in the course of the disease, when treatment can make a great deal of difference and may prevent more severe consequences.

Many people also postpone seeking medical treatment because of the mistaken idea that there is little that can be done for these diseases. In truth, there is a great deal that can be done to treat arthritis. Today's approach to diagnosis and treatment is more sophisticated than in the past, and over the last twenty years we've developed an array of effective and powerful drugs that are far superior to what was available previously. Exercise regimens and physical and occupational therapy have also improved. Prompt diagnosis and treatment is key to halting the progress of disease. Once a joint has been damaged, it usually cannot be repaired. And therein lies the tragedy of deferring medical care.

This book should not replace your physician, nor would I recommend that you try to diagnose your own illness. As a matter of fact, one of my first suggestions is that you consult a doctor, if you have not already, if you suspect you have arthritis. It's essential that you find a qualified physician with whom you can build a trusting relationship. Good patient-physician rapport is an important part of your treatment. In my own practice, there is a great deal of give-and-take between me and my patients. The things I learn about my patients' lifestyles and beliefs help me to make more intelligent treatment decisions with them. For example, if I know a patient's arthritis is aggravated by his staying on his feet for many hours on the job, I may work with him to see if we can modify his workday. If I'm considering a course of treatment that involves injections and a patient tells me that she has a strong aversion to needles, I may try to find an equally effective drug that can be taken orally.

This book will give you a basic understanding of your condition so that you can work together with your physician most effectively. You are the only one who can report your symptoms or follow your doctor's recommendations regarding medications. A better understanding of the benefits and risks of various treatments will help you and your doctor develop an individualized treatment plan that's right for you.

If you, a family member, or someone you know has recently been diagnosed with arthritis, you may be confused by the unfamiliar and often imprecise terminology surrounding this medical condition. You probably have a great many questions about the causes of arthritis and may wonder about the prognosis. I'll discuss these issues in depth later in this book. First, however, I think it will be helpful for you to have a broad overview of arthritis.

What Is Arthritis?

Arthritis comes from the Greek words *arthron*, meaning joint, and *itis*, meaning inflammation. Literally, then, arthritis means an inflammation of the joints. This definition seems simple and straightforward enough, and most cases of arthritis do involve an inflamed joint. However, many types of arthritis involve no inflammation at all. In common usage, arthritis has come to mean any aches and pains in the bones, joints, and muscles; indeed, almost any pain outside of the head, chest, or abdomen. I have found that patients use the word *arthritis* to describe conditions as varied as bursitis, tendonitis, back pain, and heel spurs; in effect, almost any painful condition is labeled as arthritis. While medically incorrect, this broad application of the term has become common usage. In this book I will also frequently use the term *arthritis* broadly for lack of a better term. As we talk about specific diseases in subsequent chapters, however, I will use more precise terminology, calling individual diseases by their specific names. This should help you talk more clearly to your physician about your particular condition.

Key Medical Terms

You may be confused by the many ways doctors refer to and categorize your condition. Here are some key medical terms you will come across in this book and in discussions with your doctor. There is considerable overlap in many of these definitions; I'll explain some of them more thoroughly later in the book.

Rheumatism.

This term comes from the Greek word *rheuma*, which means flux. The term derived from the ancient Greek theory of disease. Physicians once believed (incorrectly) that arthritis was caused by substances called humors that flowed from the brain to the joints and other parts of the body to produce pain. Today the term *rheumatism* is an imprecise one with several possible medical meanings, although it is frequently used as an umbrella term to describe conditions that cause pain and swelling in joints and in surrounding supportive tissues, ligaments, and muscles. Doctors may also use the term to refer to such inflammatory diseases as rheumatoid arthritis and systemic lupus erythematosus. Because of the confusion surrounding its meaning, the term *rheumatism* is used less and less frequently. However, a specialist in the diagnosis and treatment of arthritis is still called a rheumatologist.

Inflammatory Disease.

Inflammation, the hallmark of arthritis, normally occurs when the body has been injured or is fighting off an infection caused by bacteria or a virus. In order to fight the invading microorganism, the body sends red and white blood cells into the affected area. The resulting inflammation is marked by redness, heat, swelling, pain, and loss of function. Many arthritic conditions, such as rheumatoid arthritis, are inflammatory. The joint linings may become thickened and tender, and the joint fluid fills with white blood cells. There is often no apparent reason for the inflammation in arthritis, and in some cases the inflammatory process itself can cause joint damage.

Systemic Disease.

Inflammatory arthritis may be *systemic,* meaning the disease is not confined to the joints but may affect other organs and tissues. Systemic forms of arthritis can cause generalized symptoms such as a low-grade fever and achiness. Rheumatoid arthritis is an example of a systemic inflammatory arthritis.

Musculoskeletal Diseases.

As the term implies, these are forms of arthritis and related conditions that affect the muscles, skeleton, and supporting tissues.

Collagen Vascular Diseases.

Collagen is the major supportive structural tissue in the body, making up ligaments, tendons, and joint structures. Diseases that affect these structures are known as *collagen diseases,* and there are several types of arthritis that fall into this category. The term *vascular* refers to the fact that many of these diseases also involve some changes in the blood vessels, often as a result of the inflammatory process.

Connective Tissue Diseases.

Connective tissues are the structural tissues of the body. Connective tissue diseases include various forms of arthritis as well as inflammatory conditions involving muscles, ligaments, and tendons.

What Causes Arthritis?

It's impossible to talk in general terms about the cause of arthritis because, as I've said, arthritis is actually more than a hundred separate diseases. Just as there are many forms of the disease, so there are many possible causes.

One common misconception is that arthritis is caused by a cold, wet climate. Numerous studies have disproven this myth. While some patients may feel better when it's warm and dry, climate itself neither cures nor causes arthritis.

Some people believe that arthritis is caused by a poor diet. A nutritious diet can help build your resistance and fight disease, but we do not yet have any scientific proof that specific foods can prevent or cause arthritis (see chapter 16).

Some forms of arthritis appear to be hereditary; others are not. Some conditions seem to involve a malfunctioning of the immune system; others result from overuse of a joint or from the wear and tear of joints over time. Still other possible causes of arthritis are metabolic disturbances, infections, environmental triggers, and injuries. I'll discuss what we know about individual types of arthritis later in separate chapters on these conditions.

Who Gets Arthritis?

Many people have the notion that arthritis is a disease only of old people. This simply isn't true. There is no one typical portrait of an arthritis patient. Arthritis can affect children, young adults, middle-aged people, and the elderly.

Anyone can have arthritis. It is not confined to a particular age group or gender, although some types of arthritis seem to affect men more than women and vice versa. Women, for example, seem more prone to rheumatoid arthritis and lupus; men are more likely to get gout and ankylosing spondylitis. In addition, certain forms of arthritis appear to have a hereditary link, and some individuals seem genetically predisposed to these diseases.

Older people are most likely to have osteoarthritis, a degenerative disease linked to the wear and tear that daily living inflicts on joints. However, all parts of the human body show some wear and tear with the passage of time. Your heart, for example, doesn't work as well when you are seventy-five as it did when you were twenty-five. In the same way, we all suffer some degenerative changes in our bones and joints as we age. Most of us eventually have some deterioration of the cartilage, the spongy material that cushions the ends of the bones where they come together in the joints. We may have some aches and pains in the joints as we grow older, but in most cases the arthritis is mild and probably nothing to worry about.

Prognosis

Since there are many forms of arthritis, it's also hard to offer a single prognosis. The arthritis that accompanies an infection may be prevented or cured with appropriate antibiotic treatment. Local conditions such as bursitis and tendonitis may be completely cured by a short regimen of rest. However, some forms of arthritis, such as rheumatoid arthritis, may be chronic: throughout your life you may have flare-ups, during which your symptoms become worse, and periods of remission, when your disease completely clears.

However, the good news is that even chronic forms of arthritis can usually be well controlled. For the vast majority of patients, medication, combined with rest, protection of joints, good nutrition, and exercise, will keep the disease in check.

Do You Have Arthritis?

Aches and pains in your joints and muscles can signal problems other than arthritis. You should *never* attempt to diagnose or treat yourself. The correct treatment for you depends upon the diagnosis your doctor makes. Some conditions respond to aspirin and similar types of anti-inflammatory drugs. Other types of arthritis require different medications.

The Arthritis Foundation, the voluntary health organization whose function is to help patients with arthritis, recommends that you consult your physician if you have any of the following:

WARNING SIGNS OF ARTHRITIS

- Swelling of one or more joints
- Early-morning stiffness
- Recurring pain or tenderness of any joint
- Inability to move a joint normally
- Obvious redness and warmth of a joint
- Unexplained weight loss, fever, or weakness combined with joint pain

You should be especially concerned if any of the above symptoms persist for more than two weeks. Other symptoms associated with arthritis include muscle pain; fatigue; muscle weakness; fever; rash; depression; sleep disturbance; and malaise.

Your doctor will want to perform a thorough physical exam and conduct several lab tests before he or she can determine whether you have arthritis, and if so, which type you have. If your doctor confirms that you have arthritis, he or she may very well refer you to a rheumatologist, a specialist in the field.

More than 90 percent of arthritis patients are seen for a handful of arthritic conditions. The two most common forms of arthritis are rheumatoid arthritis and osteoarthritis. Other common conditions include ankylosing spondylitis, gout, and systemic lupus erythematosus.

I will discuss these and other conditions separately in later chapters. However, I think I should first talk about how a normal joint functions. When I speak with my patients, I find that the best way to explain their condition is to start with a look at the healthy joint and at the changes that may take place when a person is affected by arthritis.

2

Joints and the Musculoskeletal System

When you are eating lunch, walking to your mailbox, or opening your car door, you probably don't give your joints a second thought. All human movement, from the dextrous touch of a surgeon to a football player's tackle, is accomplished through the precise and coordinated movement of your joints. Only when they become inflamed or injured, as they can with arthritis, do you begin to appreciate the jobs that they normally perform.

Since most forms of arthritis involve the joint and its surrounding tissues, it's important to understand the basic structure and functions of the normal joint and what happens to that joint when you have arthritis.

Types of Joints

The human skeleton is a hard, dense framework that supports your skin and muscles and protects your delicate internal organs. It's amazing, really, that this rigid structure should allow us such a variety of complicated movements. The more than 200 bones that comprise the human skeleton are connected by nearly 150 joints. These joints permit motion in any number of directions.

A joint, or articulation, is the place where two or more bones come together. Joints are categorized by the degree of motion they allow. Some joints don't allow any motion at all. For example, the tough, fibrous joints in the skull called sutures connect the skull bones, but are not designed for movement. Other types of joints allow only limited movement, such as those in the pelvis. A third class of joints allows free movement, as with those joints in the hip, wrist, or neck. Most of the joints in the body are free-moving joints. While arthritis can affect many types of joints, the free-moving joints are the most frequent target.

Joints are also categorized by the direction in which they move. Here are some of the major categories of joints.

Gliding Joint.

A gliding joint permits a slight gliding movement. The gliding joints that connect the vertebrae in your spine help you bend and stretch and give your back its flexibility.

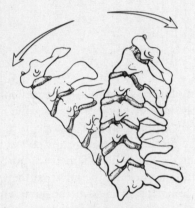

GLIDING JOINT

Hinge Joint.

Make a fist and watch the way your fingers bend at the joints. The joints in your finger are called hinge joints. Like door hinges, they allow movement to and fro, but only in one direction. Elbow and knee joints are also hinge joints.

HINGE JOINT

Ball-and-socket Joint.

This type of joint permits movement in all directions. The upper end of this joint is round, like a ball, and fits into a cup-like socket. Your shoulder is a ball-and-socket joint and is the most freely moving joint in the body. You can move your arms up, outward, and back, or rotate them in circles. Your hips are also ball-and-socket joints.

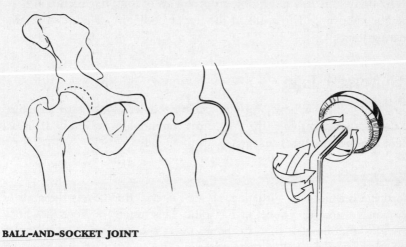

BALL-AND-SOCKET JOINT

Saddle Joint.

This type of joint is so named because opposing bones are concave and convex and resemble a saddle. Saddle joints can move up and down and side to side, but cannot rotate. Your wrist and thumb are examples of saddle joints. When you hold your arm tightly so that it's completely stationary and then try to rotate your wrist, you can see that it's your arm, and not your wrist, that allows the rotation.

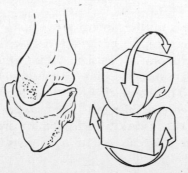

SADDLE JOINT

Joints are also described as weight-bearing or non-weight-bearing. The major weight-bearing joints are the ankles, knees, hips, and vertebrae in the spine. They bear the brunt of mechanical stress and are most likely to show the effects of the wear and tear of time. In general, the more weight a joint must sustain, the more damage it is likely to experience. The ankle is an exception to this rule. Although it bears the full weight of the body, it is less susceptible to problems of joint degeneration than the knee above it. The joints in the upper body are called non-weight-bearing joints.

The Normal Joint

Now that you know how joints are categorized, let's look at the structure of the free-moving joints, the ones most commonly involved in arthritis. Here are the structures that make up these joints.

Cartilage.

Cartilage is a smooth, glistening, elastic material that covers the ends of the bones where they meet at the joint. This tough, resilient substance provides a cushion so that the bones don't rub against each other. Its smooth, slick surface allows bones to slide over each other, and gives the joints flexibility. Cartilage is a spongy, compressible material that can absorb shock. Much of cartilage is composed of water, and about half is made up of collagen, a substance composed of long protein molecules woven together to give it a fabric-like structure. Collagen, like its relative gelatin, can change form when compressed and then spring back into shape when the weight is released. Bend the cartilage in your nose and ears and you'll see how resilient it is.

Joint Capsule.

The ends of the bones and the cartilage are completely encased in a sealed capsule called the joint capsule or the synovial sac. Thick, cord-like fibers called ligaments help form the outside of this capsule and are anchored to the bone on either side of the joint. They help to keep the bones in the correct alignment. The movement of the joint results from the action of muscles, highly specialized tissues whose capacity for contraction and relaxation allows all body work. Muscles, in turn, are attached to bone by tendons, which, like ligaments, are strong, fibrous bands.

Synovial Membrane.

The inside of the joint capsule is lined with a thin, delicate, velvety lining called the synovial membrane. In a healthy joint, the synovial membrane is only one or two cells thick and is rich in blood vessels and nerve endings. The synovial membrane produces a clear, viscous fluid that fills the space inside the capsule. (The word *synovial* means like an egg and is so called because the fluid produced resembles raw egg white.) Synovial fluid lubricates the joints and nourishes the cartilage, which has no blood supply of its own.

Bursae.

These are small fluid-filled sacs that lie outside the joint. Like the synovial membrane, bursae produce a lubricating liquid that helps muscles, tendons, and bones to slide over one another.

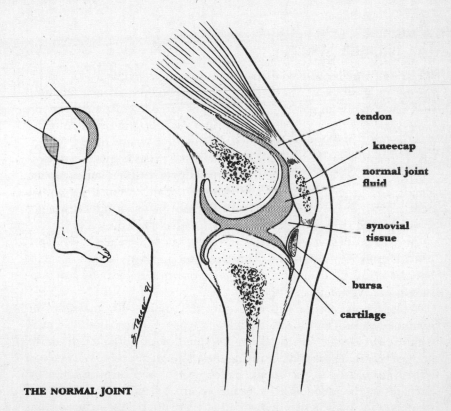

tendon

kneecap

normal joint
fluid

synovial
tissue

bursa

cartilage

THE NORMAL JOINT

Inflammation

Arthritis is a group of diseases that affect structures in and around the joint—i.e., synovial membranes, cartilage, bones, bursae, muscles, tendons, and ligaments. The suffix -*itis* means inflammation, and most forms of arthritis involve some joint inflammation. In medical school, students are taught that the classic signs of inflammation are *rubor, calor, tumor, dolor,* and *functio laesa*—redness, heat, swelling, pain, and loss of function, respectively. Rheumatoid arthritis is a good example of an arthritic disease that is often accompanied by inflammation.

Since inflammation figures so prominently in many forms of arthritis, a general understanding of its cause and purpose is important. A joint that's red, tender, and warm to the touch feels that way because it is involved in a complex set of events triggered by your body's immune system.

The Immune System

We are all familiar with sunburned skin that looks red, feels hot, and is painful to the touch. The inflammation of sunburn is your immune system's response to skin damage caused by ultraviolet light. When you bang your arm and it swells up, you are also triggering your immune system. Inflammation may also be a response to a wound or to a foreign microorganism in the body. It is a sign that your immune system is working. Other signs of immune system activity are fever, chills, swollen glands, and generalized aches and pains. Once the immune system has done its job, destroying the foreign substance or repairing the wound, these physical signs abate, and you begin to feel like yourself again.

Perhaps the best way to understand the immune system is to compare it to an army. It protects your body from an opposing force of harmful bacteria, viruses, fungi, and other microorganisms. Such foreign substances are known collectively as antigens.

White blood cells, or leukocytes, are the soldiers that make up the immune system. There are many different types of white blood cells, each with its own specific role to play in blocking foreign substances from the body or searching out and destroying these foreign invaders. White blood cells are stationed in the lymph nodes, spleen, and thymus; they also circulate in the blood. The immune system differs from other organ systems in the body in that many of its cells are not rigidly organized, but are capable of patrolling throughout the body to look for and repair injury in various ways.

The immune system has a variety of methods of recognizing foreign substances, the most exquisitely sensitive of which is the production of antibodies. Antibodies are proteins individually tailored to destroy a specific foreign substance. Over your lifetime, your body may produce as many as 10 million different types of antibodies. Each antibody is uniquely designed to bind with a foreign antigen in a lock-and-key fashion.

When antibody and antigen lock into each other, they activate a series of proteins called the complement system. The complement proteins in turn trigger the release of other chemicals that help destroy the foreign invaders and call forth even more white blood cells to join the battle. Complement proteins are consumed during the process of fighting an infection. In some forms of arthritis, a test to measure complement levels can help the physician assess how active your disease is.

The immune system is very efficient. Once it encounters an antigen, it stores a picture of it in its memory. Should you encounter the antigen again, your immune system will be able to recognize and destroy it more quickly. In other words, you will have built up an immunity to the disease. Vaccines for such diseases as polio, measles, and diphtheria have been developed in recognition of this principle. A weakened or a slightly altered form of the bacteria or virus may be administered, just enough to stimulate your body to produce antibodies against it, and in this way you may acquire an immunity to that disease.

The White Cell Arsenal

The immune system is very intricate, with a complex system of coordinated events and checks and balances. Many specialized white blood cells are involved. The following are some of the members of the white cell arsenal:

B Cells and T Cells.

The B cells are directly responsible for the production of antibodies. Their work would not be possible without the assistance of a variety of other cells called T cells. Helper T cells stimulate the B cells to produce antibodies. Suppressor T cells tell the immune system that its job is complete and that it should switch off. Killer T cells directly attack cells infected with viruses. Still other types of T cells make hormone-like substances called lymphokines, powerful chemical secretions that trigger the body's immune response. Some of the discomfort you feel when you have an infection or an inflammation is caused by the presence of lymphokines. Interferon, one type of lymphokine, appears to prevent viral attacks.

Macrophages.

Other white blood cells called phagocytes, or scavenger cells, engulf and destroy any antigen particles in the blood. One type of scavenger cell, the macrophage, also secretes monokines, potent chemical substances that help bolster and regulate the immune system response. Interleukin 1 is a type of monokine. Its secretion may result in symptoms of fever and inflammation. Another type of monokine, tumor necrosis factor, has actions similar to interleukin 1. It also appears to promote the destruction of tumors in the body. Monokines are very potent and have very powerful systemic effects.

Neutrophils.

When a wound fills with pus, it's largely due to the presence of neutrophils, circulating white blood cells that destroy bacteria and remove cell debris and solid substances from the blood. Their powerful enzymes can be very destructive. In some types of arthritis, when there is an infection in a closed joint space, the activated neutrophils may even destroy tissue.

To illustrate what happens when the immune system is activated, let's imagine that you have an infected finger. Once the immune system has been alerted to the foreign bacteria, blood containing antibodies rushes into the area to do combat. The white blood cells, including many neutrophils, accumulate, causing the formation of the dense, cloudy liquid called pus. The neutrophils in turn produce materials that increase blood flow to the area, enabling other white cells to join the attack. This blood flow also causes inflammation, so your finger becomes red, tender, and warm to the touch. The blood vessels become leaky so that white blood cells can seep out of circulation into other body tissues. This leakage makes your injured finger swell. Once the battle is over and the infection neutralized, the redness, swelling, and heat disappear, and your finger looks normal again. Sometimes fiber-like tissue replaces some of the tissue lost through injury or infection, leaving you with a permanent scar.

The Role of Immunity in Arthritis

The immune system is supposed to *protect* the body, so how can it be involved with the onset of arthritis? Inflamed and swollen joints are the hallmark of a group of diseases classified as inflammatory arthritis. In this group of diseases, the body for no apparent reason reacts as if it were being invaded by a foreign microorganism. Scientists believe such inflammation may result from a malfunctioning of the immune system. The body seems to attack itself, mistaking its own healthy tissue for foreign antigens. It develops what is known as autoimmunity (from the Greek *autos*, meaning self). Perhaps some kind of infection or unusual bacterium or virus has lodged in the joint, but for some reason the immune system can't get rid of the invader, so the swelling in the joints doesn't go away. So far, in most forms of arthritis, no one has been able to identify such a microorganism.

The Arthritic Joint: An Overview

Joint inflammation is just one cause of arthritis. There are other forms of arthritis, however, such as osteoarthritis, that are noninflammatory and do not appear to activate the immune system. Let's examine briefly the other ways a healthy joint and the tissue surrounding it may be affected by arthritis.

Cartilage Degeneration

Some forms of arthritis are caused by a wearing away of the cartilage that normally cushions the ends of the bones. A certain amount of wear and tear to the cartilage over time is normal, and most people will show some cartilage degeneration in their later years, though they won't necessarily notice any arthritic symptoms.

When the normally glistening cartilage wears down, it becomes dull and opaque, and its smooth surface may become fissured, cracked, and uneven. As the cartilage continues to wear away, the bones it covers may thicken, cysts may form, and the joint space may become narrower. Sometimes the bones try to repair themselves by forming structures called spurs, which make the joint look enlarged. Cartilage degeneration in the finger joints may make them look knobby.

Osteoarthritis is an arthritic disease that involves cartilage degeneration as a result of the normal process of aging or from a previous injury to the joint. In addition, some people appear to have a hereditary defect that allows their cartilage to wear away at a faster rate than normal.

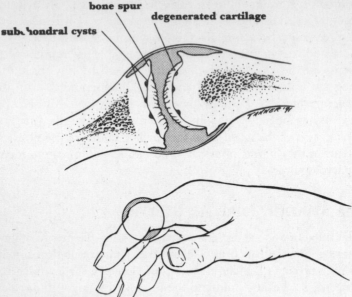

CARTILAGE DEGENERATION

Synovitis

Synovitis—an inflamed joint lining—is a classic sign of inflammatory arthritis. If you looked inside a joint with rheumatoid arthritis, for example, you would see that the normally smooth, thin, inner membrane has become thickened and swollen. Both the joint fluid and the synovial lining have been infiltrated by white blood cells. The joint fluid has expanded and looks like pus, and in severe cases, the white blood cells inside the joint have produced substances that can wear away the bone's protective cartilage to form gaps or breaks called erosions. Without prompt and appropriate therapy, the cartilage loss may progress to the point where the ends of the bones are exposed and begin to rub together. The supportive tendons and ligaments may also be weakened, so the joint slips out of position and its function is impaired. This is not an inevitable part of inflammatory arthritis, however, and in most cases the disease does not progress to this point.

Diseases of Attachment

An enthesis is an attachment, a place where tendons and ligaments are anchored to the bone. In certain forms of arthritis these attachments, as

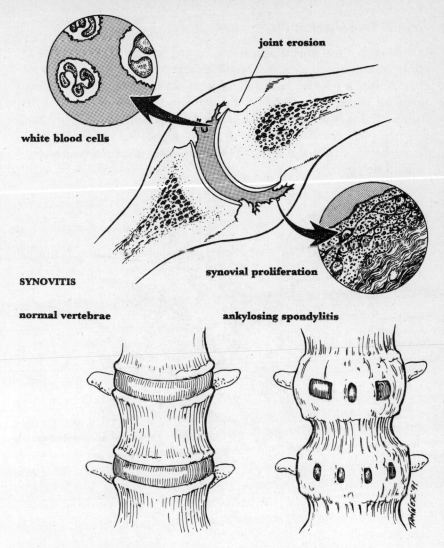

joint erosion

white blood cells

synovial proliferation

SYNOVITIS

normal vertebrae   ankylosing spondylitis

DISEASES OF ATTACHMENT

well as the joints, become inflamed. As a result, ligaments and tendons become thickened and scarred, and in some cases, rigid or bony. The bones in the joints may grow into one another, eventually becoming fused. The result is stiffness and loss of mobility.

Ankylosing spondylitis is an arthritic disease of attachments that affects the vertebrae of the spine.

Crystal Deposition

When you put too much sugar into a cup of water, the water becomes saturated and the excess sugar crystallizes and settles to the bottom of the glass. A similar reaction occurs in the joints when levels of certain blood chemicals become too high. Crystals form in the joint and irritate the synovial lining, causing a very severe local inflammation. White blood cells rush to the site, causing the joint to become swollen, red, and painful. Gout, the most common crystal-induced disease, is caused by monosodium urate crystals.

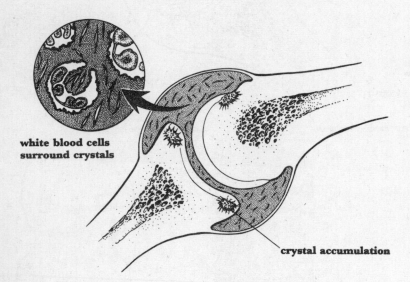

white blood cells surround crystals

crystal accumulation

CRYSTAL DEPOSITION

Infectious Arthritis

A joint may become the target of infectious arthritis when an infection in another part of the body travels through the bloodstream to the joint, where the infectious organism multiplies in the rich nutrients of the synovial fluid. An infection can also enter the joint directly, through a wound.

Infectious arthritis is not a common disease. Most cases of infectious arthritis occur in people who have preexisting arthritis, usually rheumatoid arthritis, or in people with preexisting joint damage or diseases that have lowered their immune response, like cancer.

One recently recognized form of infectious arthritis is called Lyme disease, named after the town in Connecticut where the original cases were recognized. Lyme disease is caused by a type of microorganism called a spirochete, which is transmitted to humans from deer ticks. The etiology of Lyme disease bolsters the theory that inflammatory arthritis may indeed be caused by a foreign microorganism lodged in the joint.

The most common form of infectious arthritis is triggered by the gonococcus bacterium, which causes gonorrhea; however, as we will see in chapter 11, this form of infectious arthritis differs in presentation and medical management from other types of infectious arthritis.

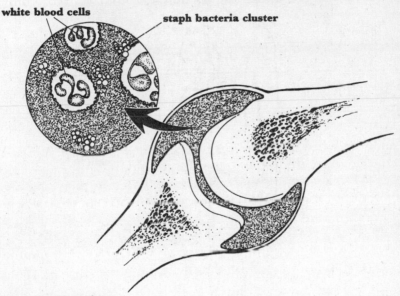

white blood cells   staph bacteria cluster

INFECTIOUS ARTHRITIS

Muscle Pain

When a joint is inflamed, the pain may travel to the nearby muscle, causing aching and tenderness in the area. Sometimes an inflamed or injured joint makes a nearby muscle go into spasm. When the inflammation is taken care of, the muscle, too, feels better. Polymyalgia rheumatica is a form of arthritis with muscle pain.

Connective Tissue Disorders

Connective tissue diseases involve inflammation of tissues that support and connect other tissues and body organs. Bone, skin, blood vessels, and cartilage are made up of connective tissue. A systemic arthritis such as rheumatoid arthritis or systemic lupus erythematosus can affect connective tissues throughout the body, causing achiness, fever, and sometimes damage to other body organs. Another form of arthritic disease, scleroderma, is considered a connective tissue disease because it can affect skin, kidneys, blood vessels, and the intestinal tract as well as the joints.

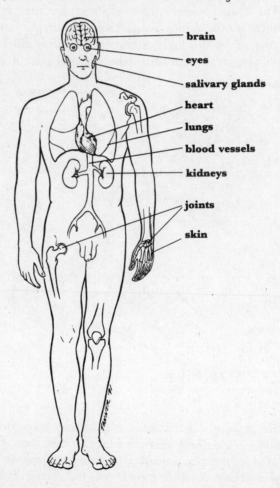

brain

eyes

salivary glands

heart

lungs

blood vessels

kidneys

joints

skin

**CONNECTIVE
TISSUE DISORDER**

3

Diagnosing Arthritis

Your joints are tender and swollen, you ache all over, and you feel stiff in the morning. It's been several weeks, and the problem doesn't seem to be going away. You know it's time to visit a doctor, but which doctor? Arthritis can cause a bewildering variety of symptoms, from joint pains, backaches, and morning stiffness to fatigue and even depression. It's understandable if you're confused about where to go for medical attention.

Finding the Right Specialist

Which physician you consult first may depend upon where you live, your insurance, and your initial symptoms. If you live in a small town, for example, you may not have easy access to various specialists. You might begin by consulting your general internist or family practitioner. If you already have a long-term relationship with a general internist or family practitioner, he or she will be familiar with your medical history and can help determine whether you need to see a specialist, and if so, where the specialists in your area are located. Of course, if you're covered by a health maintenance organization (HMO), it will probably have its own established procedures for referral.

The first specialist you might want to consult is a rheumatologist. Rheumatologists are fully trained in general internal medicine and have an additional two to three years of training focused entirely on arthritic diseases. This specialist can evaluate and treat a variety of problems, including arthritis, inflammatory diseases of muscles, blood vessels, and other connective tissues, and painful conditions of the musculoskeletal system. Since many forms of arthritis go on beyond the joint to affect other organs in the body, a rheumatologist is qualified to evaluate a wide variety of illnesses.

Many cases of joint pain seen by a rheumatologist turn out to be noninflammatory, resulting from some mechanical problem, such as a sports injury. In such cases, the rheumatologist may refer you to an orthopedic surgeon, a specialist skilled in operating on joints.

Arthritis doesn't always begin with painful joints. One of my lupus patients, for example, first came to see me because she was having abdominal pains. Another, with scleroderma, had Raynaud's phenomenon, an extreme sensitivity to cold that made her hands turn blue and numb. If your arthritis begins with these less typical symptoms, you may not realize that your problem is in fact due to arthritis. As a result, you would probably first consult specialists other than a rheumatologist. For example, if you felt a weakness or pain in your extremities or suffered from bad headaches—less common signs of arthritis—you would probably first consult a neurologist, a specialist in diseases of the nerves. Some types of arthritis, such as psoriatic arthritis and systemic lupus erythematosus, can cause skin rashes, which might send you to a dermatologist, or skin specialist. If you have an aching jaw and are having problems chewing, you'll probably want to bring it to the attention of your dentist.

Some people choose to consult a chiropractor, a nonphysician whose practice is based on the premise that misalignment of the spine can cause disease. I consider this an alternative form of medicine, not based on the same principles that are accepted by internal medicine.

Many of these specialists may be good first choices, depending on your symptoms. After a review of your medical history or a physical exam, your physician has to decide whether he or she has the expertise to do the workup, or whether you need to be referred to another specialist, particularly a rheumatologist.

Does this mean that everyone with arthritic disease needs to see a rheumatologist? In the best of all possible worlds, I think that everyone with a serious joint problem should at least have a consultation with a rheumatologist to assure a correct diagnosis and establish an overall plan for therapy. A rheumatologist deals with arthritic conditions on a daily basis, has a great deal of experience in diagnosing and treating these diseases, and has the most up-to-date information on your condition. After the initial consultation, another physician, whether it be your family practitioner, internist, or orthopedic surgeon, can administer your care.

The rheumatologist can then be consulted as needed; however, some forms of arthritis are best managed by rheumatologists because of the knowledge and experience required for their diagnosis and treatment.

If you don't presently have a physician and don't know how to go about locating one, call your county medical society or the local branch of the Arthritis Foundation.

The Patient-Doctor Partnership

Arthritic conditions are usually chronic, so you and your physician are likely to form a lifelong, frequently close relationship. I think it's important that you like your doctor and have some rapport with him or her. Some of the decisions you have to make together may be difficult—to start therapy with a potentially dangerous medicine, or to replace a joint by surgery, for example—so a relationship based on trust and empathy is important.

With many acute medical diseases, the decisions are fairly black and white: if you have pneumonia, you need antibiotics in order to get better; for appendicitis, you need surgery to avoid serious complications. However, arthritis, like other chronic illnesses, has no one treatment, and decisions have to be made on an individual basis. Some of my patients will live with their disease for thirty or forty years. As their physician, I have to understand their lives and design therapies compatible with those lifestyles. I have to look at the whole patient, including his mental outlook.

To give you an example, Ed, a fifty-five-year-old patient of mine, had a hip problem which I felt necessitated surgery. When I presented this option to him, he said no. Ed was very frightened about having surgery and said he'd prefer to wait a year and see if he could get along using a cane. I respected Ed's feelings and we are continuing to work together to help him function as well as he can without the surgery.

Margaret, a sixty-five-year-old woman with an advanced form of rheumatoid arthritis, was faced with deciding whether to embark on a regimen of Plaquenil or of gold injections, both potent drugs. We talked at length about the relative advantages and risks of these therapies. Gold therapy would require intramuscular injections and the drawing of blood every week to monitor possible side effects. Plaquenil has the rare but potentially serious side effect of retinal damage, which can lead to visual impairment. Margaret didn't like the idea of weekly injections and blood drawings, but because she already had cataracts, she was concerned about even the slightest possibility of any vision loss. Together we decided that gold injections were the better option for her.

My patients and I are in a long-term partnership that often requires open communication and a lot of give-and-take. I think a physician should allow you plenty of time to air your concerns. At Duke, we believe strongly that to understand a patient and his or her life requires extra consultation time, especially in initial evaluations. We recognize that arthritis is a very complicated disease with many possible treatment options, and that patients often need detailed explanations and information in order to make informed decisions.

But treatment and decision-making are a two-way street, and things go better when you too take some responsibility in your own care. When I encourage patients to stop smoking and drinking or to lose weight in order to relieve the pressure on their joints, I am often frustrated. I told one of my patients, Jim, a three-hundred-pound salesman, that he might need a knee operation and that the extra stress caused by his weight only exacerbated his problem. I explained to Jim the importance of diet and sent him to our dietician, who recommended a weight reduction plan. Nevertheless, by the next office visit, he'd gained five pounds!

I've seen such scenes repeated many times. But after many years of working with patients, I have come to realize that there is a lot more involved in rheumatology than just dealing with a person's medical symptoms. I am trying now to work with Jim to help reinforce a change in his lifestyle patterns. It's very difficult to change lifelong habits, and such changes can't be accomplished automatically.

To help your physician and yourself, you might want to read up on your illness so you'll have a better understanding of the disease process. You should be forewarned, however, that a lot of information you will get from the media and via word of mouth can be inaccurate or misleading, especially the type of literature that holds out false promises for easy cures. Contact your local Arthritis Foundation chapter for accurate, accessible literature on arthritis. I've provided other sources of information in the resources section of this book.

Bring your past medical records on your first visit to the doctor, along with a list of the medications you may already be taking. I also recommend you bring a list of any questions you have. It's easy to get flustered during an office visit and then find later that you've forgotten to ask something very important.

Diagnosing the Problem

No single diagnostic test can ascertain whether you have arthritis. Aches and pains in your joints or muscles can be caused by a variety of different diseases. The diagnostic process follows an orderly path, including a detailed medical history, a thorough physical exam, and a series of laboratory tests. Results from all three will give your doctor a very good indication of the exact nature of your problem.

The Medical History

The medical history is the story of your disease as well as a complete review of your medical problems and current lifestyle. Your doctor will want to collect basic information about you, including your age, sex, marital and family status, place of residence, and occupation. Some of these areas may seem unrelated to arthritis, but they give us insight into you as an individual and the potential impact of arthritis on your life. Certain forms of arthritis appear to run in families, so a detailed medical history will include questions about the occurrence of arthritis among your parents, brothers, sisters, and children.

Your physician should ask you about your chief complaint, the symptom that brought you into his or her office in the first place. Joint pains are most common, but you may also be bothered by other arthritis-related symptoms, such as fatigue, fever, headache, and weight loss. Sometimes arthritis can be a clue to other problems, such as glandular, skin, or bowel disease; and this will lead to another line of questioning.

If the problem centers around your joints, your doctor will want to have the following information:

- Which of your joints hurt?
- When and how did the pain start? Was there an injury or accident?
- What was the pattern of disease? Did the pain spread quickly to many joints, or was the progression slower, involving one joint at a time?
- What makes the pain come on?
- What makes the pain better?
- What time of day is the pain the worst?
- Do your joints lock or give way?
- Do you feel stiff in the mornings?

Since many forms of arthritis are inflammatory and systemic, your doctor may also ask you the following:

- Do you have fever?
- Have you lost weight?
- Do you get tired? If so, at what time of day?
- Do you have symptoms of depression—e.g., sleep disturbance, bowel problems, loss of social interest?

After gaining a sense of your general symptoms, your doctor will formulate more specific questions to help pinpoint the type of arthritis you might have. For example, if I suspect that a young man has ankylosing spondylitis (AS), an arthritis that primarily affects the joints in the spine, I'll ask him more specific questions about his back pains, and whether he's having any eye or bowel problems, both of which are associated with AS. If a young woman complains to me that she has a fever and joint pain, I'll ask her if she's having any pains in her chest and abdomen. Is she losing any hair? Does she have any skin rashes? These latter symptoms point to the possibility of lupus.

I also like to know whether a patient has been previously diagnosed as having arthritis, and if so, what the specific diagnosis was. Did your previous doctor simply tell you that you had arthritis, or were you told that you had a specific type of arthritis, such as gout or rheumatoid arthritis? Most doctors take their colleagues' diagnoses seriously, so this type of information provides important background. If you've brought along the records from previous office visits, laboratory tests, and X-rays, your physician can avoid unnecessary or duplicate testing. It's to your advantage to bring as much information as possible to this consultation.

Your doctor must know about any previous medications you have taken or are currently taking for your arthritis. Did they work? Did you experience any serious side effects? If you stopped taking them, what was the reason? Show your doctor the list of all the drugs you are taking and/or bring in your medicine bottles, since their labels will provide relevant information.

The medical history will also include questions about your general health (hospitalizations, surgery, immunizations, transfusions, and allergies) and health-related habits (diet, smoking, drinking). Your doctor will undertake a very detailed review of symptoms in all your major organ systems, regardless of your current complaints, to ensure he or she doesn't miss anything important.

Physical Examination of the Joints

I can tell a lot about a patient's physical condition before the physical exam is even conducted, and therefore I like to watch the way a patient gets out of a chair and walks toward my examining room. Does he appear comfortable in a sitting position, or when rising? Does he limp? When he gestures or moves, does he look as if he is in pain? By watching these actions, I can learn a great deal about the nature of his joint pain. A patient with rheumatoid arthritis often gets stiff when he sits in one position for too long. This is known as the gel phenomenon. He may rock or push himself from the chair to a standing position and walk hesitantly. Another patient might hold a swollen wrist or elbow protectively to prevent pain.

Such observations are a good complement to the physical exam. If a patient appears to be in pain, I may structure the examination to minimize patient movements that could cause discomfort. If you're afraid your exam might be painful, don't hesitate to tell your doctor so he or she can modify it as necessary.

Since symptoms of arthritis may not be restricted to the joints, your doctor will give you a full physical exam, including an assessment of your blood pressure, pulse, heart, and lungs. I'll skip over the finer points of the general physical and focus on how an arthritis specialist examines your joints.

First, your doctor will try to establish the pattern of arthritis by checking the following:

- How many joints are involved? Arthritis can be broken down into conditions that are monoarticular (involving one joint), oligoarticular (few joints), and polyarticular (many joints).
- Is the involvement of joints symmetric? Does it involve the same joints on both sides of the body?
- Are large joints (knees, hips, and shoulders) and/or small joints (fingers, feet, and toes) involved?
- Is there involvement of the spine as well as peripheral joints of the arms, legs, feet, and hands?

Your physician will begin the examination by systematically examining all of your joints on both sides of your body, often checking your hands first. Hands are considered the calling cards of arthritis because they are involved in so many forms of the disease. Your doctor will inspect each joint visually, then carefully touch, or palpate, them, from the hands, wrists, elbows, and shoulders, to the knees, ankles, and small joints of the feet.

Sometimes when a patient's arthritis is very active, even the smallest amount of pressure can be very painful. If your doctor sees that your joints are red, hot, and tender, he or she will go very gently and apply the least amount of pressure. When there is less evidence of arthritis, your doctor will apply more pressure, to be sure he or she doesn't miss any subtle signs of inflammation.

Your doctor will check for synovitis, an inflammation of the joint lining. Synovitis may be hard to detect early on, when the joint may be tender only to the touch, without much redness and swelling. As inflammatory types of arthritis progress and the joint lining becomes more obviously inflamed, the cells there multiply and thicken. This is called synovial proliferation. The abnormally thickened joint lining feels boggy or rubbery and can be quite tender. In some cases, this thickening is easily visible, appearing almost as a lump under the skin.

Some types of arthritis do not involve synovitis. Your doctor will check to see if the swelling in your joints is caused by growth of excess bone or accumulation of fluid. In osteoarthritis, for example, he or she will examine the small joints of your fingers for bony enlargements called Heberden's or Bouchard's nodes.

Your doctor will then examine the joints of your hips and spine. These joints are difficult to palpate because of their location, so your doctor will try to judge whether they're inflamed by asking how much pain you feel and by gauging whether the movement of these joints has been affected. For example, one type of arthritis, ankylosing spondylitis, can cause the vertebrae in the spine to fuse and thus limit mobility. To assess your spinal mobility, your doctor might ask you to bend and touch your toes or to stand against a wall and try to lean your back against it. When the joints in the back are unaffected, the vertebrae move apart as you bend; with arthritis, the back loses flexibility, and the bones can remain rigid. To see if your neck is affected, your doctor will ask you to bend it up and down, and left and right. Your doctor will also check your chest expansion by measuring your ribs with a tape measure before and after you take a deep breath.

By the time your doctor is finished with this part of the physical, he or she will usually have a good idea about which joints are involved.

Range of Motion

Your doctor will next try to determine the extent to which the motion of your joints has been limited. A joint may lose some of its function as a result of severe inflammation or from such mechanical problems as the rupture of a tendon or ligament or damage to the cartilage. Your doctor will systematically assess the range of motion of all of your joints. The range of motion is usually expressed in terms of degrees of motion, considering the possible range of a joint's movement as an arc of a circle. For example, the elbow joint can normally be fully extended to a straight line, or 180 degrees. A limitation of movement might be expressed as a 30-degree lack of extension.

Your physician will then evaluate your joint motion as it relates to your ability to perform everyday tasks. He or she may ask you to oppose your index finger and thumb, make a fist around his or her fingers, or reach your arms up. This will tell your doctor whether you're able to button clothing, open a bottle of medicine, or reach a plate on a high shelf. If the range of motion of your joints is limited, you may find it difficult to feed yourself, shop, or even comb your hair. Your doctor can then tell a great deal about the impact of the disease on your daily life.

Deformities

Many forms of arthritis produce easily recognized deformities. For example, severe cases of rheumatoid arthritis can produce characteristic changes in the shapes of the fingers. They may become crooked (swan neck or boutonniere deformity) or drift to the side (ulnar deviation), or the thumb may be bent out of shape (hitchhiker's thumb). Some of these deformities are fixed, or permanently locked into position by fibrous tissue. Others are reversible and movement is still possible in the joint. These distinctions will help your doctor diagnose your disease and prescribe the proper treatment.

Other Physical Signs

Sometimes physical signs outside the joint, in other parts of the body, can help your doctor pinpoint which type of arthritis you have. Changes in the skin are often the most important indicators of arthritis. Nodules, or painless lumps about an inch wide, are typical of rheumatoid arthritis and may appear anywhere under the skin, but most commonly near the elbows, at the place where you rest them against the table. Another type of lump called a tophus may form under the skin as a result of crystal deposits common in gout. It's not always possible for your physician to distinguish a nodule from a tophus just by feel.

Skin rashes may present additional diagnostic clues. Patches of scaly, red skin accompany psoriatic arthritis. Lupus patients may have a butterfly-shaped rash over the nose and cheeks.

Systemic types of arthritis, such as rheumatoid arthritis, cause changes in the blood vessels that are clearly apparent. Fingertips may look red, as if they were dipped in paint. The blood vessels in the palms become more prominent, actually visible through the skin. Dilated blood vessels may appear at the base of the fingernails. Your doctor will check for all of these signs.

The Follow-up "Joint Count"

The physical examination helps your physician not only to diagnose your arthritis but also to assess how active it is and to plan a treatment regimen. When your doctor counts the number of swollen and painful joints you have, he or she can tell how active your arthritis is and whether or not it's responding to therapy. Your doctor will perform this joint count on many visits and with increasing speed as he or she becomes better acquainted with you. After a while your physician will be able to look at just a few key joints (signal joints) and gauge the intensity of inflammation, although a complete exam should be performed each time.

Laboratory Studies

The medical history and physical exam should allow your physician to make at least a tentative diagnosis, but even "textbook," or "classical" cases that seem fairly clear-cut need to be confirmed by laboratory tests.

The number of laboratory studies you need will vary, depending on the findings of the medical history and the physical exam. If I suspect that a patient's arthritis is caused by another underlying condition, such as a metabolic problem, I may order extensive testing. But generally speaking, only a few key tests are in order.

The main objective of laboratory tests is to determine which type of arthritis you have and whether there's significant inflammation present. No single laboratory test can tell this with exact certainty. Lab findings can only be suggestive of or compatible with a diagnosis of a given disease.

Similarly, there's no precise test that can measure how active your disease is. Laboratory findings are interpreted in light of the medical history and physical exam. Together, these sources of information help your doctor make an accurate diagnosis.

Several blood tests are commonly performed in the initial evaluation of arthritic diseases. The blood for all these tests can be drawn during one visit, with one needle stick (usually several small tubes are needed—each tube is the equivalent of about 5 to 10 milliliters, or a few tablespoons of blood). The blood is then sent to various laboratories for examination. Some of these tests take minutes to perform, others take hours, and still others take days. In most cases, your doctor should have all the results within a week.

Complete Blood Count (CBC).

Blood consists of discrete cell types (red blood cells, white blood cells, and platelets) suspended in a thick, colorless fluid called plasma. Each cell type can be rapidly counted by an automatic machine.

The process of inflammation can cause certain typical changes in a person's blood count: The red blood cell count may go down (anemia), the white blood cell count may go up (leukocytosis), and the platelet count may be elevated. While anemia may accompany inflammatory arthritis, it can also be caused by other things, such as blood loss or iron and vitamin deficiency, so a low red blood cell count does not always mean you have inflammation. In the same way, a high white blood cell count can be the result of an infection. Only when other possible causes have been ruled out by the medical history, physical exam, or other tests can the doctor interpret the blood abnormalities as a sign of possible inflammation. Even then, there are exceptions to the rule. In lupus, for example, there is intense inflammation, yet the white blood cell and platelet counts can be strikingly low.

Chemistries.

Blood plasma contains proteins (antibodies, clotting factors, enzymes), salts, and other dissolved materials. Tests that measure the concentration of various chemical substances in the plasma are called chemistries. For example, the presence of a high level of creatinine, a waste product in the blood, may mean that the kidneys aren't working properly. This can be due to certain types of inflammatory arthritis that affect kidney function. More often, though, disturbances of kidney function are the result of high blood pressure, aging, or other diseases. Certain drugs used to treat arthritis may affect kidney functioning, so a test to measure creatinine level may alert your doctor to possible side effects or help him or her adjust your drug dosages during treatment.

Another blood chemistry measures the amount of uric acid in the plasma. High levels of uric acid are associated with gout. This test has its limitations, however, because many people with high uric acids don't have gout, and conversely, many gout patients have normal uric acid levels. You can see why a diagnosis of gout should not be based on uric acid levels alone.

Erythrocyte Sedimentation Rate (ESR, or Sed Rate).

If a sample of your blood were left to stand undisturbed in a tube, the red blood cells would gradually settle to the bottom. When inflammation occurs, your body produces certain proteins in the blood that make your red blood cells clump together. These heavier cell aggregates fall faster than normal red blood cells. The distance that the red cells fall in one hour is known as the sedimentation (sed) rate or ESR. The more inflammation you have, the more clumping substances you have in your blood, and the faster your blood settles. In healthy individuals, blood settles at a rate of up to 20 millimeters in an hour (the rate is a bit higher for older people). With inflammatory disease, the rate can exceed 100 millimeters per hour. So the ESR gives us a good indication of whether you're experiencing inflammation, but since inflammation can be caused by conditions other than arthritis, this test alone is not diagnostic.

Urinalysis.

Blood and/or protein in the urine signal a disturbance in kidney function. This problem may be the result of inflammation or the side effect of certain drugs.

Rheumatoid Factor (RF).

The discovery of the rheumatoid factor in the 1940s was a milestone in the field of rheumatology. RF is an antibody found in unusually large amounts in the blood of patients with rheumatoid arthritis (RA). Some scientists think that RF may cause the disease, but others think it is more likely the body's response to infection and inflammation. Whatever the reason for its existence, the presence of RF in the blood is extremely useful in the diagnosis of rheumatoid arthritis. About 80 percent of RA patients have RF in their blood. Usually the higher the concentration of RF, the more severe the rheumatoid arthritis.

This test for arthritis is not without its problems, however. First, it can take many months for RF to show up in the blood, so if a patient is tested early in the course of the disease, this test won't be revealing. For this reason, if an RF test turns out to be negative, I'll often have the test repeated at a later date. Second, there are patients who have all the symptoms of RA, but who lack this factor in their blood: these people are called seronegative. (Some doctors suspect that in such cases another disease may masquerade as RA.) And finally, RF can occur in response to inflammatory or infectious diseases other than RA, though the amount is usually lower. While perhaps not perfect, the RF test is one of the best tools we have in the diagnosis of RA.

Fluorescent Antinuclear Antibody (FANA).

This test is one of the most important and also one of the most confusing in rheumatology. A curious feature of patients with certain rheumatic diseases, especially lupus, is that they make antibodies to the command centers of the body's cells, the nucleus. These antibodies are called antinuclear antibodies (ANAs). To test for these antibodies, a patient's blood serum is placed on a microscope slide containing cells with easily seen nuclei, and then a substance containing a fluorescent dye is added that binds to the antibodies. Under a microscope, the abnormal antibodies can then be seen staining or binding to the nucleus. While this is an elegant and sensitive test, it is unfortunately not standardized. Consequently, different laboratories use different procedures and sometimes get different results with the same blood sample. A change in the FANA test may not reflect a change in the patient's condition, but rather in the laboratory used for analysis. You can see why it is so important that a physician be familiar with the laboratory that is performing the test.

Over 95 percent of patients with lupus have a positive FANA test. However, patients with other diseases, including rheumatoid arthritis, can also have positive FANA tests. Indeed, with certain test methods, 50 percent of RA patients will test positive for FANA. A positive FANA test, then, does not necessarily mean the patient has lupus. To diagnose lupus, you need to look at other criteria as well.

LE (Lupus Erythematosus) Test.

This related antinuclear antibody test is not commonly performed anymore, although its discovery opened up the whole field of antinuclear antibodies. The test is technically difficult and cumbersome, and only 50 percent of lupus patients have positive LE cell tests, which means it won't identify 50 percent of patients as having the disease. In addition, 10 percent of RA patients have a positive LE test.

Both RF and FANA reactions can occur in healthy people. Both occur rarely in the young but are found in as many as 5 percent of the elderly. No one knows exactly why this is so.

Anti-DNA and Anti-Sm.

Patients with lupus have antibodies to DNA (deoxyribonucleic acid, the material of heredity). It is unusual to find such antibodies in anyone who does not have lupus, so this is very useful for diagnosis. The levels of anti-DNA frequently rise and fall with disease activity, making this test a good monitoring tool. By gauging anti-DNA levels, the physician can tell how severe the disease is and perhaps increase the frequency of monitoring and look for changes in the condition so that therapy can be adjusted appropriately.

Lupus patients also have antibodies to Sm, another substance found in the cell's nucleus (Sm is an abbreviation of the name Smith, the patient in whose serum the antibody was first discovered). These antibodies also occur in lupus patients only. There's no clear relationship between the severity of lupus and levels of anti-Sm. This test is therefore not useful in monitoring the activity of the disease, and is usually not repeated during the course of treatment.

Complement.

The complement system consists of a complex set of blood proteins that are key to the body's defense system. These proteins remain inactive in the blood until an antibody binds to an antigen and activates the complement components. The complement system in turn produces factors that help destroy bacteria and summon white blood cells to combat the invasion of foreign material. These reactions consume complement, so depressed levels indicate that a great deal of immune complex formation or antibody binding with antigen is going on within the body. Lupus patients often show depressed levels of total complement. However, the same is true with some infectious diseases such as hepatitis or bacterial endocarditis (an infection of the heart lining). Complement may also be low in diseases called vasculitis (an inflammation of the blood vessels). Complement testing may be useful in monitoring how active a lupus patient's disease is, but it alone is not proof of the diagnosis.

Examining the Joint Fluid

Though arthritis affects the joints, doctors seldom perform joint tissue biopsies (removal of a small piece of tissue for examination under the microscope). Joint biopsies do not usually give us enough diagnostic information to be worthwhile.

Analysis of the synovial fluid that fills the joint, however, can provide a great deal of valuable information. It can tell us with certainty whether the crystals that cause gout are present or if there is an infection in the joint. To remove the joint fluid, your doctor will first sterilize the skin around the joint with iodine and anesthetize the area, usually with a freezing solution. He or she will then insert a needle similar to those used to draw blood into the joint, and, depending on the joint, will draw out anywhere from a few drops to a few tablespoons of fluid. This is called tapping a joint. If the joint is very swollen, your doctor will remove larger amounts of fluid to help relieve pain. This is an outpatient procedure, and there may be some discomfort.

Your doctor will then look carefully at the fluid. Synovial fluid from a normal, healthy joint is usually clear, although the fluid can also be clear if you have degenerative arthritis, the kind that involves a wearing away of the cartilage that cushions the ends of the bones. After a major injury, fracture, or bad cartilage tear, there may be some blood in the fluid. The fluid in the joints of patients who have inflammatory or infectious arthritis is usually cloudy and pus-like, because it contains a large number of white blood cells.

If your doctor is at all suspicious about joint infection, he or she will search for microorganisms in a sample of synovial fluid. The fluid is treated with a special dye called Gram's solution and then observed under a microscope. Bacteria that have been stained by this dye can then be easily seen. This method gives results right away. However, a laboratory culture of the fluid, in which bacteria are allowed to multiply in special nutrients, is also performed to allow detection of rare organisms not easily seen with a Gram's stain. If bacteria are present in joint fluid, the fluid is considered infected. Although joint infections are not common, examination of the joint fluid for bacteria is a worthwhile precaution because it's sometimes difficult to tell the difference between joint inflammation and infection.

The laboratory also performs a cell count to determine precisely the number and kinds of white blood cells in the joint fluid. Joint fluids that are clear and contain few cells are called noninflammatory. Joint fluids that contain large numbers of white blood cells are called inflammatory.

Finally, your doctor will examine the joint fluid for crystalline materials, such as those that cause gout and pseudogout. These crystals appear brightly colored under a polarizing microscope. The presence of such crystals signifies a definitive diagnosis. Examination of crystals should always be performed for patients with undiagnosed arthritis.

Analysis of joint fluid therefore allows your doctor to classify your arthritis in one of three categories—noninflammatory, inflammatory, or infectious.

X-rays

X-rays are a key diagnostic tool in rheumatology because they allow the clinician to see the swelling of soft tissue or the accumulation of fluid in a joint; bone problems, such as bone loss in rheumatoid arthritis; and changes in the surfaces of a joint.

Those joints that are the most painful or inflamed are the ones I'll generally target for an X-ray. This may be a difficult choice for some diseases, such as rheumatoid arthritis, in which many joints are involved. In such a situation, to avoid unnecessary expense and radiation exposure, your doctor may decide to X-ray only your hands and feet because they are so commonly involved; X-rays of these areas will give your doctor helpful information about the type of arthritis you may have, especially about joint erosion. Sometimes the joint selected for X-ray may seem strange to you. For example, if you come in complaining of knee pain, your doctor might X-ray your hips. This is because pain in the hip often travels to the knee.

X-rays are particularly helpful in helping your doctor distinguish between the two most common arthritic diseases, osteoarthritis and rheumatoid arthritis. Each of these looks very different on an X-ray. Osteoarthritis causes a narrowing of the joint space. The irregular wearing away of protective cartilage makes the joint space appear uneven. Other visual evidence of osteoarthritis includes thickening of bone, formation of cysts under the cartilage, and bony growths called spurs. In contrast, rheumatoid arthritis causes a uniform narrowing of joint space, loss of bone density around the joint, and swelling of the tissues. In more advanced cases of RA, when joint damage has occurred, there will be a wearing away or erosion of the bone at the end of the joint, which may look under X-ray as if a bite has been taken out of the bone. The appearance of bone erosions on X-rays will help your doctor make important decisions about drug therapy.

X-rays are often taken for baseline purposes so your doctor can see whether your disease is progressing and how it is responding to treatment. They may also be taken when surgery is being considered, to assess the extent of joint damage.

X-rays can also be helpful in diagnosing ankylosing spondylitis and the related conditions called spondyloarthropathies by allowing your doctor to judge inflammatory changes around the sacroiliac joints.

Sometimes dye is injected into a joint space before taking X-rays. This dye is radiopaque—that is, it cannot be penetrated by X-rays—and therefore appears as a light area on X-ray film. The dye outlines features of the joint and allows your doctor to see if there has been any mechanical damage to joint structures, such as a torn cartilage.

Arthroscopy

If you have severe pain or swelling in your knees or shoulders, your doctor may perform an arthroscopy. An arthroscope, a fiberoptic instrument about the diameter of a straw, allows the physician to see inside a joint and determine whether there is any damage to the bone or cartilage. The arthroscope is inserted through a small incision. Its flexibility enables the doctor to see the entire interior of the joint. The procedure is often done on an outpatient basis and anesthesia may be general, local, or spinal. Arthroscopy is often used to diagnose and treat various sports-related injuries. It can also be used for minor surgical repairs, such as the removal of small pieces of torn or loose cartilage. In that case, another small incision will be made through which the surgeon operates, and a third incision may be made for drainage. Arthroscopy, however, is not a routine procedure for the diagnosis of arthritic conditions.

Tissue Typing

Several years ago, there was a great deal of excitement about tissue typing—the analysis of tissue to determine its pattern of genetic markers—as a diagnostic tool for arthritis. It was discovered that some common arthritic diseases are associated with the presence of genetic markers called human leukocyte antigens (HLA). Most people with ankylosing spondylitis, for example, have an HLA marker known as HLA-B27.

Another HLA marker, HLA-DR4, is associated with rheumatoid arthritis. The problem with using tissue typing as a diagnostic tool is that many perfectly healthy people who have no symptoms of arthritis also have these markers. Most people with HLA-B27, for example, do not have arthritis. The chances of having a positive test result for this marker will vary among different ethnic and racial groups. There is an 8 percent chance among whites that the test will be positive. Blacks have a 3 percent chance. Many physicians therefore hesitate to use tissue typing and feel it has little, if any, place in routine diagnostic work. Although my own research at Duke involves the genetics of arthritis, I rarely use HLA typing for clinical purposes. The information obtained can be ambiguous and may lead to overdiagnosis. Recently, there has been interest in using HLA markers to help determine the likelihood of disease progression and the need for more aggressive therapy. The value of tissue typing for these purposes is still untested.

Other Diagnostic Tests

Since arthritic diseases often affect parts of the body other than the joints, other diagnostic tests may include biopsies or special tests of other tissues and organs. When the eyes are inflamed, as they are in ankylosing spondylitis, Reiter's syndrome, and childhood arthritis, a special eye examination called the slit-lamp exam will be conducted. This is a painless procedure during which an ophthalmologist shines a light into your eye while looking through a magnification scope. For more unusual and rare types of arthritis, kidney, liver, artery, muscle, and nerve biopsies may be performed, depending upon the organs affected. In most cases, however, the more simple diagnostic procedures described in this chapter will provide your doctor with enough information to make an accurate diagnosis.

Should You Get a Second Opinion?

You may also want to get a second opinion. I think many doctors appreciate second opinions, especially before embarking on therapy with potentially serious side effects. In my own practice, I often seek second opinions from colleagues with specialized expertise. I'll often refer my rheumatoid arthritis patients to an orthopedic surgeon early on if they look like possible candidates for future surgery. I feel the surgeon should get to know these patients and should be an integral part of their treatment plan.

Because arthritic diseases can affect a person's work and lifestyle, I often refer patients to physical and occupational therapists as part of an initial evaluation. Those of us in the Duke program feel this team approach to medicine is most helpful for you.

Putting Together the Diagnosis

Though the preceding list of tests may seem long and complex, you will probably need to have no more than a few of them performed to complete your diagnosis. To illustrate, let's look at the case of Betsy, a fifty-five-year-old who came to my office complaining of swollen joints in her hands, generalized achiness, and morning stiffness. The pattern of symptoms Betsy described and a physical examination of her affected joints led me to suspect that she had rheumatoid arthritis. I ordered ESR, RF, and FANA tests, which revealed a high sed rate and a high RF, but a negative FANA. These results pointed to a diagnosis of rheumatoid arthritis. I then took X-rays of Betsy's hands, which confirmed the initial diagnosis.

In another case, a nineteen-year-old college football player came into my office complaining of swelling in his left knee. The physical examination showed no indication of any other joint involvement, and it was a good guess that this swelling was related to a sports injury. A blood count and a sed rate test came back normal, and I sent the young man to an orthopedic surgeon, along with a note saying that if the surgeon felt this wasn't a sports-related injury, we might think about doing further testing to see if this wasn't a symptom of ankylosing spondylitis.

After a thorough physical examination, your doctor should have a good idea about other tests that will be needed to confirm the diagnosis. Most of these tests will be blood tests and may require only a single trip to the laboratory. You'll probably have the results back within a week. Then together, working as partners, you and your doctor can use these results to discuss what the probable course of your disease will be and what treatment options are available.

PART TWO

What Kind of Arthritis Do I Have?

4

Rheumatoid Arthritis

Mary was forty-two years old when she first began to notice a nagging discomfort in her joints. First her wrists and fingers bothered her, and then her knees. The pain came and left. Mary sometimes felt achy all over, as if she had the flu. She noticed that her joints felt worse in the morning, but that if she took a hot shower, she felt better.

With two school-aged children and a secretarial job, Mary didn't have much time to dwell on her aches and pains. She took some extra-strength aspirin and tried to brush her discomforts aside. She joked to her husband about being over the hill.

Over the next few weeks, however, the pains became more constant, and Mary's fingers became swollen. She felt so stiff in the morning that it was hard to get out of bed. The stiffness wore off in an hour or two, and by the time she got to the office, she was able to get through the day and type without too much pain. But she decided it was time to consult a doctor.

Mary's family physician referred her to a rheumatologist, who did a thorough physical exam and conducted several lab tests. He told Mary that she had rheumatoid arthritis.

Mary remembered an aunt whose fingers were misshapen from arthritis. She was concerned that this might happen to her.

Like Mary, many patients come to my office concerned about their diagnosis. Younger patients can't seem to believe they have arthritis. Isn't that supposed to be a disease that old people get? They are full of questions: Will they be able to work, take care of their families, keep up with their outside interests? Will they end up crippled by the disease? Some are so fearful they don't consult a doctor at all until their symptoms are quite severe. "After all," explained one of my patients, "you really can't treat arthritis anyway. So why bother?"

These widespread misunderstandings about rheumatoid arthritis—or RA—are unfortunate, especially when they keep people from coming for treatment. It is true that a small percentage of people with RA may have more serious complications. But this is one disease in which early intervention can make a big difference. As a physician, I find it discouraging that people wait, sometimes for years, before seeking medical care. While doctors can't make any definite promises as far as the course of this disease is concerned, we can provide excellent medicines that may slow or prevent more serious complications.

The vast majority of people with RA have mild to moderate symptoms that can be kept under control. With proper medication, physical therapy, and rest, most patients lead essentially normal, productive lives.

What Is Rheumatoid Arthritis?

Rheumatoid arthritis is an inflammation of the synovial membrane, the thin tissue that lines a joint. No one knows exactly why the joint linings become inflamed, but most people with RA suffer a mild to moderate amount of swelling and pain as a result of this inflammation.

Normally, inflammation is part of a protective response by the immune system. The inflammatory process helps your body fend off infection and heal injuries. But the inflammation in RA seems to occur for no apparent reason. The immune system is activated and sends white blood cells to the joints as though there were an infection present. Sometimes the joint inflammation becomes so intense that it damages protective cartilage, bone, and tissue. RA is sometimes called an autoimmune disease because the body seems to be mistaking its own tissues for a foreign invader and attacking itself. However, we don't really know the exact cause of RA, or if this is a proper designation.

Your rheumatoid arthritis may never progress beyond the initial swelling and inflammation of the joints. In fact, I've known many patients who have had a mild form of RA for ten to twenty years, and there's no reason to believe that their condition will get worse.

In a small percentage of patients, the disease may progress to a more serious stage. Over a long period of time, the inflamed tissue can grow and produce substances that may eventually damage the cartilage and bone in the joints, so movement of the joints becomes painful. The continued damage to cartilage, bone, and ligaments may lead to severe pain and deformities, which is why RA is sometimes called crippling arthritis.

As RA advances, the cells of the joint lining begin to multiply rapidly, and the normally thin, smooth synovial membrane becomes thickened, rough, and swollen, forming a mass of tissue called a pannus that can be seen and felt. This thickening process is called synovial proliferation.

Physicians at one time thought that there was a similarity between the rapid division of synovial cells and the growth of cancer cells. They mistakenly called the thickening membrane malignant synovium. We now know that the cells growing in the synovium are normal, not cancerous. Their growth is caused by the inflammation process.

If you examined the fluid in an arthritic joint under a microscope, you would see that the inflammation attracts an invasion by white blood cells. The joint fluid, infiltrated by these cells, expands and looks as if it is filled with pus. A large number of white blood cells called leukocytes become very active in the joint, producing enzymes and other substances that can damage protective cartilage. If untreated, RA may over the years wear away the cartilage, leaving bony surfaces unprotected.

Though the effects of RA are most clearly seen in the joints, RA is a systemic disease and can affect the body as a whole. For example, some people run a low-grade fever, are fatigued, or have muscle aches and pains. In fact, many RA patients describe themselves as feeling "sick all over." Rarely, this form of arthritis can affect such organs as the skin, muscles, lungs, and heart.

To summarize, RA can progress in three main stages: inflammation of the synovial lining; the rapid division and growth of cells; and the resulting destruction of cartilage and bone. I'd like to emphasize here that only a minority of people with RA will progress through the last stages of the disease. In fact, most patients have a controllable form of RA that never moves beyond pain and swelling in the joints.

Who Gets RA?

Rheumatoid arthritis is the most common form of inflammatory arthritis. An estimated 0.3 to 1.5 percent of the U.S. population have it. It is found in all racial and ethnic groups and can affect anyone at any age. I've seen children as young as three and elderly people as old as ninety-five with RA. Most cases of RA, however, are diagnosed in people in the middle years of life, between the ages of thirty and fifty, and the prevalence generally increases with age. The odds of getting RA also increase if you are female: Women are two to three times more likely than men to have RA. Heredity likely plays some role in increasing a person's susceptibility to this disease (see chapter 20).

What Causes RA?

Although scientists have been studying this disease for many years, its exact cause remains elusive.

Since the inflammatory process is the body's response to a foreign invader, many scientists believe the inflammation in RA is a reaction to some as-yet-undetected infection, perhaps a virus or bacteria, that is lodged in the joint. At one time, physicians surgically removed internal organs, such as the gallbladder, in the belief that they were sources of infection that could "seed" the joints. This approach was not successful.

Despite years of investigation, no infectious agent has yet been found in a rheumatoid joint. But there still remains great interest in searching for unusual microbes. Possibly the bacterium or virus that causes arthritis alters the body's immune system and then disappears from the body before arthritic symptoms appear.

Another hypothesis is that an invading virus or bacterium may give off a protein similar to the body's own joint tissue. The body may have a great deal of difficulty distinguishing between the invader and its own tissues. In its effort to destroy the invader, the body may mistakenly turn against itself.

Since RA seems to run in families, a genetic predisposition to the disease may help explain why some people get RA while others do not. If someone in your family does have RA, however, that doesn't mean you're automatically going to get it, too. Genetic transmission of RA appears to be a complex process. Of susceptible individuals, only a minority ever develop disease. In animal research at Duke, we've found that *at least* two genes are involved in the transmission of RA to offspring. In addition, there may be some factor in the environment that plays a role in the development of this disease.

There is so much variation in the symptoms of people who have rheumatoid arthritis that some physicians wonder whether it is actually a single disease or instead is a collection of separate conditions that share some features in common.

Early Warning Signs and Symptoms

The joints affected by RA, the amount of swelling and discomfort, and the progression of the disease vary a great deal from person to person. Though the disease does follow a general pattern, it is unlikely that your experience with rheumatoid arthritis will be exactly like anyone else's. You may have several of the symptoms mentioned here, but you aren't likely to experience all of them.

The first sign of RA is synovitis, an inflammation of the synovium, or joint lining. You may feel this as a nagging achiness in your joints. The small joints of the fingers, wrists, and feet are commonly affected early on, but any joint can be the site of the first symptoms.

Often the disease comes on so gradually, over a period of weeks or months, that it's hard for you to pinpoint when symptoms first began. You may notice a feeling of weakness or a recurring tiredness before you feel any joint pain. Less typically, the disease may start out violently, with an overnight explosion of many painful and swollen joints.

The amount of joint pain and swelling is also very individualized. Many find the swelling only moderately annoying and say that it comes and goes. They may be able to continue their work and leisure activities with little disruption. Others report that the pain is severe and constant from the start, and that they need to alter their lifestyles.

While RA may begin in one or two joints, it generally spreads to many joints of the body, both large and small. Typically the fingers, hands, wrists, elbows, shoulders, knees, ankles, and feet are involved. The jaw and neck are also commonly affected. RA usually settles into the joints in a symmetrical fashion, so if your right shoulder or wrist is inflamed, the left one will be too.

Arthritic joints are usually tender and swollen, and may even appear red. The inflammation brings an increased blood flow to the area, and you may find your joints hot and puffy to the touch. The inflammation can get better or worse over time. A sudden worsening of the inflammation is called a flare of the disease. The causes of flares are not understood, but some patients report an increase in pain related to the weather, especially the cold, or to stressful conditions, such as a death in the family, a divorce, or the loss of a job.

Sometimes the pain and swelling will decrease or disappear, either temporarily or permanently. This is known as a remission. These periods of relief from the disease can last from weeks to years. Approximately 10 percent of RA patients will have a complete remission during the first year of the disease.

Sometimes a remission occurs naturally, without treatment; but many times the remission is a result of therapy. I have seen wheelchair-ridden patients who had endured much discomfort undergo complete remissions, after which they were able to resume many of their normal activities.

Though there may be a lot of variation in the duration and severity of symptoms, if you and your doctor develop a good relationship, you can work together to anticipate possible changes in your condition. That's why I personally like to follow patients over a long period of time. If I know that a patient has more trouble with his arthritis in the winter than in the spring, I may suggest that we hold off on making major changes in therapy until I'm sure this is not simply the usual worsening brought on by the cold weather. If I know that there's a family upset and that this may worsen the condition, I try to work along with the family to reduce the stresses and help to prevent a possible flare.

As I mentioned, RA is a systemic disease. Its effects may be felt throughout the body. For example, many people say that they feel stiff in the morning and have "trouble getting going." The stiffness is not usually described as feeling painful. It is more like the morning-after achiness you may feel when you have indulged in strenuous exercise. A hot shower usually helps to alleviate the discomfort.

Morning stiffness usually eases off with time, and physicians use the number of hours it lasts as a measure of how severe your arthritis is. The stiffness may last as long as two to three hours. If the stiffness lasts less than fifteen minutes, it is likely that your condition is improving and that you are in remission. If the amount of morning stiffness is increasing, your condition may be getting worse.

You may also find that you become stiff when you sit in the same position for any length of time. This sensation, which feels as if your muscles have solidified, is called the gel phenomenon. Moving your body at regular intervals helps you to avoid this stiffness.

Fatigue, another common symptom of RA, usually occurs in the afternoon. Fatigue is very likely your body's reaction to substances released into your bloodstream by the activated immune cells. Like morning stiffness, fatigue may be a barometer of your current condition. The earlier in the day you begin to feel fatigued, the more serious your condition may be. Many people complain of a flu-like achiness, and some run a low-grade fever. Some people report a loss of appetite, depression, weight loss, anemia, or cold, sweaty hands and feet.

Firm, painless lumps called rheumatoid nodules may appear under your skin. These can appear anywhere, but are typically found on the elbows, where you rest them against the table. They may come and go.

Muscle pain is another frequent complaint. It is unclear whether the muscles themselves are directly involved by inflammation or whether the muscle pain is caused by inflammation in neighboring joints.

Rheumatoid arthritis may affect the glands in the eyes and mouth that produce tears and saliva, resulting in a feeling of dryness or grittiness in the eyes or in a dryness of the mouth. This condition is called Sjögren's syndrome, or sicca, meaning dryness.

Advanced Physiologic Changes

If you are in the early stages of RA and are undergoing therapy, there is a good chance that you will never be faced with the physiologic changes that occur in the later, more severe forms of the disease. However, you should be aware of the possible complications.

As RA progresses, it can cause damage to cartilage, tendons, ligaments, and bone. On X-rays, this damage can be seen as a narrowing of the joint space (from cartilage loss) and erosion of the bone, usually on the edges of the joint. These erosions make the bone look as if a bite has been taken out of it.

When tendons and ligaments and their attachments are damaged, the alignment of the joints is affected. Fingers may become misshapen, drawing up into positions that are called swan neck and boutonniere deformities. The fingers may drift to the side (ulnar deviation), and the wrists too may become dislocated.

If your neck is involved, you may experience headaches and unnerving popping and cracking sounds. Damage in the feet can sometimes make walking severely painful as the small joints become partially dislocated, causing the ends of bones to absorb the shock of each step.

Pain, inflammation, and erosion of bone and surrounding tissue may permanently limit the joint's full range of motion. It may become hard to perform simple tasks, such as grasping a fork, combing your hair, or buttoning a shirt.

If your knees and hips are affected, walking may become painful and precarious. The rheumatoid knee can be unstable, locking or giving way during walking, thus increasing the likelihood of falls.

In rare cases, fragile skin and inflammation of the small blood vessels can lead to skin ulcers.

A person suffering from advanced RA may experience a general decline in health and be more susceptible to infections. In addition, his or her bones may weaken from disuse. However, most people with RA won't experience these more advanced symptoms, and early treatment can often be extremely effective in preventing them.

How Is RA Diagnosed?

There is no single diagnostic test that can tell your doctor whether you have rheumatoid arthritis. In making a diagnosis, your doctor will try to gather information from your medical history, physical exam, and several laboratory tests and X-rays.

In taking your medical history, your doctor will ask you for details about the onset of your symptoms. Do you have morning stiffness, and if so, how long does it last? How severe is the pain and swelling in your joint? Is the swelling present in the same joint on both sides of your body? The presence of these symptoms for at least six weeks is a strong indication of RA.

Your doctor will also conduct a complete physical exam, checking for evidence of tenderness and swelling in the joints and for the presence of rheumatoid nodules. You will be asked to move your joints so your doctor can observe whether pain and swelling is limiting their range of motion.

There are many laboratory tests that can help diagnose RA. However, the following three tests are the most commonly used.

Rheumatoid Factor (RF) Test.

There is an antibody known as rheumatoid factor that appears in unusually high amounts in the blood of many people with RA. The RF test, also known as the RA latex test, measures the amount of this factor in the blood. Generally speaking, the higher the concentration of rheumatoid factor in the blood, the more severe the rheumatoid arthritis appears to be.

The RF test is extremely useful, but it has several drawbacks. First, rheumatoid factor is not always present during the early course of the disease, often taking several months to appear in the blood. So while you may indeed have RA, this test can come out negative if done too early.

Second, you may have RA, yet never have any measurable signs of rheumatoid factor in your blood. Some 20 percent of RA patients test negative for rheumatoid factor. Even though they lack this factor, their disease follows the same pattern as that of patients who test positive for RF.

Finally, rheumatoid factor can be found in the blood of people with diseases other than rheumatoid arthritis, including those with other forms of arthritis and some infectious diseases.

I am always very interested in the results of the RF test. If one of my patients tests negative for rheumatoid factor, I may repeat the test later. I am also likely to pursue the diagnosis further in order to rule out any of a number of diseases such as gout or lupus that can cause similar symptoms.

Despite its drawbacks, the RF test is the most commonly used in diagnosing RA. Since rheumatoid factor eventually shows up in the blood of most RA patients, it provides the physician with a key piece of information.

Erythrocyte Sedimentation Rate (ESR).

Informally known as sed rate, this test is not as specific a diagnostic tool as the RF test. It can reveal only if there is inflammation present in the body.

The sed rate is the rate at which red blood cells fall to form a sediment at the bottom of a tube. A sample of your blood is placed in a substance that prevents clotting, and is left to sit for one hour. If during that time the red blood cells settle rapidly to the bottom of the tube, that is a sign of inflammatory disease. (Inflammatory substances make red blood cells clump together, so they are heavier and fall faster.) The more rapidly the cells fall, the more severe the inflammation. Of course there are many conditions other than RA that can cause inflammation. So the ESR is just one small clue that the physician may use to interpret the whole picture.

Red Blood Cell Count (RBC).

This blood test will show if you have anemia, a common symptom of arthritis.

Depending on the results of these tests, your doctor may order other blood tests. In addition, he or she may take an X-ray of your joints. X-rays can be very useful in the detection of early bone and cartilage loss, before any deformity has taken place. However, such losses may not show up during the first few months of the disease. Your physician may therefore wish to take X-rays early on to serve as a baseline to determine progression and later damage, should it occur.

Your physician may also wish to examine the joint fluid for evidence of inflammation or infection. Joint fluid is removed by inserting a needle into the joint. This is done under a local anesthetic, as an office procedure.

The hardest time to diagnose RA is early on in the disease, since rheumatoid factor may not be apparent in the blood during the first year and rheumatoid nodules may also take months to develop. In addition, the erosion of bone and cartilage won't show up on X-rays right away. Your doctor may need to examine you a number of times over several months before an accurate diagnosis can be made.

Prognosis

It is difficult to make predictions about the outcome of an individual case of RA, but I can say that the overall prognosis for RA is generally good. RA is usually a lifelong disease, but most people diagnosed as having RA respond to medication and can generally go on with their normal activities, able to lead active professional and family lives.

There are many excellent therapies today that were unavailable in the past, and only a small number of patients develop deformities or have to limit their lifestyles. Mercifully, only a very small number eventually become confined to a wheelchair or a bed.

About 10 percent of patients have a complete spontaneous remission, usually within the first year. Since the condition clears up so quickly and completely for this group, some physicians suspect that these patients may have had some other condition that has been confused with RA.

RA and Childbearing

RA commonly affects women in their childbearing years, and some of my patients worry about whether this condition will affect their ability to have a family. Fortunately I'm able to reassure them that there is no evidence that RA affects fertility or causes damage to the developing fetus. Pregnancy, in fact, seems to improve the condition. Most women with RA who become pregnant notice a marked decrease in the pain and swelling of their joints, at least during the pregnancy.

I must caution you, though, about taking medications while you are trying to conceive or during pregnancy. It's important that you consult your doctor about any medications that could cause problems. An expectant mother being treated for RA must have close medical supervision throughout her pregnancy.

Physician Evaluations

When trying to predict the course of an individual's condition, I usually rely on some key facts from the medical history, physical examination, and laboratory tests. You may want to use this information as a point of discussion with your doctor when you are deciding treatment options.

Seropositive versus Seronegative.

Patients who have rheumatoid factor in their blood are called seropositive. The higher the concentration of rheumatoid factor, the more severe the arthritic condition seems to be. This doesn't mean that seronegative patients are home free. As I mentioned earlier, it's possible to be seronegative and to have a serious form of RA.

Nodular versus Non-nodular Disease.

Nodules are accumulations of inflammatory cells and usually appear in the more intense and persistent cases of RA. As a general rule, people with nodular disease are more likely to have joint damage and deformity.

Erosive versus Nonerosive Disease.

People who have joint erosions—the wearing away of cartilage tissue and bone that can be seen on X-rays—are most likely to suffer later deformities.

Deforming versus Nondeforming Disease.

Deformity is the dreaded and irreversible end result of rheumatoid disease. Some people have a severe bout of RA lasting months or years and develop deformity at that time. The condition may then go into remission, either because of medication or due to the natural course of the disease. With the inflammatory process under control, further damage may be prevented. However, prior deformity and damage cannot be undone. Unprotected bony surfaces rub against each other, making movement painful. People with erosive and deforming disease are therefore likely to have continued pain, even if they have no further inflammation, unless they have corrective surgery.

Duration of Disease.

It's impossible to predict the course of RA for each individual. Generally speaking, the longer someone has a serious form of the disease, the worse he or she is expected to do. Diseases associated with aging tend to make more severe RA symptoms worse. However, if your condition is generally quiet and easy to manage, that's the way it could stay. I've had patients who have had RA for ten or more years without any progressive changes for the worse, and I've had patients with severe RA who have even gone into complete remission. Again, there is no reason to assume that your case of RA will necessarily get worse with time.

Other Predictive Factors

There are several other factors that can influence the outcome of a patient's disease:

Sex.

Rheumatoid arthritis generally affects men more severely than women.

Age of Disease Onset.

The older you are when the disease strikes, the milder your symptoms are likely to be. If you develop RA after you reach the age of fifty, your disease is likely to have a more benign course than if you develop it earlier.

Educational Status.

More highly educated people with RA seem to do better. This is true for many chronic diseases, and the reason is likely complex, since level of education is also related to income and lifestyle, among other factors. More educated people may have better access to care, seek help earlier, or comply better with their treatment programs. They may have less physically demanding white-collar jobs and better resources for modifying their lifestyle so that they get the proper amount of rest. For example, one of my patients, a carpenter, was unable to give up demanding physical labor, even though his joints were aching. We both knew the activity would make him feel worse, but he had to continue working to support his family. In contrast, another of my patients, a college professor, was able to modify his schedule and get sufficient rest during the course of his workday.

Genetic Makeup.

There is evidence that RA is linked to hereditary factors. The presence of a genetic marker—HLA-DR4—may increase a person's risk for RA. Not everyone with HLA-DR4 gets rheumatoid arthritis, but the marker has been found more than twice as often in adults with rheumatoid arthritis than in adults without RA. This marker, found on the body's white blood cells, helps the body distinguish between its own cells and foreign substances.

Psychological Outlook.

RA has long been considered a psychosomatic illness. This doesn't mean that the disease is "all in your mind"; rather, this means that it is affected by your mental outlook. Many of my patients tell me that a recent episode of stress in their lives made their RA worse. So this may be a good time to look at your life and try to clear up unresolved problems. It's also a convincing argument for being optimistic about your condition. Patients who maintain a positive outlook tend to get more involved in their own care and seem to do better physically. Those who are depressed and consumed by their illness may experience more complications. Since mental outlook plays such an important role in this disease, I've presented some suggestions for dealing with stress elsewhere in the book (see chapter 17).

Physician/Patient Partnership.

Informed patients who take an active role in educating themselves about their illness generally fare better. I like to inform my patients about their condition and the possible treatment options. I believe they'll do better, and together we can make better decisions about therapy. My patients also help me understand their needs, and thus I can better manage their care around these areas of concern. One of my patients didn't respond to a daytime medication schedule because he worked nights and the medication didn't take effect when he needed it most. Together we worked out a better medication schedule so that he could work more efficiently. Another patient, a tax accountant, felt overly stressed when the April fifteenth deadline loomed. Together we rescheduled his elective surgery for a quieter time of the year.

Make a list of your personal concerns and discuss them with your doctor. The more you learn about RA and the various treatment options available to you, the more intelligently you can participate in choices about your care, and the more in control you will feel over your life.

Treatments for RA

RA symptoms vary from person to person, and so do recommended therapies. Fortunately, excellent therapies have been developed over the past fifty years. In the last ten years alone, nearly half a dozen new, more effective medications have become available. Surgery to remove diseased synovium or to replace joints with man-made prostheses are additional alternatives now available to people with more severe forms of RA (see chapter 18). These developments are all very encouraging.

The aim of RA therapy is to reduce inflammation and pain, to keep joints as flexible as possible, and to prevent or minimize joint damage. Here at Duke, we use a basic program that has been used successfully at many treatment centers throughout the country. Most people can follow this basic program with good to excellent success. Briefly stated here, the key components of the Duke Program are:

1. Relief of inflammation through nonsteroidal anti-inflammatory drugs (NSAID) (see chapter 14).
2. Sufficient and regular daily periods of rest (see chapter 15).
3. Physical therapy and joint protection (see chapter 17). This includes regular gentle exercises to maintain joint mobility by extending the joint through its full range of motion. Joint protection entails learning new ways to perform everyday tasks to minimize stress on the joints and protecting the joints through splinting and other measures.
4. Pain relief, through medications, physical therapy, and improving your mental outlook (see chapters 14 and 15).
5. Bolstering your general health with proper nutrition, gentle exercise, and a positive outlook (see chapters 16 and 17).

Beyond the Duke Basic Program, there is no one uniform treatment for RA. Treatments will vary, depending on an individual patient's condition.

Medications

The art and science of rheumatology is knowing when to give which drugs so that you can get the maximum benefit with the least amount of risk. When I prescribe medication, I ask myself several questions: Is the disease active? Is the patient in pain because of inflammation? Are the joints being damaged by the progression of the disease?

Generally speaking, if a patient has very severe symptoms, and it looks as if his or her RA is progressing to a more advanced stage, we may decide together to accept the risks of the more powerful, but potentially harmful, drugs. On the other hand, I will usually treat milder forms of the disease more conservatively.

I don't have any set pattern that I apply to every patient. RA patients can have flares and remissions, and I may add or subtract various drugs from the therapy regimen as the patients' needs dictate.

If you have RA, your doctor will probably prescribe an NSAID such as aspirin as a first step, because these drugs are very effective and do not usually have serious side effects. If these don't work or the disease progresses, your doctor may recommend more potent medications. Some of these work within days or weeks while others may require several months to take effect and entail great patience on your part. In more severe cases of RA, the benefits of taking these drugs outweigh their possible side effects, and patients will always be very closely monitored while undergoing drug therapies.

The following are the three main drug groups (for a fuller discussion on individual drugs, see chapter 14).

Nonsteroidal Anti-inflammatory Drugs (NSAIDs).
These drugs reduce inflammation and alleviate its symptoms, including swelling, pain, and fever. While some—for example, aspirin or ibuprofen—can be purchased over the counter, they are generally prescribed for RA in doses much larger than you would normally take on your own. Most NSAIDs require a doctor's prescription.

There are many types of NSAIDs. They differ in frequency of administration, potential side effects, and cost. Your doctor will work with you to determine which drug or combination of drugs should work best for you. Both prescription and nonprescription NSAIDs require close supervision by a physician to assure appropriate dosage and safe use.

Remittive Drugs.
These are slow-acting drugs that may take weeks or even months to produce an effect. They have a variety of different actions and effects on the immune system. Included in this category are gold salts, penicillamine, and antimalarial drugs. Drugs that affect cell growth (called antimetabolites or cytotoxic drugs) are also considered remittive drugs, and include methotrexate, Imuran, and Cytoxan. These drugs were originally developed to treat cancer but now have many uses where inhibiting cell growth is desired. Imuran and Cytoxan are commonly used to suppress immune activity in a variety of diseases other than RA.

Steroids or Corticosteroids.

These powerful drugs act quickly to suppress inflammation. They are related to cortisone and can cause serious side effects if given in high doses for prolonged periods of time. Steroids are therefore prescribed in the smallest possible doses for the shortest time possible.

Follow-up Visits

How often you have to see your doctor depends on the severity of your condition and the type of medication you may be taking. I like to see my patients regularly, to monitor closely the progress of their condition and the effectiveness and safety of the treatment I've prescribed. I see some of my patients as frequently as every week, while others may not come into the office more than a few times a year.

When a patient starts on a remittive drug, such as gold, he or she may need to come in weekly for a blood test and injection. Once the gold therapy has been established, he or she will need to come in only once every three to four weeks. Treatment with methotrexate, another remittive drug, requires a laboratory evaluation every two to four weeks. On the other hand, many of my patients do very nicely on the Duke Basic Program and may only have to see me once every few months. They may also visit physical therapists, occupational therapists, and dietitians as part of follow-up care.

Years ago, patients were commonly hospitalized for rheumatoid arthritis so they could rest for several weeks at a time. This period away from the stress of home life and work often led to dramatic improvement. While rest is still a valuable tool in treating RA, overcrowded hospitals can no longer justify the use of their beds for nothing more than a period of bed rest. Today you will most likely be treated as an outpatient. Hospitalization for rheumatoid arthritis is reserved for times when severe inflammatory symptoms fail to respond well to therapy. A few days in the hospital with complete bed rest, corticosteroids by injection, and intensive physical therapy can make a world of difference for a patient in flare. Surgery, of course, also requires hospitalization.

Surgery

Surgery may be required in advanced cases involving severe pain and disability and a lack of response to other therapies. Surgery is used most commonly to correct joint deformities and relieve pain.

RA Outlook

We understand more about treating RA today than we did in the past, and we're learning more each year. Promising research in the areas of immunology and genetics may eventually unlock the mysteries of this disease.

We are learning through research that NSAIDs offer more benefits than most scientists at first suspected. In addition, as many as fifteen to twenty drugs have been discovered to treat RA—an impressively large arsenal.

There have also been dramatic new improvements in joint replacement. Even those whose joints have been completely immobilized by the disease should have hope: The surgical replacement of damaged joints with artificial ones is now highly successful in reducing pain and restoring function. Hip, knee, hand, shoulder, elbow, and ankle joints can now be replaced with man-made parts.

Although the media is paying a great deal of attention to joint replacement, the really good news is that with today's treatments, most RA patients do not progress to the more severe forms of the disease that might require such surgery. Through a combination of rest, exercise, joint protection, pain relief, and drugs, you can usually lead a full life with RA.

RHEUMATOID ARTHRITIS (RA)

A chronic inflammatory disease that is systemic (i.e., affects the entire body). The synovial membrane that lines the joints becomes inflamed. In severe cases, the disease damages cartilage and bone, leading to crippling deformities.

CAUSE: Unknown, but scientists suspect that some kind of infection and a hereditary predisposition to the disease are involved.

SYMPTOMS: Painful, swollen joints—usually striking symmetrically, in joints on both sides of the body. Also, early morning stiffness; flu-like achiness; fatigue; pain on prolonged sitting; low-grade fever; rheumatoid nodules; muscle aches.

WHO GETS IT? Can strike anyone at any age. Women are two to three times more likely to get it than men. Onset is usually between ages thirty and fifty.

DIAGNOSIS: There is no one definitive test. Diagnosis is based on medical history, a physical examination, several blood and laboratory tests, and X-rays.

TREATMENT: Nonsteroidal anti-inflammatory drugs (e.g., aspirin and ibuprofen), rest, exercise, pain relief. In severe cases, more potent drugs and/or surgery may be necessary.

PROGNOSIS: Generally good. Most people with RA can control their symptoms and lead normal lives. Ten percent go into a complete remission during the first year.

5

Osteoarthritis

Sarah experienced occasional aches and pains in her back for years, but had always shrugged them off and gone on with her active life, which included golf, swimming, and volunteer work at a local hospital. Then about five years ago, when she reached the age of seventy-two, her knees started to hurt, and her back pains grew quite bad. Sarah belongs to a golf league and became very upset when the pain became so acute that she was sometimes unable to walk the greens or to play past the sixth hole.

It was about that time that Sarah also noticed some changes in the shape of her hands. Her knuckles became enlarged, and she had to have her wedding ring enlarged so that she could slip it on and off her finger. Though she didn't have much pain in her hands, they sometimes felt stiff, so it was hard for her to get a good golf grip or to open jars at times.

Sarah's joints sometimes felt stiff in the morning, but after she began to move them around, they felt better. She noticed also that when she sat still for too long, as she did at church services, her joints seemed to freeze up on her.

The physical changes in her fingers and the increasing stiffness in her joints finally prompted Sarah to seek a consultation at Duke's rheumatology clinic. I examined Sarah's joints and conducted several laboratory tests and X-rays. It was quite evident from her medical history and test results that she had osteoarthritis. I started Sarah on a daily regimen of aspirin to relieve her discomfort and recommended a program of daily exercise that would keep her joints limber and strengthen her muscles.

On most days Sarah feels fine. She does her prescribed range-of-motion exercises every morning under a heat lamp in her bathroom. She discovered that the warmth from the lamp helps ease the stiffness in her joints. She's had some episodes in which the pain was severe enough to require her to walk with a cane. She's also had to switch from aspirin to another nonsteroidal anti-inflammatory drug that doesn't irritate her stomach so much. Overall, though, she says she's in "pretty good shape." At seventy-seven years old, she continues to be very physically active. She golfs and swims laps several times a week, and fills her days with volunteer work. As she herself says, "Osteoarthritis can be annoying, and it's hard to keep a good attitude when the pain is bad. But I've learned to live with it. If you don't keep moving, you're a goner."

Osteoarthritis (OA) is the most common form of joint disease. When people say they have arthritis, they usually have this condition.

OA probably results from the wear and tear on our joints over many years of living. If we live long enough, there's a good chance that most of us will develop some form of osteoarthritis. The most common symptoms are stiffness and pain in one or two joints. The symptoms will not necessarily change or grow worse, but they are usually lifelong. Even in cases where the symptoms do grow more severe, as they did for Sarah, the disease can usually be well controlled.

What Is Osteoarthritis?

The word osteoarthritis is a little bit misleading. Literally, *osteon* means bone, and *-itis* means inflammation. Yet osteoarthritis is not really an inflammation of the bone. In fact, there may be little or no inflammation involved in this disease at all.

Osteoarthritis is caused by a change in the nature of the cartilage, the smooth, fibrous tissue that normally cushions the ends of the bones. As the cartilage degenerates, the bones at the ends of the joints thicken, and extra bony growths called spurs, or osteophytes, may form. As a result of these changes, the joint does not function as well, and movement may be stiff and painful. The cartilage breakdown may or may not cause joint inflammation.

Some people confuse osteoarthritis and rheumatoid arthritis, but they are two very different diseases. Rheumatoid arthritis (RA) is an inflammatory disease. It causes tenderness, pain, and swelling of the joints and surrounding tissue. RA is also systemic, meaning that it can travel throughout the body and cause such generalized symptoms as fever, an overall achiness, and anemia. With OA, the joints are not usually inflamed; if they are, the inflammation is comparatively mild. OA is exclusively a joint problem, and does not travel to other parts of the body or affect other organ systems. It does not cause fever, achiness, or anemia. OA, like RA, is a chronic condition, which means that its symptoms may persist for a long time. However, they do not necessarily grow worse over time.

You can see why the term osteoarthritis does not accurately describe what is going on in this disease. Doctors use several medical terms for OA that are somewhat more precise:

Osteoarthrosis.
A disease or a condition involving bony changes around the joint. This definition is more accurate because it does not suggest inflammation.

Degenerative Joint Disease (DJD).
A disease caused by the degeneration or breaking down of a joint component. This refers to the breakdown of cartilage, a major event in OA. Some physicians like to use this term because, again, it does not imply inflammation is involved.

Hypertrophic Arthritis.
Hypertrophic means extra growth, referring to the growth of excess bone or bone spurs typical of the joints of some OA patients.

While these terms may be more accurate in describing the disease, most people still use the term osteoarthritis, and we will, too.

Who Gets Osteoarthritis?

Over 16 million people in the United States have osteoarthritis. The disease usually affects older people, and most people do not show signs of OA until they are at least forty. The prevalence of the disease increases with age, and by the time we reach the age of sixty, well over half of us will have some signs of degeneration in our joints. By the time we enter our eighties or nineties, just about all of us have some evidence of osteoarthritis on X-ray, though we may have no noticeable symptoms.

People in occupations requiring repetitive motions may be more likely to develop OA. Ballet dancers, concert pianists, and pneumatic drill operators, for example, place a lot of stress on their joints. A machine-shop operator who for thirty years ran machinery that required repetitive hand motion developed OA in his fingers. One carpet layer got OA of the knee because he was always jamming his knees into corners to smooth down the carpets. A fair number of farmers whom I treat have OA in their hands from a lifetime of hard physical work. I call it "farmer's hand."

Athletes who overuse and abuse their joints are also more likely than the rest of us to develop osteoarthritis. Baseball pitchers and football players, for example, subject their joints to much abuse. Joe, an avid thirty-six-year-old tennis player, is a good example. He injured his knee playing tennis and had to have surgery. He was told not to overtax the knee again. But Joe didn't listen to this advice. Instead, he continued to play long and strenuous sets of tennis and then tried to ice his knee to lessen the pain. Eventually he developed osteoarthritis in that knee.

Whenever a joint is imperfectly aligned, it is also more prone to develop OA. Some people are born with slight congenital deformities in their joints that may predispose them to OA. Other times the misalignment may be caused by a previous injury or break in the joint.

Overweight individuals are also more likely candidates for OA because of the added stress they impose on their joints.

Some types of OA appear to run in families, so there may be a genetic component to this disease.

What Happens Physiologically?

All forms of OA involve a breakdown of cartilage. As I've already mentioned, most of us will experience some degree of cartilage degeneration over the course of our lives. When I examine older patients in the hospital for other reasons, I frequently find evidence of osteoarthritis—knobby enlargements in the finger joints, for example, or limited neck motion. In most cases, these symptoms will be mild or moderate. Many people who have osteoarthritis have no symptoms at all.

Cartilage is made largely of water and a tough, fibrous substance called collagen. Because of its components, cartilage is normally resilient and can spring back into shape. The spongy cartilage in a healthy joint helps absorb shock and cushion the bones so they glide over one another and allow the joints to move smoothly and effortlessly.

The cartilage has no blood vessels and cannot nourish itself, but it is highly absorbent. It keeps itself healthy by soaking up the nutritious synovial fluid that normally fills the joint space. The normal movement of a joint helps the cartilage fill and empty itself of synovial fluid, thus taking in nutrients and cleansing itself of waste products.

In OA the normally smooth cartilage becomes softened and dull. It begins to lose its elasticity, and its surface may become worn in spots. It also thins out, so it can't absorb as much synovial fluid. Consequently, the bones move closer together, and the joint space narrows. Eventually the cartilage may grow so thin in spots that the bones begin to rub against each other; as they do, tiny pits, fissures, and cracks develop in them.

As the body tries to repair the damage, the ends of the bones thicken and spurs form, resulting in bony enlargements around the joints. Cysts may form in the bone beneath the cartilage, and sometimes pieces of cartilage or bone break off and float around in the joint fluid, irritating and inflaming the synovial membrane, the thin, delicate membrane that lines the joints.

When the cartilage wears away and the joints become stiff and painful to move, your tendency will be to try not to use them. You might favor one hand over another, for example, or unconsciously adapt your movements so you don't use an affected limb at all. While this adaptation is natural, it may only exacerbate the problem. If you don't use a joint, you weaken the muscles and ligaments that surround it. This can make the joint even stiffer. A prescribed program of gentle exercises can help to break this cycle, and is an important part of our program at Duke (see chapter 15).

In extreme cases, when the entire cartilage is worn away, the bone may be completely exposed. This can make it very painful to move your joints.

What Causes OA?

For many years, osteoarthritis was considered purely a result of the aging process. As with other parts of the body, the joints wear out with the passage of time. More recently, scientists have identified other factors that contribute to this disease. There is now a clear distinction made between two types of osteoarthritis—primary and secondary.

Primary OA is the cartilage breakdown associated with the normal process of aging. It is the wear-and-tear type of arthritis that eventually happens to us all to some degree. There is no apparent cause for this type of OA.

Secondary OA is a breakdown in cartilage that seems to have an apparent cause. It can occur in a joint years after an injury such as a fracture or sprain. If the injured joint doesn't heal properly, it may become misaligned and cause later problems. One of my patients, for example, fractured her ankle ice skating when she was in her mid-thirties.

Since then she has had a nagging soreness in her ankle, especially when she plays sports or does a lot of walking. X-rays now show evidence of early OA.

Secondary OA can also be caused by a previous inflammation that changes the functioning of a joint. For example, patients with RA, an inflammatory joint disease, may be more prone to develop OA in that joint, too.

Excessive stress on a joint over time is another cause of secondary OA. Obese people who place extra weight on their joints seem more prone to OA in their hips and knees.

In addition, some people may be born with a misalignment of the joint. This congenital problem may not be apparent when the person is young, but may predispose him or her to arthritis in later life.

Overuse of a joint over a lifetime can also cause secondary OA, which is why professional athletes and people in certain occupations seem to be more prone to the disease.

Scientists also suspect that there is a hereditary predisposition to some forms of OA. The type of OA that causes knobby enlargements of the fingers, for example, seems to be passed down to females in a family.

Some people appear to have the type of metabolism that causes their cartilage to wear out faster than normal. Sometimes osteoarthritis is a sign of an underlying disturbance in hormone balance or mineral metabolism. OA may accompany such conditions as acromegaly (caused by too much growth hormone), hyperparathyroidism (too much calcium in the blood), and hemochromatosis (too much iron in the blood).

Signs and Symptoms

Most people don't experience any symptoms of OA until they are in their forties or fifties. OA usually affects only one or a few joints, but can affect many. The joints most commonly involved are the knees, hips, fingers, neck, and lower back. It's interesting that the knuckles, wrists, elbows, shoulders, and ankles usually do *not* develop signs of OA, unless they have been injured or used excessively. If OA was caused by simple wear and tear, you would expect these body parts to be affected more often.

OA symptoms vary a great deal from person to person. Most often, the disease comes on gradually, causing an annoying soreness or stiffness that tends to be dismissed as a minor nuisance. The pain is often mild or moderate and may come and go, rarely interfering with daily living. Often OA doesn't advance beyond this stage.

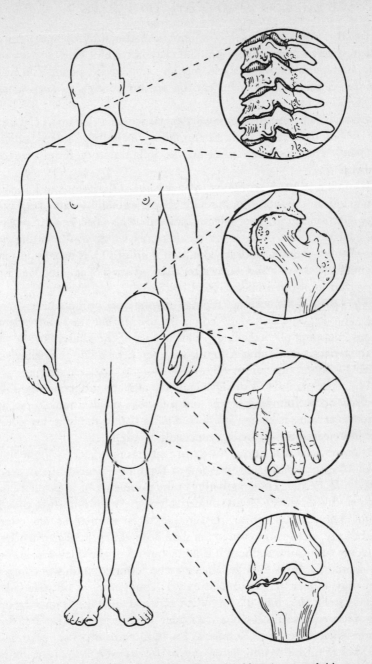

At its common sites of involvement (neck, hips, fingers, and knees), osteoarthritis causes joint space narrowing and spur formation.

On the other hand, some patients find the stiffness and pain grow progressively worse, making it difficult to climb stairs, carry heavy objects, sew, or type. When knees and hips are involved, walking can become painful. Sometimes the pain can be serious enough to keep a person awake at night.

Less typically, some patients will experience a sudden onset of pain with more obvious signs of joint inflammation, including redness, pain, and swelling. This condition is known as inflammatory or erosive osteo-arthritis.

If you have OA, it's common to have some stiffness in your joints when you get up in the morning, but with proper stretching exercises, you can ease the stiffness out. Your affected joints may also become stiff when you hold them in one position for too long, as when you're sitting at the theater or working at a desk. The joint pain of OA is usually less at the beginning of the day and worse after a day's worth of activity. Resting the overtaxed joint often makes it feel better.

You may feel a crackling (crepitus) in your knee or hip when you move the joint. Patients frequently complain to me that they can hear their bones "popping and cracking." This is part of the change in the joint's characteristic functioning. Often I can even hear a faint crackling sound when I examine the joints.

While the pain of OA usually centers in and around the affected joints, pressure on surrounding nerves and muscles can occasionally radiate to other areas. This is known as referred pain. OA in the hips, for example, can be referred down the leg, especially to the knee.

Deformities due to bony growths are common, especially in the fingers. A knobby enlargement in the joint of the finger nearest the fingertip is called a Heberden's node; growths in the middle joints are called Bouchard's nodes (both nodes are named after the men who first described them). These nodes appear most frequently in women, usually after the age of forty, and seem to run in families. Sometimes these growths appear suddenly and cause redness and pain, but often they develop gradually and painlessly. Bony enlargements may be confined to only one finger, or they may appear in several. Naturally, the appearance of these enlargements can be alarming. Though their physical appearance may be upsetting, Heberden's and Bouchard's nodes are not progressive and do not seriously interfere with the normal functioning of a person's hands.

Other deformities may be caused by the uneven erosion of the cartilage. The cartilage on the inside of a joint may be more worn away than the outside, for example, and the result can be misshapen joints, such as bowlegs, that make motion more difficult.

How Is OA Diagnosed?

The diagnosis of osteoarthritis proceeds along the same path as that of rheumatoid arthritis (see chapter 4). Your doctor will first take your complete medical history and perform a thorough physical exam, then order the appropriate laboratory tests and X-rays.

My major goal in diagnosis is to establish that a patient indeed has OA as opposed to an inflammatory form of arthritis such as RA, or another form of arthritis, such as gout. Therefore, I'll usually order the rheumatoid factor (RF) test, erythrocyte sedimentation rate (ESR, or sed rate), and a red blood cell count (RBC). Laboratory tests for OA generally show a lack of rheumatoid factor, a normal sed rate, and a normal red blood cell count.

Laboratory tests, however, do not always give clear-cut answers. Sometimes people with OA, especially older individuals, have other unrelated medical problems that can lead to a low blood count or high sed rate. Inflammatory forms of OA sometimes produce a higher-than-normal sed rate, although the rate is not usually as high as it is for patients with RA. In addition, people over sixty years of age frequently have sed rates twice as high as those for younger people. The reasons for these results are unclear.

As osteoarthritis progresses, X-rays can help your doctor determine whether you have OA. Osteoarthritic joints show a narrow, uneven joint space, spurs, thickened bone, and the formation of cysts underneath the cartilage. The X-ray portrait for RA is very different: The narrowing of the joint space is even, bone is less dense, and there is swelling of the soft tissues. When X-rays are performed very early in the course of these diseases, these distinctive differences may not yet be evident. Your physician may therefore suggest follow-up X-rays in order to assess the progress of your disease.

Sometimes your doctor will want to examine your joint fluid by inserting a needle into the affected joint and withdrawing a sample. The procedure can be done in his or her office with a local anesthetic. OA joint fluid is usually clear, containing few inflammatory cells.

As a consultant rheumatologist, I occasionally see patients whose referring physicians have difficulty distinguishing between osteoarthritis and rheumatoid arthritis, especially in the cases of older patients, in whom the presentation of RA may be somewhat different. Given the similarities in the initial symptoms of RA and OA, this is not surprising. Your doctor wants to be completely sure of the right diagnosis, because treatment may be quite different for each disease. For example, remittive agents (see chapter 14) should not be used in OA because they can do nothing to improve the condition and they have potentially serious side effects.

If your doctor is still confused about your diagnosis after the lab tests and X-rays, he or she will probably want to observe you over the next few months. Usually these conditions will eventually "declare themselves": Their characteristic features will become more obvious, and follow-up lab tests and X-rays will show a clearer pattern of disease.

Treatment

Many people with osteoarthritis don't seek medical help. They think the aches and pains they feel are a normal part of the aging process, and therefore they just put up with the condition. That's a shame, because there are good treatments for OA that can bring relief and help you live more comfortably.

Part of the problem, as I see it, stems from misconceptions picked up from the media. Advertisements and commercials directed toward the "arthritis sufferer" suggest that people can diagnose and treat themselves with over-the-counter pain relievers such as aspirin and ibuprofen. These advertisements do an injustice to the consumer because they do not stress the importance of medical evaluation, especially when symptoms are chronic and persistent. No one should accept constant pain as a normal component of aging, and people should know that there *is* help, even for mild cases of OA.

The aim of treatment in OA is to reduce pain and increase joint mobility. This is accomplished through the use of drugs, rest, exercise, physical therapy, and joint protection. Sometimes your doctor will also help you modify your everyday activities.

Drugs

As with rheumatoid arthritis, treatment for OA usually relies on a group of drugs called nonsteroidal anti-inflammatory drugs (NSAIDs). Aspirin is one of the most effective drugs in this group, but there are many others to choose from, each with its own benefits and disadvantages.

Most NSAIDs have both painkilling and anti-inflammatory actions, but you get these actions at different doses, depending on the drug. For example, if you have osteoarthritis and feel pain in your joints, but have no signs of inflammation, I would want to treat the pain alone, and the dose of aspirin I would prescribe would be on the order of eight tablets a day (two tablets four times a day). On the other hand, if you were suffering from the inflammation that often accompanies RA, I would prescribe a much higher dose.

Lower doses of NSAIDs are, of course, preferable—they are less expensive, safer, and less toxic. For example, aspirin in very high doses can cause such side effects as hearing problems, tinnitus (ringing in the ears), and stomach upsets. By reducing the dosage, we minimize the chance of ulcers, stomach bleeding, and other stomach-related disorders.

Also, if relieving the pain of osteoarthritis is the major goal, then I might want to recommend acetaminophen preparations such as Tylenol. This is an effective analgesic, but does not treat inflammation. Acetaminophen is very safe and lacks some of the more serious side effects of other NSAIDs, especially stomach upset and kidney problems.

Low-dose aspirin and acetaminophen are much less expensive than the newer NSAIDs. This is especially important for many of my older patients, who are frequently on medication for other problems and find the cost of medicine to be a financial burden. Also, OA affects mostly older people, who frequently have other health problems, such as decreased kidney function and heart failure, which increase the risks involved in taking NSAIDs.

It's hard to know how much inflammation is involved in OA, so my usual approach is to prescribe the simplest analgesic therapy, usually low-dose aspirin. If that is not effective, I'll prescribe higher doses or switch to one of the newer NSAIDs that have a more potent anti-inflammatory action. If the more potent drugs work, it probably means that inflammation may be what's causing the pain.

The drug I choose to prescribe will also depend on the individual patient's preferences and on his response to treatment. Some people respond more favorably to one NSAID than another.

Whatever drug your doctor prescribes, he or she will probably aim for the lowest dose that provides acceptable relief. That sometimes means no medication at all. Osteoarthritis may come and go, the symptoms becoming more or less severe at certain times, and your doctor can adjust dosages or try new drugs as the situation arises.

Sometimes the advice I give sounds like the stereotyped doctor's response: "Take two aspirins and call me if it's not better." So why, you may wonder, do you need to consult a rheumatologist? It's easy to forget that anything as common and readily available as aspirin is actually a powerful drug. When you take aspirin or any drug over a long period of time for a chronic condition such as arthritis, you need to be under a physician's guidance. Also, treatment of osteoarthritis often involves more than a trip to the pharmacy. The advice your doctor can give you on proper rest and exercise, physical and occupational therapy, and regular monitoring of your condition may help keep your arthritis under better control.

Since OA does not appear to affect the immune system, the more potent remittive drugs, such as gold, penicillamine, methotrexate, and Plaquenil, have no role in its treatment. Neither does another class of drugs, corticosteroids, which include cortisone and prednisone. Occasionally, however, your doctor may inject a corticosteroid into a painful joint that seems to have become inflamed.

In a few cases, joint pain from OA can become so extreme that it hinders sleep or limits normal activities, and a more powerful painkiller that contains a narcotic may be called for. Narcotics are addictive, and are usually given in the smallest amounts for the briefest period of time. As long as patients are educated about these hazards, and the drug is prescribed in a time-limited fashion, they can be used safely. Narcotics are best used as a temporary measure, for example, while a patient is awaiting surgery.

Weight Loss

There is now good evidence that excess weight can cause joint problems. When a patient with OA is overweight, he or she places an additional burden on joints that are already weakened. I often counsel my overweight patients on the importance of weight reduction. I realize that losing weight may be easier said than done. It's hard to change old habits, and it's especially difficult to lose weight when your joints hurt so much that you've cut down on your normal level of activity. Many people eat out of frustration or boredom. But a healthful diet is extremely important to your improved condition.

I recently treated an overweight patient with OA in his knees. Although I talked to him many times about the necessity of losing weight, he continued to overeat, and in fact put on even more pounds while under my care. Eventually he had a heart attack. Following heart surgery, he joined the Duke University Preventive Approach to Cardiology program

(DUPAC), and started on a diet modification and exercise program. He learned how to cut fat out of his diet and began to swim and exercise regularly on a stationary bicycle. Not only did he lose a great deal of weight, but he can walk farther, he's no longer short of breath, and his joints don't bother him anymore. If you're overweight, you may find that you too can reap many additional benefits from a sensible diet.

Joint Protection

Sometimes during a flare-up, you may need to relieve the stresses on your affected joints. Crutches, walkers, and canes can help tide you over those periods.

Exercise

When your joints hurt, you tend not to want to use them too much. As I mentioned earlier, however, this inactivity may be harmful in the long run. Joints that aren't used tend to stiffen up, and the surrounding muscle may in turn grow weaker. Exercise strengthens the muscles and helps keep joints flexible. It also keeps your bones strong, improves your cardiovascular fitness, and gives you a feeling of well-being.

Gentle stretching exercises performed each day can help you to maintain or increase the range of motion in stiff joints. If you have access to a pool, doing water exercises designed especially for people with arthritis is an excellent way to loosen up your joints, as the water supports your weight and doesn't allow your joints to be taxed. Isometric exercises, in which you tighten the muscles in your body without moving your joints, may also be helpful. At Duke, an exercise regimen is an important part of our arthritis program (see chapter 15).

On the other hand, be careful not to exercise to the point of pain or to add stress to already weakened joints. Check with your doctor to see if the exercises you are currently doing are good for your joints; you may have to modify or abandon them altogether. Your doctor should be able to offer good suggestions on which exercises are best for you. Your local Arthritis Foundation also offers exercise programs.

Sometimes poor posture can place added stress on your joints. A physical therapist can help you improve your body mechanics so that you will learn how to sit, stand, bend, and lift heavy objects in ways that put the least stress on your joints.

Surgery

Occasionally, pain from OA can be so severe and constant that life becomes unbearable. In such cases, joint replacement surgery, the most commonly performed surgery in cases of OA, represents one of the biggest advances in arthritis treatment over the past two decades. Sometimes a damaged joint can be totally removed and replaced by a prosthesis; however, other procedures involve more limited replacement or joint realignment (see chapter 18 for a fuller discussion). Hip and knee joints are the two most frequently replaced joints.

Richard, a sixty-five-year-old bank executive, had OA in both hips. For many years he'd been a very active skier and tennis player, but the pain had grown so bad that he'd had to give these sports up. An energetic businessman who traveled quite a bit, Richard got to the point that he couldn't carry his own suitcases at the airport. Eventually he had trouble walking and even sleeping. The pain interfered with his work, and he had to take a lot of time off.

Richard and his physician decided to go ahead with the surgery, and both of Richard's hips were replaced with man-made joints. For Richard, the surgery has meant a new lease on life. He is now back at work. He can't ski or play tennis anymore, but he enjoys walking and swimming.

Surgery is often very successful in OA because the disease is usually confined to one or a few joints, and it doesn't involve any other organs. With your painful joint replaced, you may once again enjoy life.

Changes in Lifestyle

Most people with OA can continue with their work and their family lives without taking any special measures. However, if your OA interferes with your work, you and your doctor may have to sit down together and evaluate the interrelationship between your arthritis and your lifestyle, a complex issue. What would the personal and financial consequences be if you had to stop work or switch jobs? Should this be a matter of disability or even liability? Is your job important to your self-esteem?

You as the patient must make the final decision on the course of action as far as your job is concerned, but you may find it helpful to talk it out with a professional and discuss possible alternatives that might minimize the economic and emotional trauma of giving up your work. There are many ways to cope with the anxieties caused by lifestyle changes, and I'll discuss these in chapter 17.

You'll also need to take a look at the sports you participate in. Sports-related injuries and overuse problems may contribute to OA. You'll need to consider which sports will minimize your chances of stressing or injuring the joint. If you have a joint problem that is preventing you from participating in a sport, you should certainly have a medical evaluation by an orthopedist or a rheumatologist. My advice is to get a medical evaluation first and find out what the problem is before you continue in the sport or try to treat your arthritis yourself.

Be flexible about your activities, too. If one particular sport, such as skiing or running, is causing a worrisome joint symptom, switch to another activity, such as bike riding or swimming. Later on, if your symptoms subside, you can try switching back. Perhaps if you participate in moderation, you'll be able to stay with the sport. If not, you may have to give it up and switch to a form of exercise that's easier on your joints.

Does jogging cause OA? We don't know yet. The enthusiasm for and broad participation in running is relatively recent, and we have not yet had sufficient time to document its long-term impact on the joints. OA can take many years to develop. As with any sport done in moderation, jogging can build bone and muscle, improve cardiovascular performance, help with weight control, and result in a general feeling of well-being.

I'm sometimes baffled by the devotion of sports enthusiasts to their activity even when it causes pain. Maybe the mastery of pain is an inherent part of athletics. As long as you're educated about the risks to your joints from various activities, you can set your own priorities in terms of risks and benefits. Only when it is undeniable that an activity is harmful would I strongly advise you to give it up. As in many aspects of medical care, you should be informed and then use your own judgment.

Osteoporosis: A Related Condition

A condition commonly considered along with osteoarthritis is osteoporosis. Osteoporosis means porous bones. It is a condition in which the bones become thin and structurally weakened so that they fracture easily. When the bones of the back are affected by this disease, your vertebrae may collapse and you may actually shrink an inch or more. You may become hunched over, exhibiting a deformity known as dowager's hump. Osteoporosis is a common cause of broken hips in the elderly.

We all lose bone as we age, but women are more susceptible than men to this disease. This is because women usually start out with less bone density than men, and then they experience a marked increase in bone loss following menopause. There is evidence that sufficient calcium intake during your adult years can help you keep your bones dense and reduce the chances for osteoporosis. Activity, especially such weight-bearing exercises as walking and bicycling, also builds bone and helps prevent osteoporosis. Conversely, inactivity may accelerate bone loss. Astronauts in space lose bone because of weightlessness; so do those who are bedridden or paralyzed and those whose limbs have been immobilized by fractures.

People with arthritis may in general be more susceptible to osteoporosis because they tend to be less active. They may also be taking cortisone-related medications, which may worsen osteoporosis. Osteoarthritis and osteoporosis can occur together in older patients and frequently interact. Sometimes lower back pain caused by osteoarthritis is thought to be due to osteoporosis. During the early stages of these diseases, it may be difficult to distinguish between them on X-rays.

While we know that exercise can slow down osteoporosis and help keep bones dense, it may be hard for a patient with osteoarthritis to be active. In addition, some patients with osteoarthritis are reluctant to move their joints because they fear they'll inflict additional damage. When a patient of mine has both osteoarthritis and osteoporosis, I try to treat the pain of OA and help him or her start or resume an exercise program to improve the range of motion and keep his or her bones as healthy as possible.

To help prevent osteoporosis, I advise my patients to make sure they have adequate amounts of calcium in their diets, including calcium supplements if necessary. Some people with OA worry that the extra calcium will make their spurs enlarge and worsen their disease. I don't know of any evidence to this effect. I think that the need to minimize the chance of osteoporosis, especially in women, overrides the theoretical possibility that calcium supplementation will add to bone growth in OA.

Prognosis for OA

The outlook for OA is generally very good. Although the disease is chronic, many people have mild to moderate symptoms that may never get any worse. Osteoarthritis can usually be controlled well through a combination of nonsteroidal anti-inflammatory drugs, exercise, protection for the joints, and pain-relief techniques. Only a minority of people develop severe pain or disabling deformities from this disease. With today's ever-improving surgical techniques, joint replacement offers hope to this group. Most people cope very well with OA, experiencing minimal disruption of their daily lives.

OSTEOARTHRITIS (OA)

A chronic degenerative disease of the joints caused by the erosion of cartilage, the protective cushioning at the ends of the bones. As cartilage degenerates, joint spaces may narrow, bones around the joint may grow thicker, and bony growths, or spurs, may form. The changes in the joint and surrounding tissues may cause stiffness and pain. Usually there is little or no inflammation involved, and the disease is confined to the joints and does not spread to any other body systems.

CAUSE: Primary OA appears to be due to the normal wear and tear of aging. Secondary OA may be caused by a previous injury, congenital deformity, previous joint damage, or overuse of a joint for prolonged periods of time. Some forms appear to be hereditary.

SYMPTOMS: Stiffness and pain in one or several joints, especially after activity. Rest usually makes the joint feel better. May be least painful in the morning and worse at night.

WHO GETS IT? Primary OA is seen mostly in older people, and rarely in people younger than forty. Women are at higher risk than men. Secondary OA can affect anyone who has had a previous joint injury or infection, who has a congenital joint problem, or who works in a profession that requires repeated use of a joint.

DIAGNOSIS: It is important to distinguish OA from inflammatory arthritis. The same tests are used for both, including a medical history, physical examination, several blood and laboratory tests, and X-rays.

TREATMENT: Nonsteroidal anti-inflammatory drugs (e.g., aspirin and ibuprofen), rest, heat applications, and exercises to improve body mechanics and joint flexibility. In severe cases, surgery may be necessary.

PROGNOSIS: Generally good. Most people have mild to moderate symptoms that do not interfere with their daily routines.

6

Systemic Lupus Erythematosus

Barbara is an outgoing and energetic twenty-two-year-old who had just started a new job as an assistant administrator in the personnel department of a large department store. This was her first job after graduating from college, and she was naturally anxious to prove herself. Barbara's cheerful efficiency impressed her new boss; she seemed always willing to go the extra mile. Then, over a three-month period, Barbara began to notice some strange symptoms that were making it difficult for her to concentrate. She ran periodic fevers, her joints hurt her, and she had pains in her chest that seemed to come and go for no apparent reason. She felt depressed and began to have trouble sleeping.

At first Barbara thought that the stress of her new job was making her nervous and run-down. But as the pain and the swelling in her joints, especially in her fingers, increased, she became convinced that something must be wrong physically. Suspecting that she had arthritis, she went to see her family doctor.

Though Barbara's fingers and hands hurt, the physical examination did not show any obvious signs of joint inflammation. Laboratory tests showed Barbara's red and white blood cell counts were a little low, and her doctor was concerned. He thought maybe this was an early form of rheumatoid arthritis and wanted to keep a close eye on the condition. He prescribed aspirin (ten tablets a day) and told Barbara to come back in a month for further testing.

Over the next month, things got worse. Barbara's hands ached constantly and she had severe chest and abdominal pains. The fevers became more frequent, and she became quite depressed. For the first time since she had started her job, Barbara had to call in sick and missed three days of work. She called her parents, who lived in a nearby city, and they became quite worried about her. They urged her to keep her next doctor's appointment.

On Barbara's next visit, her doctor ordered a more complete battery of laboratory tests. This time the tests told a different story. The new laboratory work and the appearance of certain antibodies in Barbara's blood pointed to a diagnosis of systemic lupus erythematosus.

What Is Lupus?

Systemic lupus erythematosus (also called lupus or SLE) is a chronic condition that usually includes joint inflammation. Unlike many other diseases associated with arthritis, however, lupus is not solely a disease of inflamed joints. Rather, it is a systemic condition that can affect the skin, blood, lungs, cardiovascular and nervous systems, and kidneys.

The word *lupus* is Latin for wolf. The disease got its name because many people who have it develop a characteristic rash on the face and cheeks that was thought to look wolf-like. *Erythematosus* simply means red, and refers to the color of the rash.

Lupus is called an autoimmune disease because the immune system, which normally helps destroy foreign invaders, seems to turn against itself and attack healthy tissues in the body. It is also called a connective tissue or collagen vascular disease because of the types of tissues it can affect.

Lupus is a challenging disease for the physician. It is sometimes called the "great pretender" because its symptoms are so wide-ranging and difficult to separate from other conditions. If one of my lupus patients has aches and fever and other signs of infection, for example, I have to figure out whether this is a manifestation of her lupus or a completely separate condition.

The drugs used to treat lupus may cause side effects that are also hard to distinguish from the symptoms of lupus. Red blood cells in a patient's urine may be evidence that lupus is affecting the kidney; on the other hand, it may be a reaction to Cytoxan, a drug that sometimes irritates the bladder. Some patients develop personality changes and don't quite act themselves. This is sometimes a reaction to corticosteroid treatment; however, it may also be a sign of lupus.

To add to these complexities, the benefits of therapy for each complication of lupus have to be weighed against the effect of the therapy on other organ systems, and against its impact on the patient as a whole.

It is not possible to discuss the intricacies of lupus in one short chapter. What I will do instead is give you a broad overview of the disease and its treatment. In reading this material, you should not be alarmed at my description of all the symptoms or complications of lupus. I can't emphasize enough that no one patient will experience all of these, and I want to reassure you that having lupus doesn't invariably mean a dire prognosis.

Who Gets Lupus?

Lupus primarily affects young women. In fact, females are about five to ten times more likely to get it than males. The disease usually begins when a young woman is in her childbearing years, between the ages of twenty and thirty, leading researchers to suspect that female hormones may predispose women to this disease or may accelerate its course. This predisposition to lupus as well as to other immune disorders may stem from some basic differences in the female immune system and from some specialized mechanisms that allow a woman to conceive and maintain a pregnancy.

Less commonly, the disease has been known to affect older people and sometimes children. Generally speaking, those who get the disease after age fifty have milder symptoms.

Lupus also strikes certain racial and ethnic groups more frequently than others. In the United States, blacks and Hispanics are at greater risk. In other countries, different ethnic minorities are at higher risk. Frequently these minorities have recently immigrated to their new country and have a lower standard of living. This seems to suggest that the environment, nutrition, and other socioeconomic factors may play some role in the disease. If you combine the factors of race and sex you get some startling statistics: a black woman in America is approximately one hundred times more likely to get lupus than a white man.

Heredity may contribute to a person's so-called relative risk for lupus, but having a blood relative with lupus doesn't necessarily mean that you will also develop the disease. The chance of developing a disease also has to do with how common that disease is to start with. Lupus is not all that common, affecting only several hundred thousand people in the United States. So if you have a one in a thousand chance of developing lupus and one of your blood relatives has that disease, your risk is liable to go up to two in a thousand, still relatively unlikely.

A number of identical twins have been reported to have lupus. This "experiment of nature" shows the powerful role heredity can play in susceptibility to arthritis. On the other hand, there have also been twin studies in which only one twin developed lupus. These studies illustrate that other factors also play a role in the appearance of this disease.

Some data suggest a curious relationship in families predisposed to lupus and other autoimmune diseases. While women in such families appear more vulnerable to immune disorders, the men may be more affected by other problems than chance would dictate. There seems to be a higher than expected number of men who stutter or who have learning disorders such as dyslexia, for example. So males in families predisposed to lupus may not be free from problems; the problems may just be expressed in different ways.

Signs and Symptoms

Probably no two patients show exactly the same signs and symptoms either at the outset of lupus or as it progresses. One patient may come to me complaining of severe headaches and skin rashes; another may tell me that she has severe abdominal and chest pains; still a third may have fever and mild joint pains.

Despite this baffling array, there are certain signs and symptoms common to the disease that will generally lead a physician to suspect lupus. The following is a rather lengthy list, and I hope it doesn't alarm you. If you have lupus, you may have one or several of these symptoms, but I want to emphasize that you are not likely to have all of them. Lupus is often mild or moderate in its course. You should, however, be aware of the many possible warning signs.

Generalized Symptoms.
The first symptoms you feel may be a generalized malaise or discomfort. You may experience a flu-like achiness, weight loss, swollen glands, fatigue, and fever—all symptoms pointing to an infection.

Arthritis.
Your joints may be painful and tender, as they are with rheumatoid arthritis. Indeed, when lupus first appears, it may be mistaken for RA, and vice versa. The most frequently involved joints are the hands, wrists, elbows, knees, and feet. Lupus does not usually damage the bone and

cartilage in the joint the way rheumatoid arthritis can, but in rare cases it can lead to some deformity.

Early on in the disease, you may experience a great deal of joint pain, yet there may be little evidence of swelling or tenderness. When other signs of lupus are not yet apparent, this joint pain can be confusing. You and your family must understand that the pain is definitely not "all in your head." It is very real. An experienced physician should be able to recognize this discrepancy and suspect a diagnosis of lupus.

Rash.

Lupus causes skin rashes on the face and on other parts of the body. The classic lupus rash is called a butterfly rash because it spreads over the patient's nose and cheeks in the shape of wings. In a type of lupus called discoid lupus, the condition stays confined to the skin.

Serositis.

A serosa is a layer of connective tissue that lines a body cavity and organs such as the heart and lungs. In lupus, the serosa may become inflamed, causing pleuritis or pericarditis (inflammation of the tissue covering the lungs and heart). This can result in severe chest pains, difficulty in breathing, and fever. Fluid can accumulate in the membranes and be visible on X-ray. Sometimes so much fluid accumulates around the heart that it impairs the heart's ability to pump blood. In such cases, the fluid has to be drained either through a needle or surgically.

The serositis may also affect tissues in the abdominal cavity and may mimic conditions such as appendicitis, which, unlike serositis, requires prompt surgery. When a patient complains of severe abdominal pains, a physician may therefore have to consider exploratory surgery. There is sometimes no other way to be sure that the pain is simply serosal inflammation.

Blood Cell Changes.

Lupus can lower red blood cell, white blood cell, and platelet counts. As a result, you may become pale, tired, and weak. You may also have an increased susceptibility to infection. Since blood platelets are necessary for clotting, a decrease in their count may cause an increased tendency to bleed after surgery.

Photosensitivity.

Some people with lupus have an increased sensitivity to ultraviolet light, and their symptoms, especially skin rashes, may worsen when exposed to the sun.

Immunologic Abnormalities.

People with lupus have abnormal antibodies in their blood called autoantibodies. Some of these autoantibodies may attack the body's own healthy tissues and cause the signs and symptoms of lupus. Identification of these antibodies in laboratory tests helps the physician to diagnose this disease (see FANA and anti-DNA and anti-Sm tests, chapter 3).

One unusual antibody found in people with lupus mimics those that the body produces when infected with syphilis and can produce false positive results in the test for syphilis. This test is called the Venereal Disease Research Laboratory test (VDRL). One young patient I saw in consultation discovered she had lupus when she applied for her marriage license and was found to have a positive VDRL. She was extremely upset and embarrassed about the test results. However, further evaluation indicated that the test result was false positive and likely due to lupus.

Hair Loss.

Some people find that they lose their hair when the disease flares, or becomes active. This is called alopecia. When the lupus improves, the hair grows back.

Raynaud's Phenomenon.

You may find that your fingers become numb, burn, tingle, and change color whenever it's cold or when you have an emotional upset. This condition is caused by a narrowing of the blood vessels in the fingers; the fingers first turn white when vessels constrict, blue as the blood pools in the fingers, and then red when the vessels open and normal flow is restored. Raynaud's phenomenon may also occur in people who do not have lupus, or it may be a part of other connective tissue diseases including rheumatoid arthritis.

Kidney Problems.

The kidneys, which separate waste products from the blood and excrete them as urine, are a major site of inflammation and injury in lupus. However, how severely they are affected varies from one person to another; often the involvement is mild.

If the inflammation damages the kidney's filtering system and too much protein from the blood leaks into the urine (proteinuria), your body's balance of fluids and salts may be affected, resulting in edema, swelling caused by the accumulation of fluid in tissue spaces. The name for this condition is the nephrotic syndrome.

Left untreated, lupus can damage the kidney's ability to cleanse the body of waste products. In extreme cases, if these poisons build up, in a condition known as uremia, you may experience weakness, nausea and vomiting, itching, and eventually changes in brain function. This kind of kidney failure may affect the body's balance of fluids and salts. Fluid retention can be so extreme that excess fluid accumulates in the lungs, causing breathing difficulties.

Uremia can be successfully treated with dialysis and, if necessary, kidney transplantation. Fortunately, modern treatment methods are designed to prevent kidney damage, and such damage is a much less common complication of lupus today.

Depression and Nervous System Disorders.
Depression is an exceedingly common symptom of lupus—over three-quarters of people with lupus show some evidence of depression. Sometimes the depression is a reaction to feeling sick or to the physical changes caused by this disease. A thirty-five-year-old bank executive who was diagnosed with lupus two years ago says that she feels down from time to time because she feels as if she's in mourning for her former healthy self.

Many people with chronic disease have such feelings, and you may feel especially troubled because lupus can sometimes cause life-threatening problems. In the early stages of the disease, lupus may be difficult to diagnose; small wonder that you may feel anxious or depressed if you've sought help from several physicians without anyone finding a basis for your physical complaints. As one of my patients said, "Everyone thought I was neurotic or crazy. It was almost a relief when a diagnosis was finally made."

Some people with lupus feel depressed because they feel constantly fatigued and can no longer keep up as well with their work or their family life. To compound this, since someone with lupus may not look sick, friends and family often don't understand what you're going through and might not offer the support you need. It's not surprising that you feel upset if the people you care about think you're being lazy or a hypochondriac.

While depression may be caused by emotional factors, it can also be caused by the physical changes in the brain and nerves. Lupus is an immune system disease, and the immune system and the nervous system are linked.

Mood changes may also be caused by the drugs being used to treat lupus. Sometimes depression is a side effect of treatment with corticosteroids, a class of cortisone-like drugs commonly used to treat lupus.

Patients, family members, and friends should be aware that people with lupus sometimes just don't act like themselves. They may seem down, withdrawn, or disinterested in things. Some have trouble concentrating. Their thought processes may seem off. One of my patients, a thirty-two-year-old artist, for example, was preparing for a big local art show. She says she sat and stared at her canvas, and although her mind knew what she wanted to paint, she could not put it onto the canvas. She felt as if some connections were missing. Others may have strange thoughts or may lose control of their feelings, such as the normally cool and collected lawyer who broke down in tears in my office when discussing why she wanted to become a partner in her law firm.

The rarer and more serious nervous system problems of lupus are called cerebritis. This term means inflammation of the brain, although it is not known that inflammation is the cause of these symptoms. This category includes seizures (also called epilepsy or fits), strokes, hallucinations, and altered consciousness, including coma. Even with powerful new X-ray techniques, we sometimes find it hard to locate specific abnormalities in patients with cerebritis, making this condition hard to diagnose.

You should discuss any emotional or neurologic disturbances with your physician. Sometimes appropriate counseling may help you and your family cope with and understand these changes. You may also want to consider joining a support group sponsored by local branches of the Lupus Foundation or the Arthritis Foundation.

This is only a partial list of possible signs and symptoms of lupus. Lupus can cause problems in many different body systems, and it's not unusual to see those symptoms change unpredictably over time. A patient can have problems with skin rashes one year, then have joint pains the next. Still later, she may have abdominal pains and anemia. Patients may worry that every new fever, ache, or pain is a sign that the lupus is getting worse. Fortunately, this is not necessarily the case, but you should report any new symptoms to your physician as soon as possible. Prompt treatment of various conditions caused by lupus can greatly improve the outcome of the disease and help keep it under control.

In some patients, lupus seems to go away, entering a long period of remission. Scientists are trying to find out how these remissions occur so that one day they may be regularly induced by treatment.

What Happens Physiologically?

When your body is fighting a virus, a bacterium, or another invading organism, your immune system normally becomes very active. An army of white blood cells is sent to the affected area to seek and destroy the foreign invader. Some of these white blood cells produce antibodies, proteins specially designed to recognize and attack a foreign microorganism. In lupus, something seems to go amiss with the immune system. The body appears to mistake its own healthy tissues for a foreign invader and begins to produce autoantibodies, antibodies that attack the body's own tissues. Autoantibodies can cause disease by either of two mechanisms: They can make a direct attack on cells of the body, such as red or white blood cells or brain cells, or they can bind tightly together with other substances in the body, such as DNA, to form an immune complex. The immune complex may circulate in the blood and settle in other parts of the body, where it activates other elements of the inflammatory system and may destroy local tissue.

What Causes Lupus?

No one knows exactly why so many autoantibodies form in lupus. It appears that lupus is caused by the interaction of several factors, including heredity, the environment, and hormones.

In the laboratory, scientists have been able to breed strains of mice with lupus, a powerful indication that there can be a hereditary component to this disease. Since the various kinds of mice that are susceptible to lupus differ in genetic makeup, it appears that more than one gene or sets of genes can predispose an individual to this disease.

Other factors may also have to be present for lupus to develop in genetically susceptible individuals. Perhaps an infection or something in the environment triggers lupus in those who are predisposed to the disease.

Lupus may also be an abnormal response to a virus, bacterium, or fungus. Work with AIDS patients argues strongly that a viral infection can cause alterations in the immune system.

Lupus patients seem to have an inherited tendency to produce abnormally large amounts of antibodies. The levels of antibodies to viruses or bacteria are generally high in lupus patients even though there is no evidence of infection in their systems. Anything that affects the immune system may trigger this tendency to abnormal antibody responsiveness; this includes hormone changes, physical or emotional stress, infection, tissue damage from exposure to ultraviolet sunlight, and the use of certain drugs. Under such conditions, the lupus patient's abnormal immune system begins to produce antibodies against his or her own body. These abnormal products can destroy tissue. The dead tissue may then further stimulate the immune system and lead to even more autoantibody production, feeding a vicious cycle in which tissue destruction leads to more inflammatory reactions, which raises the level of antibody production.

Given this possible model for the disease, why should lupus vary so much from one person to the next? Why, for example, does one person with lupus have skin rashes and painful joints while another has kidney damage, nervous system disorders, and heart disease? One theory is that there is an undetermined interplay between the disease process, the environment, and a patient's inherited characteristics. Investigation into all of these possible factors will help scientists to determine more effective treatments for and methods of prevention of lupus.

Drug-induced Lupus

The form of lupus I have so far been discussing is called idiopathic, meaning that we do not know its cause. But there is another form of this disease with an identifiable cause—drug-induced lupus. Patients who are taking certain medications for other conditions may develop lupus-type symptoms. The two most common causes of drug-induced lupus are hydralazine (Apresoline), a drug prescribed for high blood pressure, and procainamide (Pronestyl), used in treating irregular heartbeat. A number of other drugs, including those used to treat tuberculosis and some anticonvulsants, may also cause drug-induced lupus. The symptoms of this type of lupus are fever, joint pain, and inflammation of the membranes that line the lungs (pleuritis) or heart (pericarditis). The kidneys are not usually involved.

Patients with drug-induced lupus will have abnormal antibodies and their FANA test is usually positive, but they show no anti-DNA antibodies (see chapter 3 for a full explanation of these diagnostic tests).

Patients with drug-induced lupus are usually older, because the medications associated with this syndrome are commonly given for diseases of older people. It affects men and women equally.

Treatment consists of stopping the drug and administering anti-inflammatory drugs. The condition is self-limited: Once the offending drug is out of your system, the symptoms should all disappear.

What if you are in the early stages of lupus and one of these drugs is inadvertently prescribed for you before your diagnosis has been confirmed? Will it affect the course of your disease? This seems unlikely. Drugs that can induce lupus don't appear to make the idiopathic form of lupus any worse.

As a rheumatologist, I find drug-induced lupus to be especially interesting because it suggests that environmental factors can cause inflammatory disease. A lot of research is being conducted to study more closely the changes in the immune system caused by these drugs. If we know that certain drugs can induce lupus, perhaps we can track down other drugs, chemicals, or dietary substances that may play a role in causing lupus or rheumatoid arthritis.

Diagnosis

Lupus can be difficult to diagnose because it is so different for each person and may range in severity from a very mild disease with few symptoms to a serious one affecting many organs. Symptoms may even vary in the same person over time.

In addition to the medical history and physical exam, your doctor will perform a number of laboratory studies to help confirm the diagnosis. These tests are described in detail in chapter 3, but I will review them briefly here.

Lupus patients generally produce high levels of abnormal antibodies in their blood, and there are several laboratory tests that can detect these antibodies; these include the fluorescent antinuclear antibody (FANA) test and the anti-DNA and anti-Sm tests. Over 95 percent of lupus patients will have a positive FANA, but the test can also be positive in a variety of other arthritic diseases, including rheumatoid arthritis. On the other hand, lupus patients are nearly the only people known to have antibodies to DNA and Sm. In addition, anti-DNA levels may rise or fall depending on the severity of the disease, and thus help the physician assess the level of disease activity. Not everyone with lupus has anti-DNA or anti-Sm; maybe half have anti-DNA and a third have anti-Sm. The two antibodies are actually unrelated, though it is possible for an individual to have both.

Other tests are less specific for lupus and will tell your doctor only that there is active inflammation going on in your body. These include the complement test (a low complement gives only a general indication of disease activity) and the complete blood count (as mentioned, lupus patients usually have low red blood cell, white blood cell, and platelet counts). The presence of active inflammation is also suggested when there is a high sed rate (the rate at which red blood cells fall to the bottom of a tube).

Still other tests indicate whether the kidneys are affected. Tests called chemistries measure various chemicals in the blood plasma. For example, a high level of creatinine, a waste product in the blood, can mean that the kidney isn't doing its job properly. A urinalysis may show that there are red blood cells, white blood cells, or protein in the urine, further evidence of kidney damage. Casts, clumps of red or white blood cells, are also signs of renal injury or inflammation.

A false positive VDRL test for syphilis is another indication of lupus. Subsequent tests for this venereal disease, using another method, will come out negative.

It may also be necessary to do specialized tests to determine whether lupus has spread to any major organ systems, and if so, how severely. Since kidneys are most often affected, tests for kidney function are most common. A sample of your urine may be tested with a dipstick (a specially treated paper strip) in your doctor's office, or you may be asked to collect your urine over a twenty-four-hour period so that your doctor can measure the total amount of protein excreted from your body over the course of the day. (This collection can be done at your home and doesn't require hospitalization.) High protein levels in the urine may indicate problems with kidney functioning.

In severe cases of lupus, a biopsy of the kidney may be necessary. A small piece of your kidney may be removed without surgery, using a long needle inserted through the skin. X-rays and ultrasound tests help the physician place the needle in the correct place. A kidney biopsy carries some risk, especially of bleeding, and is performed only when kidney involvement appears to be serious and the use of powerful immunosuppressive drugs is being considered. These drugs have serious side effects, and your doctor needs to be absolutely sure that inflammation is actively damaging your kidney before he or she starts you on such a course of therapy. A kidney biopsy usually requires hospitalization and bed rest for a day afterward.

Depending on your symptoms, your doctor may want biopsies of other tissues (e.g., skin, lung membrane); a spinal tap to evaluate inflammation in the nervous system; brain wave recordings; and detailed X-rays of various body organs, often using the sensitive testing afforded by computerized axial tomography (CAT) and magnetic resonance imaging (MRI) scans. If heart involvement is suspected, you may need an electrocardiogram or echocardiogram.

Your doctor may also need to do testing to rule out other conditions that may cause the same symptoms as lupus—for example, infections and drug side effects. Every time you experience new symptoms, they must be individually evaluated. Lupus patients treated with immunosuppressive drugs are subject to infections and need frequent follow-up tests to make sure they stay healthy.

Lupus is hardest to diagnose early in the disease, so if you come to your doctor's office with one isolated symptom, it could be months or even years before the diagnosis is definitive. In the interim, patients may have to suffer uncertainty as well as symptoms of the disease.

Sometimes patients don't easily fit into one or another arthritis category. They may, for example, have features of both rheumatoid arthritis and lupus, and their condition is sometimes called overlap, mixed, or undifferentiated connective tissue disease. Over time, symptoms become more distinctive, but it is not unusual for a patient's disease to start out being called rheumatoid arthritis, later be termed an overlap syndrome, and then finally be diagnosed as lupus.

Treatment

Treatments for lupus vary, depending upon which organ systems are affected and how severe your symptoms are. Treatments also change as your condition improves or grows worse over time, or as new symptoms develop. In my own practice, I like to say that I do not treat lupus; rather, I treat the arthritis of lupus or the kidney disease of lupus, and so on. In this way, I match the therapy with the symptoms of the disease.

You must keep your doctor apprised of any new developments so that your treatment regimen can be altered or reevaluated as necessary. You will probably be asked to see your physician frequently—perhaps every few weeks or months—so he or she can determine the activity level of your disease and monitor your drug therapy. Frequent monitoring generally makes it possible to keep your symptoms under control.

In general, the less severe the disease, the more conservative the drugs used to treat it. Milder forms of lupus can usually be treated with non-steroidal anti-inflammatory drugs (NSAIDs) such as aspirin and ibuprofen, which help reduce the pain and inflammation or reduce fever.

When you have a potentially serious involvement of a major organ system, your doctor will usually prescribe corticosteroids, drugs related to the hormone cortisone. These are quick-acting and highly effective in reducing inflammation, but they are potent drugs with serious side effects, so their use must be very carefully monitored. Corticosteroids are a mainstay of lupus therapy, being used by about two-thirds of lupus patients; however, they are best when used in the lowest possible doses for the shortest possible period of time.

Antimalarial drugs such as chloroquine and hydroxychloroquine (Plaquenil) are useful in treating the skin disease and arthritis of lupus. Because impairment of vision is a potentially serious side effect, people using these drugs must have frequent eye checkups (usually every six months), and they should discontinue therapy if any signs of eye problems develop. If a patient is properly monitored, however, such complications are rare.

Immunosuppressant drugs are used in the most extreme cases, especially with kidney involvement, when corticosteroids don't seem to be effective. These very potent drugs suppress the immune system and may have serious side effects, which can include lowered blood counts, increased susceptibility to infection, sterility, severe bladder inflammation, and cancer. Patients on these drugs therefore require frequent monitoring. Given the serious nature of these side effects, a kidney biopsy will sometimes be performed before administering these drugs, to make certain the kidney disease is caused by active inflammation, not by some other condition (see page 99). However, there is a certain amount of controversy over the best timing for a kidney biopsy and whether this type of information can be obtained by other types of testing.

Other therapies for lupus are tailored to individual problems. For example, if you're depressed or have more serious neurological symptoms, you may need specific medications to treat those problems. (For a more detailed discussion on drug and X-ray treatments, turn to chapter 14.)

In addition to drug treatments, you should limit your exposure to sunlight, which can aggravate lupus and make symptoms worse. Wear protective clothing such as hats, scarves, and long sleeves when you go out in the sun, and use sunscreens and sunblocks with an SPF of 15 or more. Also, try to avoid going out in the sun between 11:00 A.M. and 2:00 P.M., when ultraviolet light is strongest. In fact, I recommend these protective measures for anyone who wants to avoid the damage the sun does to the skin. Sometimes ointments or creams containing cortisone can help alleviate rashes caused by lupus.

A change in your diet may help control the progression of renal disease. Keep your blood pressure as low as possible (your doctor can make specific dietary recommendations to help you do this) and avoid too much salt and protein in your diet.

If you have lupus, you may find that you tire more easily than you used to. It's important that you learn how to pace yourself and conserve your energy. If you can, try to incorporate several brief rest periods into your day. This may mean cutting back on your hours at work or restructuring your workday, if possible. You may need more sleep now than you did before, and while you may be able to continue all of your normal activities, you may find you have to slow down. Check your priorities; keeping yourself well-rested so you can enjoy your family and friends is probably more important than being the most demanding housekeeper or relentless executive. Try to enlist your family to help out with household chores.

Some patients say that relaxation techniques help them alleviate the stress that so often accompanies a chronic illness (see chapter 15).

Pregnancy and Lupus

Since many people with lupus are women in their childbearing years, they naturally want to know if lupus affects their ability to conceive and bear a healthy child. I'm happy to report that the chances of having a normal pregnancy and a favorable delivery are generally good. Many of my lupus patients have had successful pregnancies and have given birth to normal, healthy babies.

Lupus does in some cases limit fertility and may result in more frequent miscarriages, but it doesn't preclude motherhood. The likelihood of a successful pregnancy appears to be influenced by the severity and activity of your disease. If you feel well and if your symptoms are controlled by medication, then your pregnancy will likely go well. On the other hand, if the disease is active and unstable, you may have more difficulty conceiving and carrying a baby to term.

Surprisingly, your lupus may actually improve while you're pregnant. However, the disease may become more active after your baby is born, and some physicians treat patients with increased dosages of steroids at the time of delivery to prevent a flare after childbirth.

In general, it's best to minimize or eliminate drugs for any condition during pregnancy, so you should discuss with your rheumatologist and obstetrician the risks versus the benefits of taking medications for lupus during pregnancy. When drugs are necessary, prednisone (a corticosteroid) seems to be well tolerated by both mother and baby and can be given in relatively high doses. It has not been shown to cause fetal malformation or to have long-term effects on children. The immunosuppressive drugs are a different story. Cytoxan can damage chromosomes, causing fetal abnormalities or miscarriage, and therefore should not be used while you're pregnant. Imuran inhibits cell growth and is also unsafe to take during pregnancy. Women requiring these immunosuppressive drugs often have more serious problems with lupus and are probably less likely to conceive.

It is possible to have a flare of the disease during pregnancy. In such cases, the lupus can be treated with increased doses of corticosteroids, and we can safely control an active flare, which we recently did in the case of a twenty-eight-year-old patient I saw in consultation. This woman had a flare during her sixth month of pregnancy, when she began to run a fever and her joints began to ache. A urinalysis showed she had red blood cells in her urine, an indication of kidney damage. She was placed on high-dose prednisone. Her renal function improved and she had a normal delivery and a healthy baby.

There is a small group of lupus patients who have trouble carrying babies to term. Some of these women are thought to have a blood-clotting problem that causes the vessels in the placenta to narrow, depriving the developing fetus of adequate nourishment. Some investigators think this problem is caused by an autoantibody. The presence of this same autoantibody may also cause miscarriages in women who do not have lupus. Treatment with corticosteroids, which lower antibody levels, and/or aspirin, which decreases the blood's clotting ability, can result in successful pregnancies. The dose of aspirin used is very low, sometimes only one per day.

Some women have an antibody called anti-Ro that in rare cases may be passed to the developing fetus, resulting in a neonatal lupus syndrome. The newborn may develop a skin rash that usually fades over time and, more rarely, may also have congenital heart block. Many normal babies, however, are born to mothers with this antibody, and it is not clear why some infants develop this disease while others do not.

If you are thinking about becoming pregnant, be sure to discuss it with your physician. You will need close medical supervision throughout your pregnancy. The ideal time to conceive is when your disease is well under control. If you do not wish to become pregnant, you should discuss with your doctor your choice of contraceptive. Generally speaking, IUDs are not advised because of the increased risk of infection. In any case, please be reassured that having lupus doesn't mean you can't have a normal pregnancy and healthy baby.

Prognosis

Although lupus may seem baffling and is sometimes very serious, it can often be effectively treated. Indeed, now more than ever, the outcome for lupus patients has improved dramatically and the more dreaded outcomes, such as kidney failure, are becoming increasingly rare. Doctors are now better aware of the risks and benefits of therapy, so drugs are used more selectively for shorter times and in lower doses. In fact, many people with lupus have a disease that can be managed with relatively low doses of medication. They can lead full lives, including having children and raising a family.

SYSTEMIC LUPUS ERYTHEMATOSUS (LUPUS, OR SLE)

A chronic systemic condition that includes joint inflammation and may involve many organ systems, including the skin, blood, lungs, cardiovascular and nervous systems, and kidneys. The name *lupus* comes from a characteristic wolf-like facial rash that often accompanies the disease. Lupus is an autoimmune disease—i.e., the immune system appears to attack the body.

CAUSE: No known cause. There may also be a hereditary tendency to have disturbed immune function. Hormones may have some influence.

SYMPTOMS: Symptoms are highly variable, as the disease can attack so many different organ systems. May begin with generalized flu-like fever and achiness; painful and tender joints; and/or a characteristic butterfly rash on the face. Other possible symptoms are chest pains, hair loss, difficulty in breathing, Raynaud's phenomenon, anemia, kidney problems, lowered resistance to infections, depression and nervous symptoms, and a false positive test for syphilis.

WHO GETS IT? Mainly young women between ages twenty and thirty. In the United States, blacks and Hispanics are at greatest risk. Blood relatives of those with lupus are also at higher risk.

DIAGNOSIS: Diagnosis is based on a medical history, a physical exam, and lab studies. Can be difficult because of variation in symptoms. FANA, anti-DNA, and anti-Sm tests identify abnormal antibodies common in lupus patients, and are helpful diagnostic tools.

TREATMENT: Varies, depending on organ system affected. Nonsteroidal anti-inflammatorics (NSAIDs) such as aspirin and ibuprofen are used to treat arthritis inflammation; corticosteroids are commonly used for more severe inflammation; antimalarial drugs may be used to treat skin disease; immunosuppressive drugs are used for the most extreme cases, those that involve kidney damage.

PROGNOSIS: Much improved over last few decades. Most have mild to moderate disease that can be well controlled with regular medical monitoring. With proper treatment, patients can live full and active lives.

7

Scleroderma

Louise, a forty-year-old lawyer, began to notice the first symptoms of scleroderma two years ago, as fall was turning to winter. She felt occasional pain in her fingers, especially on cooler days. Once while she was in the frozen food section of the supermarket, her hands turned white and numb and then a bluish color. She could barely feel her fingers. After she left this part of the store, she began to rub her cold fingers; they became bright red and very painful.

Louise's mother had Raynaud's phenomenon, an extreme sensitivity to cold, so she wasn't too alarmed. She had seen these symptoms before. But over the next twelve months, new symptoms developed. The joints in Louise's fingers became tender and painful and her hands became puffy. The skin over her fingers and hands grew thick and felt tight. Painful sores began to develop on her fingertips, and these healed very slowly. Louise made an appointment to see her family internist.

The physician was most concerned by the changes in the texture of Louise's skin and in her reaction to the cold. Blood studies made the diagnosis of rheumatoid arthritis unlikely. Louise's skin changes led the doctor to suspect scleroderma. He ordered a special X-ray to evaluate Louise's ability to swallow and a test to measure her lung function. Both returned abnormal, providing evidence that this was in fact scleroderma. Louise was then referred to me for further evaluation and treatment.

While scleroderma is one of the more serious arthritic diseases, I reassured Louise that it can be treated. Warming measures and medications can often control Raynaud's phenomenon and frequent monitoring can help forestall other potentially serious complications.

We were able to control the pain of Louise's arthritis and the symptoms of Raynaud's phenomenon with the use of a nonsteroidal anti-inflammatory drug. She returned to my office every three months for regular examinations to make sure that the disease was not progressing. Over this past year, Louise's symptoms have remained in good control. She has been able to continue in her law practice and still participates in her regular activities.

What Is Scleroderma?

Scleroderma is a relatively rare form of arthritis that affects approximately 50,000 to 100,000 people in the United States. Its name comes from the Greek *sklero,* meaning hard, and *derma,* meaning skin. Many people with the disease develop areas of thick, rigid skin on their faces, fingers, and arms. This disease is also medically known as progressive systemic sclerosis (PSS). This name aptly describes the disease, which may involve a progressive hardening of tissue (sclerosis) that can affect many body sites, including the joints, skin, heart, kidneys, intestinal tract, and lungs. However, some doctors prefer the name systemic sclerosis, because not every case of this disease is progressive.

Scleroderma is called a collagen vascular disease. Collagen is the fibrous substance that gives resilience to skin and bones and that supports and joins other tissues in the body. In scleroderma, the body makes too much collagen, and the excess is deposited in the skin and other body organs, resulting in hardness and tightness of the skin and possible organ dysfunction. The disease can also cause the abnormal growth of cells lining the blood vessels, which in turn can cause vascular problems, such as the extreme sensitivity of the fingers to cold as seen in Raynaud's phenomenon.

There is a localized form of this disease that stays confined to a small area of skin. It doesn't involve internal organs. This localized scleroderma normally doesn't develop into the systemic form of this disease.

In this chapter, when we talk of scleroderma or progressive systemic scleroderma (PSS), we will be referring to the more generalized form of the disease that may affect not only the skin but also many organ systems throughout the body.

Though signs and symptoms of PSS vary from one individual to another, there are two overall patterns of this disease, each with a different prognosis. A milder form of the disease, called the CREST syndrome, has a generally more favorable outcome. CREST is an acronym that describes some common symptoms of this syndrome (although not everyone with CREST syndrome develops all of these symptoms):

C   Calcinosis: deposits of calcium in the skin or muscle.
R   Raynaud's phenomenon: an extreme sensitivity to cold that causes fingers to burn, tingle, and change color.
E   Esophageal dysmotility: muscle problems in the esophagus, causing difficulty in swallowing.
S   Sclerodactyly: thickening of the skin of the fingers and hands.
T   Telangiectasias: widening of the capillaries that can be seen through the skin.

As a group, people with this syndrome seem to do fairly well and are able to lead relatively normal lives. The CREST syndrome is less likely to spread to other organs. Fifty percent of people with scleroderma have the disease in its more limited form.

The other, more severe pattern of scleroderma may lead to generalized involvement of many internal organs, including the heart, gastrointestinal tract, lungs, and kidneys. It should be noted that the differences between the two patterns of PSS are not always clear-cut. Fortunately, we've made good progress in treating the more serious forms of scleroderma. Frequent monitoring of patients enables doctors to intervene with drugs and treatments that may prevent complications.

Who Gets Scleroderma?

Scleroderma is a rare disease. It can affect people of any age and sex, but is most common among women between thirty and fifty years old. The incidence of scleroderma increases with age, and it rarely occurs in children. This disease does not appear to run in families.

Warning Signs and Symptoms

As with so many other forms of arthritis, symptoms of scleroderma can vary from person to person. This disease may be mild and spread slowly, or it can progress rapidly and involve many organs. In most cases, however, the onset of scleroderma is gradual.

Arthritis and Muscle Pain.
Scleroderma often begins with pain and swelling in the joints, especially in the hands, and consequently it may be confused with rheumatoid

arthritis. You may also experience muscle weakness and actual inflammation, as in polymyositis (see chapter 10).

Raynaud's Phenomenon.

Patients with scleroderma will almost invariably experience Raynaud's phenomenon early in the course of their disease. However, I'd like to emphasize here that Raynaud's phenomenon can occur by itself, or with other forms of arthritis, such as rheumatoid arthritis or lupus. It can also occur as a result of occupational use, especially in people who use vibrating equipment, such as jackhammers. If you are experiencing Raynaud-like symptoms, this does not necessarily mean that you have scleroderma.

A person with Raynaud's phenomenon is extremely sensitive to the cold and to emotional upsets. His or her fingers burn, tingle, and become numb; they also turn characteristic colors—first white, then blue, then red. These color changes are caused by a narrowing of the blood vessels in response to cold or stress. The narrowed blood vessels don't allow enough blood through, so the fingers turn white. The blood that's left in the tissues loses its oxygen and the fingers turn blue. Eventually the blood vessels open and red, oxygen-rich blood rushes back in, causing the fingers to turn red.

Raynaud's can be annoying and painful. Patients have told me that they cannot pick items out of the freezers in the supermarket, reach into their own home refrigerators, or even wash vegetables under cold running water without suffering discomfort in their fingers. Cold weather may make it difficult for them to enjoy being outdoors.

Skin Changes.

Patients may also experience edema, or a puffiness and swelling of the tissues in the fingers and hands and sometimes the feet. The fingers may become swollen and sausage-like, losing their natural creases, and the tendons and the veins on the backs of the hands will no longer be visible. A hand swollen by edema may be stiff and hard to use.

After several weeks or months, the edema may change to thick, hardened skin. The skin feels taut and may look shiny. It may also change color, either darkening or losing its pigmentation. Sometimes hair stops growing on the affected skin and the sweat glands may also stop functioning. The skin may also become rough and dry, as may the underlying tissues. Sometimes your doctor will put a stethoscope over the tendons in your hand and listen as he or she moves it. The tendons will actually make an audible sound, like leather creaking.

The hardening of the skin and of other tissues around the joints can cause the joints to lock into a bent position. This is called a flexion contracture.

In the milder, more limited forms of systemic disease, the thickening of the skin may be confined to the fingers and hands. In the fingers it is called sclerodactyly. In more severe cases, the thickening may spread rapidly to the forearms, upper arms, face, chest, and abdomen. If the skin draws tight around the mouth, it may be hard to open the mouth to chew and the skin around the lips may look furrowed. Affected skin may remain thickened for several years and then thin to some extent for most people.

Another common sign are telangiectasias, fine, spidery networks of dilated blood vessels that become visible below the skin. These may appear on the fingers, face, lips, and tongue. They may come and go, or grow lighter or darker. One patient reported that her telangiectasias seemed to grow darker and more apparent at various times in her menstrual cycle. She said these blemishes made her feel self-conscious, because they resembled acne. Telangiectasias can be camouflaged somewhat with makeup.

Later in the disease there may be calcinosis, small, frequently painful collections of calcium under the skin. These may appear on the fingers, forearms, elbows, and knees.

Digestive Problems.
Digestive problems are common in people with scleroderma. Collagen may be deposited in the muscle tissue of the esophagus, the long, muscular tube that conveys food from the mouth to the stomach. This may impair muscle functioning, causing difficulty with swallowing, irritation of the lining of the esophagus, and heartburn. The large and small intestine can be damaged by deposits of fibrous tissue, leading to poor digestion.

Other Organ Involvement.
In more advanced cases, fibrous deposits in the heart can lead to irregular heartbeats or even heart failure; the kidney can become damaged by severe hypertension, and blood vessels leading to the kidney may become blocked by fibrosis, the formation of scar tissue. Lung capacity may also become reduced.

In extremely rare instances, the disease attacks the internal organs first, without any prior warning signs. Such people do not have any of the joint or skin changes typical of scleroderma.

Clearly, scleroderma can be potentially serious and life-threatening. The range of possible symptoms makes it very important that you keep in close touch with your physician and report any new problems as they arise. Many patients can control their symptoms with medication and timely treatment.

What Happens Physiologically?

There are two basic changes going on in the body of a person with scleroderma: Excess collagen is being produced and deposited in various tissues and organs throughout the body, and blood vessels may become narrowed and damaged.

Collagen is a springy, fabric-like material composed of fibrous threads. It is a major component of connective tissues, the tissues that join and support other tissues and parts of the body. Cells called fibroblasts produce collagen. In scleroderma, the fibroblasts produce too much collagen. The excess collagen is deposited in the skin and other organs, where it hardens and can cause the organ to malfunction.

At the same time, scleroderma causes changes in the walls of the blood vessels. These become narrow and make it hard for blood to pass through. The endothelial cells that line the blood vessels may become damaged, so the blood supply to various body organs is cut off and the organs can no longer function well.

What Causes Scleroderma?

It is not known what triggers excess collagen production or why blood vessels become damaged. Perhaps there is some disturbance in the body's natural immune system that causes the body to produce antibodies that attack its own healthy tissues. Indeed, we do find that some patients with this disease have abnormal antibodies that attack components of the cell's nucleus. In addition, many scleroderma patients have inflamed joints or muscles, further evidence that something is amiss with the immune system. Perhaps disturbances in the immune system damage blood vessels and stimulate the fibroblasts in the skin and elsewhere to make too much collagen. The replacement of healthy tissue by fibrous scar tissue is one of the hallmarks of scleroderma.

When the immune system is activated, it produces lots of substances other than antibodies that can promote the formation of fibrous tissue. One such substance is called transforming growth factor beta (TGF-B). Experts in the field are taking great interest in studying this hormonal growth substance and its relationship to scleroderma.

How Is Scleroderma Diagnosed?

As in other forms of arthritis, there is no single test for this disease. The diagnosis of scleroderma is based on an in-depth medical history, a thorough physical exam, and often several laboratory tests and X-rays.

Frequently, scleroderma can be diagnosed by a medical history and physical examination alone. The skin of the fingers, hands, face, neck, or trunk, usually on both sides of the body, may show the thickening, tightening, and hardening so typical of this disease. If the medical history reveals the presence of Raynaud's phenomenon as well, scleroderma becomes a likely diagnosis.

It's more difficult, however, to diagnose scleroderma earlier in the disease, before any skin changes become apparent. When a patient complains to me of pain, swelling, and tenderness in a joint, for example, I may suspect rheumatoid arthritis. Some patients complain of extreme muscle weakness and pain, and I'll have to rule out other diseases, such as polymyositis, that share these symptoms.

Sometimes patients have a variety of symptoms that do not conform to the usual diagnostic categories and together are known as mixed connective tissue disease. This may mean they have elements of several types of arthritis, including scleroderma, lupus, and rheumatoid arthritis.

The diagnostic workup for scleroderma usually includes X-ray studies, to see whether the condition has affected the esophagus and gastrointestinal system. You may be asked to swallow barium, a white, chalky liquid that outlines the esophagus and allows the physician to see how it's functioning.

In addition, your pulmonary (lung) function may be tested to see whether there are any changes caused by scarring. In this test, you'll breathe into a machine that records the amount of air you exhale and the rate at which you breathe.

You may also have an arterial blood gas test. This can involve some discomfort, since your blood must be drawn from an artery through a special syringe. An examination of the levels of various gases in your blood will give an indication of how well your lungs are functioning. In addition, you may also have an electrocardiogram and other tests to measure your heart's performance.

Occasionally, your doctor might do a skin biopsy to see if your skin is producing more collagen than normal. However, many doctors prefer not to do biopsies because they can get sufficient information for diagnosis with other tests.

Muscle biopsies can yield important diagnostic information that has an impact on treatment. There are two basic forms of muscle disease in people with scleroderma. One is myopathy, in which there is muscle weakness without signs of inflammation; the other is myositis, in which muscles are inflamed. A biopsy can tell your doctor whether you have muscle inflammation. If so, treatment with steroids may be beneficial.

Your doctor may also perform blood tests for rheumatoid factors to rule out the presence of rheumatoid arthritis, and antinuclear antibodies to identify certain abnormal antibodies in scleroderma. However, the antinuclear antibody tests may be omitted because doctors can often get the necessary diagnostic information in other ways. (For a detailed description of tests, see chapter 3.)

Help for Raynaud's Disease

While scleroderma can't be cured with drugs, your doctor can use many approaches to relieve some of its symptoms. If you have Raynaud's phenomenon, for example, you can be careful to keep your body warm and to protect your extremities from exposure to the cold. During the cold winter months, wear several thin layers of clothing rather than one or two thick layers, since the layers trap body heat and will keep you warmer. Perspiration can cool your body down on cool days, so make sure the material next to your skin is absorbent. Cotton or woolen socks and underwear are more absorbent than those made from synthetic materials such as Orlon or nylon. You may want to wear thermal socks that are lined with cotton, or a few pairs of socks rather than one thick pair, in order to keep your feet warmer. You should also protect your fingers with mittens, which trap the body heat a lot better than gloves. Since most of your body heat is lost through the head, you should always wear a hat in cold weather.

Some of the people I see have devised novel ways of keeping their extremities warm. One woman at our clinic said she discovered that a gel packet designed to keep skiers' hands and feet warm works well for Raynaud's. She simply shakes the packet and inserts it into the lining of her gloves. Many wear cooking mitts or gloves when removing items from the freezer at home, or use tongs when handling chilled or frozen foods. Others use warm water to rinse vegetables or when hand-washing their clothes.

Cigarette smoking can trigger Raynaud's by causing your blood vessels to constrict, thereby reducing the amount of blood circulating to your fingers. Of course smoking is bad for your heart and lungs, which may also be affected by scleroderma. So if you smoke and have been diagnosed as having scleroderma, here is yet another reason to kick the habit.

If these simple precautionary measures are insufficient, there are drugs that can help prevent your blood vessels from constricting. The most frequently prescribed drugs are antihypertensives, commonly used in the treatment of high blood pressure. Nifedipine (brand name Procardia) is the current choice of many physicians. Antihypertensive drugs do have a variety of side effects, though; these include dizziness, drowsiness, and low blood pressure.

Another way of treating Raynaud's is biofeedback, a method by which patients learn to control various bodily processes not normally thought of as being under voluntary control, including blood pressure, body temperature, heart rate, and muscle tension. During a biofeedback session, you will be attached by electrodes to a machine and shown how to use signals from the machine to alter your body processes. You'll learn how to use relaxation and visualization techniques to open up your blood vessels and help blood flow into your fingers. After a while you will be able to practice these same techniques at home, without the use of machines.

Since stress is a trigger for Raynaud's, it's helpful if you try to avoid stressful situations. Of course that's easier said than done; but if you can't change the stress, perhaps you can change the way you react to the stress. You may want to learn various relaxation techniques, such as those described in chapter 17.

Scleroderma may be especially stressful because it is a relatively rare and serious disease, and others in your life may not be able to understand what you are going through. One thirty-six-year-old woman I saw in consultation complained that having a disease that no one's ever heard of made her feel very isolated. Even her husband, who really wanted to help, didn't know how to be supportive. After talking with a psychologist, she eventually sorted out her feelings and now feels more in control and positive about her life. The disease will never be her friend, she says, but she's learned to live more comfortably with it.

Some people reap great benefits by talking their feelings over with others who are in a similar situation. If you are interested in a support group, your local Arthritis Foundation may be a good place to start. Your friends, family, and clergy can also offer emotional support. You may also find it helpful to discuss your problems with a social worker or counselor.

Skin Care

You may be bothered by thickened, dry skin. Excessive bathing can dry your skin, so keep baths and showers brief. Try also to avoid using harsh soaps, caustic detergents, and household chemicals, or at least wear rubber gloves while using them. Moisturizing lotions, creams, and bath oils may help replenish your skin's natural oils. Consider using a humidifier during the winter months when indoor heat can dry out your skin.

Skin ulcerations, which may form at your fingertips, may be treated with drugs to assure good blood flow and with measures to protect the skin from injury or abrasions. Sometimes your doctor will prescribe antibiotics to clear up any infection and heal the ulcer.

Exercise and Joint Protection

In more serious cases of scleroderma, joint contractures may limit your range of motion. Your natural impulse may be to keep those swollen joints still. However, to prevent further loss of function, you should stay active. Your doctor can prescribe some gentle daily range-of-motion exercises to help prevent loss of flexibility and to encourage blood flow to the area. A physical therapist can help reduce the stresses on inflamed joints by teaching you new ways to perform such everyday tasks as lifting, opening doors, or getting out of a car. Temporary splints might also be helpful.

Digestive Aids

If you are having problems with your esophagus, you may need to alter your eating habits to improve your digestion. It helps if you chew your food extremely well and avoid foods such as meat and dry bread, which can be difficult to swallow. Try eating five or six small meals throughout the day rather than three large ones, and make sure to drink plenty of liquids along with your meals, so it's easier for you to swallow.

You can treat heartburn with measures that prevent the stomach contents from backing up into the esophagus. For example, you can keep your head elevated, especially at night, with extra pillows or blocks. Your doctor may recommend taking an antacid to reduce the acidity of your stomach and the irritation to the gastrointestinal lining. Lying down immediately after eating a large meal can cause stomach acid to back up, so avoid taking a nap immediately after dining. Also, try to eat your heavier meals during the day rather than late at night, close to your bedtime.

If your esophagus has become severely scarred, it may have to be dilated. This is not a surgical procedure; in fact, it can be done in your doctor's office. Various size metal dilators are passed through the esophagus. Though it may make you uncomfortable, this procedure usually brings relief.

In advanced cases of the disease, the gastrointestinal tract may become so damaged that you may find it difficult to absorb the necessary nutrients from your food. In such instances, your doctor can prescribe a specially prepared diet that can be easily absorbed.

Sometimes poor digestion can be caused by an abnormal growth of bacteria in the intestines, and your doctor can prescribe an antibiotic to clear up the problem.

Advanced cases of scleroderma may affect the heart, lungs, and kidneys. In each of these instances, treatments will be tailored to the organ system involved.

Drug Treatments

Which drugs your doctor chooses for you will depend on your symptoms and which of your organs are affected. There is, unfortunately, no treatment proven to reverse the skin disease or fibrosis of internal organs. However, there are a variety of drugs that can treat symptoms and keep the disease under control.

Your doctor may prescribe nonsteroidal anti-inflammatory drugs (NSAIDs) such as aspirin or ibuprofen to treat the arthritis symptoms of scleroderma. Corticosteroids are not routinely used in the earlier stages of scleroderma, but may be useful for treating more serious complications, such as inflammatory muscle or lung disease.

Hypertension is a common complication of scleroderma and can lead to serious kidney damage, so it's important that your doctor check your blood pressure frequently. Renal failure used to be a real danger in advanced cases of scleroderma. However, with the many different hypertensive drugs available to keep blood pressure under control, this problem is becoming much more rare.

Over the years, many different drugs have been tried to prevent the progression of the disease and fibrosis. It has been difficult to prove the benefits of any of these drugs, but right now there is a good deal of interest in penicillamine (Depen, Cuprimine), a remittive drug also used in the treatment of rheumatoid arthritis (see chapter 14).

Penicillamine is a slow-acting drug that seems to work by modulating the immune system. There have been encouraging reports that penicillamine can slow the progression of the scleroderma, but this chronic disease requires many years of study, so we don't yet know enough about penicillamine's long-term value.

Some physicians are recommending treatment with penicillamine in more severe cases of scleroderma, even though the final verdict on its benefit is not yet in. But given the number of potentially serious side effects (including blood and kidney problems, mouth ulcers, and rashes) associated with its use and the difficulty in proving its benefit, penicillamine is not being used routinely right now.

Prognosis

Scleroderma is a serious systemic disease with possible life-threatening complications. The prognosis for this disease, however, continues to improve. For example, kidney failure due to severe high blood pressure used to be a major complication. Now, with the use of effective antihypertensive drugs, it's less common.

As mentioned above, there is currently interest in penicillamine, which may be able to slow the progress of this disease, but further testing of this drug is necessary before we can fully understand its long-term benefits.

Currently, there are no drugs that have been proven to stop or undo the fibrosis that is the hallmark of scleroderma. Researchers are currently looking at ways to modify the actions of hormone-like substances produced by cells in the immune system, the goal being better control of the excess production of cartilage. In the meantime, if doctors monitor their patients frequently, they are often able to treat various symptoms successfully. Many people with scleroderma are able to manage their disease and live relatively normal lives.

SCLERODERMA (PROGRESSIVE SYSTEMIC SCLEROSIS, OR PSS)

A relatively rare systemic disease in which the body manufactures too much collagen. Excess collagen may be deposited throughout the body in the skin, joints, blood vessels, and other organs. Skin deposits cause a characteristic thickening and hardening of the skin.

CAUSE: Unknown, but may be due to some disturbance in the body's immune system.

SYMPTOMS: Highly variable. Some common early symptoms are arthritis and muscle pain; Raynaud's phenomenon; and edema, followed by hardening and tightening of skin. Other possible signs: telangiectasias (dilated blood vessels visible through the skin); digestive problems; small, hard collections of calcium under the skin. Severe cases may involve the heart, kidneys, and lungs.

WHO GETS IT? This rare disease can affect people of any age and sex. It is most common among women between thirty and fifty years old, and it is rare in children. It does not appear to be hereditary.

DIAGNOSIS: Based on medical history, physical exam, X-rays, and lab studies. Characteristic skin changes and a history of Raynaud's are strong indicators.

TREATMENT: Nonsteroidal anti-inflammatory drugs (for arthritis symptoms); corticosteroids (for serious inflammatory complications); and antihypertensives (for Raynaud's phenomenon and for control of high blood pressure). Penicillamine may be able to slow progression of scleroderma, but is still being tested.

PROGNOSIS: Much improved with frequent monitoring and use of antihypertensives to help prevent possible kidney failure. Many people are able to control symptoms and live relatively normal lives.

8

Ankylosing Spondylitis

In order to help pay his college expenses, Jim, a twenty-year-old student, spent the summer working for a building contractor. His job involved a lot of physical exertion, and he often had to lift heavy pieces of lumber. Toward the end of the summer, Jim noticed a nagging pain in his lower back. The back pain and stiffness felt worst in the morning, but eased off over the course of the day. Jim felt quite sure the pain stemmed from his summer job, although he couldn't pinpoint a particular incident that might have caused an injury. He tried using a heating pad to treat himself, but that didn't work. A friend recommended a chiropractor who performed spinal manipulation, but this didn't relieve the symptoms either. Jim then consulted a local physician, who prescribed muscle relaxants that decreased the pain somewhat. With school beginning in a few weeks, Jim began to worry about his back pain and whether it would interfere with studies and with the college sports that he enjoyed. He decided to consult an orthopedic surgeon, who ordered X-rays of his lower spine. The X-rays showed definite changes around the sacroiliac joints, and the surgeon referred Jim to the rheumatology clinic at Duke University.

During the medical history, Jim mentioned that he had a grandfather with arthritis and a sister with eye problems. His physical examination did not reveal anything except for a decrease in the mobility of his spine. When I asked him to bend over and touch his toes, his fingertips could reach only as far as three inches from the floor. I ordered additional X-rays, which confirmed my suspicion of inflammatory sacroiliac disease. All the laboratory tests came back negative. On the basis of this information, I made the diagnosis of ankylosing spondylitis and prescribed a nonsteroidal anti-inflammatory drug and a program of physical therapy.

Jim's back problems have subsided substantially since he began drug treatment and therapy. I advised him to take it easy for a while and to

119

avoid vigorous physical activity until his back feels better. As long as he feels okay, Jim can continue to participate in sports and all of his other normal school activities. A physician cannot make any firm promises when it comes to ankylosing spondylitis, but I feel that Jim has a good chance of doing quite well.

What Is Ankylosing Spondylitis?

Ankylosing spondylitis (AS) is a chronic inflammatory disease that primarily affects the sacroiliac joints, the joints that connect the spine to the pelvic bones, and the spine. The tendons and ligaments become inflamed at the place where they are anchored to the bone. These attachment sites are called entheses, and AS is sometimes referred to as an enthesopathy, or a disease of attachment structures. It is also known as Marie-Strümpell disease, a name derived from the European physicians who first identified it in the late 1800s.

The name ankylosing spondylitis aptly describes what can happen in *advanced* cases of this disease. Ankylosing means freezing or stiffening of a joint. Spondylitis means an inflammation of the joints in the spine. The attachment structures of the sacroiliac joints and vertebrae may become inflamed, resulting in a process called ossification—the formation of bone-like material. Bony bridges can form between vertebrae and permanently fuse the spine into a stiff and inflexible position. The name AS is somewhat misleading, however, because most people do not develop the bony bridges of more advanced disease. More commonly, AS involves inflammation of the sacroiliac joint, with back pain and stiffness. The vast majority of people are not disabled by AS.

Spondyloarthropathies

AS is part of a larger group of diseases that all have similar symptoms, and in order to talk about AS you need at least a brief introduction to these other conditions. The diseases in this group include ankylosing spondylitis, Reiter's syndrome, psoriatic arthritis, and arthritis with inflammatory bowel disease.

As a group, these interrelated diseases are known as seronegative spondyloarthropathies. This is quite a mouthful to say, but the name actually tells a lot about the disease group. The term *seronegative*, for example, tells you that blood tests for patients with diseases in this group come out negative for rheumatoid factor (RF). This is an important point, because a negative RF test helps your doctor to distinguish between these diseases and rheumatoid arthritis (see chapter 4). The word *spondyloarthropathies* means that the disease involves the joints of the spine.

Some of the characteristics shared by seronegative spondyloarthropathies include:

- Inflammation of the sacroiliac joints and of the attachment structures that anchor ligaments and tendons to bone.
- A tendency to run in families (they are all associated with a genetic marker called HLA-B27).
- Arthritis in peripheral joints, including arms, legs, feet, and hands.
- Involvement of other tissues, including tissues of the skin, eyes, bowel, and genital/urinary tract.

There may be an overlap of symptoms among the diseases in this group. In fact, the symptoms of ankylosing spondylitis and Reiter's syndrome are sometimes so similar that they are hard to distinguish. It would be perfectly sensible to discuss Reiter's syndrome in this chapter, along with AS. However, Reiter's syndrome often occurs following an infection of the bowel or genital/urinary tract; for this reason, I have included it later in the book, under the discussion on infection and arthritis (see chapter 11).

Who Gets AS?

Ankylosing spondylitis is primarily a disease of young men in their twenties and thirties. Women who get AS seem to get it in a milder form, and this sometimes makes it more difficult to diagnose. AS is more common among whites than blacks, and it also seems to run in families. People with such bowel diseases as ulcerative colitis and Crohn's disease and with psoriasis, a skin disease, may have more of a risk of developing AS. The Arthritis Foundation estimates that approximately 300,000 people in the United States have AS.

Signs and Symptoms

As in other arthritic diseases, symptoms can vary greatly from one person to another. Ankylosing spondylitis usually begins gradually, with discomfort in the lower back. However, AS can also start with problems in the joints of the knees, hips, and shoulders, and even in the small joints of the hand. This is especially true for women, who usually have a milder form of the disease and less typical symptoms. When peripheral joints (arms, legs, feet, and hands) are involved, it can be difficult to distinguish between rheumatoid arthritis and AS in the early stages of the disease.

Some of my patients first notice backache symptoms after having had an injury or fall, or after overextending themselves, as when shoveling snow or lifting heavy objects. One of my patients, Linda, the thirty-two-year-old mother of an infant and a toddler, complained of backaches that began after the birth of her second child. She attributed them to all of the lifting and bending she was doing to care for her children. Similarly, Alex, a nineteen-year-old patient, blamed his persistent backaches on the physical rigors of military basic training, which he had just completed. From their medical histories, I learned that Linda had been experiencing recurrent unexplained bouts of uveitis, an inflammatory eye disease that sometimes occurs in AS patients. Alex mentioned that two of his relatives had ankylosing spondylitis. X-ray studies subsequently confirmed that both of these patients had the characteristic changes of AS. Injury or back strain probably doesn't cause AS; rather, these events probably make patients aware of an already existing problem in the spine.

During World War II, when there was a big boost in the recognition of this disease, a large number of soldiers were identified as having AS. It must have seemed at the time like an epidemic; in fact, while treating war-related injuries, doctors were picking up on many previously undiagnosed cases of ankylosing spondylitis.

Many patients have only mild or moderate pain as a result of their AS, but others find the pain more intense. Pain can be constant or it may come and go, with periods of remission that may last for weeks. The discomfort is usually worse at night, and some patients say they have trouble finding a comfortable sleeping position. Morning stiffness is quite common, but the back pain usually eases once you begin to move around.

You may also experience sciatic-like pain radiating down your legs. These symptoms can also occur with a slipped disc, but the medical history, physical exam, and X-rays should enable your physician to distinguish between these conditions.

Other joints may also be affected, including the hips, knees, shoulders, and small joints. If the area around your ribs is affected, you may feel a tenderness there.

Muscles around the inflamed joints in AS may react by tightening up protectively. When they contract for too long, the result can be tenderness and muscle spasms around the affected joints.

AS is a systemic disease, which means that it may affect areas outside of the joints. AS may cause mild fever, fatigue, weight loss, loss of appetite, skin problems, and inflammatory eye conditions that cause redness, pain, and tearing. Less commonly, AS may cause heart and lung problems.

Not everyone with AS will have all of these symptoms. With appropriate medicine and physical therapy, AS usually won't progress to an advanced form. However, in a few patients the bony growth between the vertebrae in the spine may cause the back to become progressively more stiff. In its advanced form, the spine may become completely fused so that the patient is permanently locked into a stooped position, unable to move the neck and lower back in any direction. The terms *bamboo* or *poker spine* have been used to describe the rigid spine of the very advanced AS patient. An increasingly rigid chest wall may also make breathing difficult.

The active phase of this disease is usually followed by a quiet phase, during which recurrences of AS are unusual. If a patient has already lost some flexibility in his spine due to bony bridges, however, there is currently no way to restore the flexibility.

What Happens Physiologically?

The back consists of a series of bones called vertebrae that are stacked one on top of another to provide a flexible column of support. Between these vertebrae are cushions of cartilage called discs that function as shock absorbers. Strong ligaments and tendons keep the bones in place and attach the muscles to the ribs and limbs. At the base of the spine is the sacrum, or tail bone, which joins the hip bones at the sacroiliac joints.

All of these structures can be affected by ankylosing spondylitis. The degree of damage to these structures varies from individual to individual, and in most cases is not severe.

AS usually begins with an inflammation around the sacroiliac joints. For many, the disease doesn't progress any further. In advanced cases, AS may go on to affect the vertebrae up and down the spine. The ligaments and tendons surrounding the vertebrae may become ossified, forming bony bridges that cause the spine to become rigid. The medical name for these bone formations is syndesmophytes. On X-ray these syndesmophytes are quite easy to identify. They differ markedly from osteophytes, the spurs or small bony growths that form as a result of degenerative types of arthritis.

If the ligaments connecting the ribs to the spine become fused, your chest may not be able to expand as far as before, but you won't necessarily

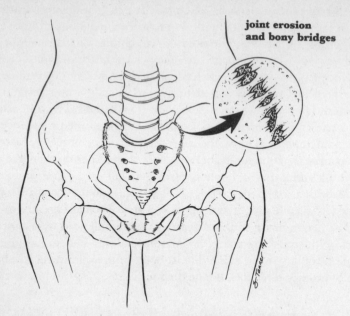

joint erosion
and bony bridges

VERTEBRAE AND SACROILIAC JOINTS: ANKYLOSING SPONDYLITIS

have trouble breathing. You may have pain in the soles of your feet caused by an inflammation of the connective tissue on the bottom of the feet (plantar fasciitis); Achilles tendonitis where the Achilles tendon is attached at the heel; and heel spurs caused by bony overgrowths. Both plantar fasciitis and Achilles tendonitis can also result from sports injuries, especially from running or jogging. So if you have this type of sports-related problem, it may not be a bad idea to see a rheumatologist, who can most easily differentiate between these conditions.

Some people with AS have problems primarily with their ligaments and tendons; others have problems mostly with inflamed peripheral joints and tend to have very little spinal involvement.

What Causes AS?

The cause of AS is unknown. The disease appears to be hereditary, however, and scientists have found a genetic marker called HLA-B27 in most of the people who have AS.

The association between HLA-B27 and AS was a very important and exciting discovery in the field of rheumatology. This genetic marker was originally identified in the sixties by researchers concerned about tissue matches between recipients and donors of organ transplants. In the early seventies, it was discovered that this marker, found on the surface of white blood cells, appeared frequently in patients who had certain types of rheumatic disease, chiefly AS and Reiter's syndrome. What is still unclear is why the diseases linked to this gene express themselves so differently from one condition to the next. Why does AS result in the formation of bony bridges in the spine, while Reiter's syndrome is more likely to cause swelling and pain in peripheral joints?

Scientists think that HLA-B27 is somehow involved in the body's immune response. It is hoped that the study of these genes will offer further clues to the cause and possible prevention and/or treatment of various forms of arthritis.

Even if you have this genetic marker, you won't necessarily be affected by ankylosing spondylitis. Many healthy people have HLA-B27 and never develop AS. Perhaps some people with this genetic marker are more susceptible to environmental factors, such as infectious agents, which can alter the immune system and cause AS.

Diagnosis

Ankylosing spondylitis is diagnosed on the basis of a medical history, a physical examination, and X-rays. There is no diagnostic test for AS, but laboratory tests help doctors exclude such other diseases as rheumatoid arthritis and lupus.

The medical history can give a good indication of AS. I will strongly suspect AS when the patient is a young male who has had low back pain for several months, morning stiffness that improves with exercise, and a family history of AS. Roy, a twenty-three-year-old computer analyst, is a typical example. Several months ago he developed a chronic lower backache. He thought the pain might have resulted from a fall he took while skiing, but the pattern of the pain and stiffness and the accompanying signs of fatigue and mild fever pointed to AS. Roy said that his father, a fifty-one-year-old businessman, was diagnosed with AS as a young man. In fact, it was his father who had urged him to see a rheumatologist. All of the facts pointed to a great likelihood of AS, and a subsequent workup confirmed Roy's diagnosis.

During the physical exam, your doctor will ask you to perform various movements to assess how much your spine has been affected. You might be asked to bend over to touch your toes while keeping your knees straight so your doctor can measure how flexible your spine is. Normal vertebrae move apart as you bend, but lose this ability with spinal ankylosis. You might also be asked to stand with your back against the wall and touch your head to the wall. In AS, the upper spine may become rigid and curve more so that you won't be able to touch your head to the wall.

Your doctor can measure your chest expansion quite simply by asking you to take a deep breath and then measuring your chest with a tape measure. You will then be asked to exhale completely, and a second chest measurement will be made. The difference between these two measurements will give your doctor a good idea of your chest expansion capacity. To see whether AS has affected your neck, you will be asked to move your neck up and down, and then turn your head to the left and the right.

X-rays can be key to the diagnosis of AS, but may be difficult to read early in the disease and require the interpretive skills of a physician experienced in this condition—frequently a radiologist, orthopedist, or rheumatologist. The sacroiliac joints are usually the first to show the effects of AS. On X-ray, they appear fuzzy because inflammation has eroded the joint surfaces. In advanced cases, you can see ossification of the tissues and the formation of bony bridges fusing the joints together. X-rays will also reveal any inflammatory changes in the vertebrae and the fusing of ligaments and tendons.

Perhaps the most controversial issue in the diagnosis of ankylosing spondylitis concerns the role of tissue typing, the process by which the patient's cells are checked for telltale genetic markers. Over 90 percent of patients with AS have the HLA-B27 marker. However, as we've mentioned, many normal people also have this marker and never develop AS. So the B27 marker may indicate a predisposition toward this disease, but is not in and of itself diagnostic. Indeed, it may be misleading to use tissue typing for diagnostic purposes. In randomized tests, there is a 1 in 12 chance that a person will test positive for HLA-B27, regardless of whether he or she has signs of ankylosing spondylitis.

On the other hand, tissue typing can sometimes be useful. For example, children sometimes get AS, but it is difficult to see changes in their sacroiliac joints on X-ray because their joints are not yet fully formed. A B27 tissue typing in such instances might help me to make a diagnosis. Similarly, X-rays may not be revealing for some people in the disease. In the early stages of AS, your doctor may prefer to avoid more extensive X-rays or bone scans, and a B27 tissue typing could give him or her some important diagnostic information.

As I mentioned earlier in this chapter, Reiter's syndrome has symptoms very similar to those of ankylosing spondylitis. During your diagnostic workup, your doctor may try to determine which of the two diseases you have. In general, Reiter's syndrome involves the peripheral joints more, the spine less; it is often preceded by a bowel or urinary tract infection. AS, on the other hand, appears primarily to affect the spine and usually occurs in previously healthy individuals. These differences, however, are not always so clear-cut. Patients sometimes have symptoms of both diseases.

Genetic Counseling

Since AS may be hereditary, should couples with a family history of the disease seek genetic counseling? The risks of inheriting this disease are relatively low, even for those who have a family history of AS. At most, one in five of those who carry the HLA-B27 marker will develop some signs of ankylosing spondylitis. Indeed, many of my patients with AS cannot recall any relative in their family with arthritis or any related diseases. Even when people do have AS, the disease can usually be controlled with medication. Most people with AS live a long, fulfilling life. Since AS occurs so infrequently and is usually not disabling, I don't see it as a reason to seek genetic counseling or as a factor in a couple's decision to have children.

Tissue typing has given medical researchers a wealth of new information about the genetic transmission of this disease and may eventually help us understand why it is that only a fraction of the people with this marker get the disease, while the others do not. Through genetic research we may eventually learn how to prevent this disease or how to treat it more effectively.

Our ability to test for HLA-B27 and to interpret X-rays with increasing sophistication has made it apparent that ankylosing spondylitis is more common than we used to think and has alerted physicians to the importance of X-ray examinations of sacroiliac joints in cases of unexplained backache. Genetic testing shows that women suffer from AS and related disorders more commonly than we thought, although they rarely have the classic bamboo or poker spine of AS. They appear to have a much more subtle version of the disease that is more similar to rheumatoid arthritis than to AS, and which primarily affects peripheral joints as opposed to the spine.

Treatment

The aim of treatment of AS is to reduce inflammation and to keep the joints as flexible as possible. Nonsteroidal anti-inflammatory drugs (NSAIDs) are the medications of choice. Most NSAIDs are effective in the treatment of AS, but the one rheumatologists most commonly prescribe is indomethacin (Indocin). Many AS patients are young when they start therapy, and may have to be on medications for many years. Indomethacin seems to be a well-tolerated drug. As any drug, it does have possible side effects, including gastrointestinal problems, salt and fluid retention, and nervous system changes (e.g., "bad feelings," nightmares, and sleep disturbances). To avoid stomach upset, patients should take indomethacin with meals, rather than on an empty stomach. Those who cannot tolerate indomethacin will usually be able to tolerate one of the other available NSAIDs. In addition, if you are having muscle spasms, your physician may recommend a muscle relaxant.

In the past, before the hazards of long-term exposure to radiation were recognized, radiation therapy was sometimes used to treat AS. In more advanced cases, X-rays were directed at the sacroiliac joints and the lower spine. Though such treatment often alleviated pain, it increased the risk of radiation-induced cancer. This treatment is no longer used.

Physical Therapy

Phsyical therapy is another important component in any AS treatment plan. Your doctor may place you on a special exercise regimen or refer you to a physical therapist. The exercises you do will be tailored to your condition and abilities. They are designed to help you to maintain as much flexibility in your spine as possible. You may be shown various stretching and muscle-strengthening exercises, as well as deep breathing exercises to help maintain flexibility in your chest and rib cage. Since AS can sometimes affect the functioning of your lungs, I urge you to give up smoking.

You must maintain good posture and keep the supporting muscles in your back strong. A physical therapist can show you how to walk, lift, sit, and stand so that your back stays as straight as possible at all times. You may also want to see an occupational therapist, who can show you how to perform work or daily activities most efficiently. The occupational therapist can also help you arrange surfaces at home and at work so that you do not have to slump or strain.

If you have a desk job, you should sit in a comfortable, straight-backed chair, preferably one with arms. The desk surface should be set at a level to keep you from having to bend too much. Try to alternate stints at your desk with periods of exercise or some other activity that gets you moving, so your joints won't stiffen up.

Special aids and equipment are available to assist those who have already lost some mobility in their necks and spines. Long-handled mops and brooms, for example, and special car mirrors can prevent unnecessary bending and straining. (For further information, see the resources section of this book.)

Good posture is important even while you sleep. To help keep your back straight, I recommend a very firm mattress (no pillows), with a plywood board between the box spring and the mattress.

While ankylosing spondylitis can usually be halted or slowed with medication and physical therapy, in rare, more advanced cases the spine may fuse into one position. Through a conscientious regimen of daily physical therapy, a patient can maintain good posture so that if his or her spine should fuse, its position will be as functional as possible.

Sports and Physical Activity

So far as physical activity is concerned, I usually encourage my patients to continue their normal activities and recreational pursuits as long as they are feeling up to it. I have many patients with mild forms of AS who continue to enjoy golf and tennis for many years. Physical exercise is usually very beneficial, both because it helps you psychologically and because it serves to keep your joints flexible and your muscles strong. You may have to cut back on vigorous movement during painful flares and then use some common sense and your own body signals as you *gradually* resume activities. A good rule of thumb is: If it hurts, don't do it. If you have any question at all about the appropriateness of a physical activity, consult your physician.

If you do have progressive spinal involvement, you may be told to limit or alter your physical activities. A stiffened spine and neck can increase your risk of physical injury, and you should avoid sports that involve a lot of bending and twisting and in which you are liable to fall or injure yourself. Your coordination and balance are not likely to be as good as before, and if you are injured, your stiffened joints may be more prone to fracture. If you have mild to moderate symptoms, swimming can be an excellent all-around conditioner. However, in advanced cases, when AS affects the shoulder and neck, this too may present problems. Many local recreational centers offer water exercise programs specially developed for arthritis patients. These can be of great benefit.

Because you have an inflammatory disease, you may tire more easily and may have to learn to pace yourself. You must learn to intersperse vigorous periods of activity with periods of rest, if possible.

NSAIDs and physical therapy often go hand in hand. The drugs can reduce painful inflammation and muscle spasms so that you can do your physical exercises. A hot shower can help you to loosen up so that your muscles and joints will feel less stiff.

AS and Sexuality

In most instances, sexuality is not affected by AS, but for some, the pain and stiffness can interfere with sexual enjoyment. This issue is not unique to those with AS. Anyone with a potential limitation in mobility, whether it is due to rheumatoid arthritis or osteoarthritis, may have concerns about sexuality. Though you may be hesitant to do so, you should discuss any concerns openly with your partner as well as your health care provider. Perhaps you and your partner can plan sexual activity for some point in the day when you hurt the least, or time it for when painkillers take effect. You and your partner should experiment together to find the positions that are most comfortable for you. A hot shower immediately before sexual relations may lessen your discomfort; in fact, if you and your partner take a shower together, it may even be incorporated into your lovemaking. For some, the physical changes of AS may alter self-esteem and feelings about sexuality. You may benefit by meeting with a counselor to discuss your feelings. (For additional advice, see chapter 17.)

Other Treatments

If you're not getting pain relief from medication, for joints other than the back, surgery is sometimes considered in advanced cases of AS. Artificial hip and shoulder replacements are having increasing success. With AS, however, joint replacement surgery is considered a last-resort therapy; the overgrowth of bony material so characteristic of the disease may also freeze the replacement joint. In very severe cases, where there is concern about chest deformity and severe respiratory problems, surgery can be performed to undo the curvature and get the spine into a more favorable position. This is difficult, major surgery which is done only rarely and should be performed only by surgeons who are experienced with this type of operation.

Since inflammatory eye disease can occur in AS, your treatment plan may involve an evaluation by an opthalmologist. Ankylosing spondylitis may also be part of inflammatory disease of the bowel or psoriasis, so you may be referred to a gastroenterologist or dermatologist.

Sometimes an important part of treatment can be just talking about your condition with other people who really understand what you're going through. You may find it helpful to join a support group or seek counseling.

Most people with AS find that it interferes little in their lives and that they are not as depressed as those with more systemic forms of arthritis. A recent applicant to our faculty, for example, had AS with a completely fused spine and neck; yet he was able to go through the rigors of house staff training. One of our radiology technicians has AS and works full-time, although he walks a little stiffly. Many of our AS patients are highly motivated young men who are very active; if anything, they may exceed their physical limitations. They work, participate in sports, and in general seem to do very well.

Prognosis

AS is one of those conditions for which there is currently a great deal of optimism. More sophisticated diagnostic techniques have made recognition of this disease much easier over the last few years. The identification of more people with the disease at earlier stages has improved the prognosis for AS significantly. Though we can make no promises as far as the course of this disease is concerned, we can often minimize and possibly prevent its progression by prompt treatment with NSAIDs, daily stretching exercises, and good body mechanics. Most people with AS have mild to moderate symptoms and lead relatively normal, active lives.

ANKYLOSING SPONDYLITIS (AS, OR MARIE-STRÜMPELL DISEASE)

A chronic inflammatory disease that primarily affects the spine and sacroiliac joints and involves enthesopathy, an inflammation of the ligaments and tendons where they attach to bone. In more advanced forms, attachment structures ossify, and bony bridges cause joints in the spine to fuse, making movement difficult.

CAUSE: No known cause, though a genetic predisposition seems to be an important factor.

SYMPTOMS: Usually begins gradually with lower back pain accompanied by morning stiffness. Pain may be worse at night. In advanced cases, spine may be fused into one position. Other symptoms may include sciatica, muscle spasms, foot pains, mild fever, fatigue, weight loss, and loss of appetite. May also cause arthritis in other joints (e.g., hip, knee, and shoulder). Chest expansion may be reduced.

WHO GETS IT? Mostly young men in their twenties and thirties. Women usually have a milder form. May appear more often in some families. Is associated with inflammatory bowel disease (ulcerative colitis and Crohn's disease), and psoriasis.

DIAGNOSIS: Diagnosis is based on medical history and physical exam. Routine lab tests are used to exclude other illnesses; tests for rheumatoid factor are negative.

TREATMENT: Nonsteroidal anti-inflammatory drugs (NSAIDs) and physical therapy to maintain flexibility.

PROGNOSIS: Generally favorable. Most have mild to moderate symptoms and lead relatively normal, active lives.

9

Gout and
Pseudogout

George, a forty-four-year-old insurance executive, is a hefty 220-pound man who eats and drinks with gusto and enjoys several martinis before dinner. He's had high blood pressure for the past five years and has been urged many times by his doctor to cut down on his drinking and lose weight. One night he attended an office retirement party, where he drank and ate with his usual zest. He went to bed feeling fine, although a bit bloated from all he had consumed at the party. Then at three in the morning he was jolted awake by the most intense pain he had ever felt. His big toe burned and throbbed, and when the sheet touched it, he felt excruciating pain. George's wife immediately phoned their family doctor, who told her to bring George to the hospital emergency room, where he would meet them. When the doctor examined George's toe, which by now was a shiny red-purple, he concluded that George had gout. He prescribed a drug called colchicine, which George was to take every hour until the pain subsided, or until George's stomach couldn't take any more. Six hours after beginning the colchicine treatment, George felt the pain ease, and by the next day he was better. His doctor told George that in order to forestall another gout attack he would have to lose some weight and cut back on his drinking.

What Is Gout?

Gout is a common form of arthritis characterized by sudden attacks that result in exquisitely painful and swollen joints. Its diagnosis and treatment is one of rheumatology's success stories. We know what causes it. We can diagnose it with virtual certainty. And we have learned how to control its symptoms and prevent future attacks. Gout is probably the best understood and most effectively controlled form of arthritic disease.

Gout comes from the Latin word *gutta*, meaning a drop. An old theory of medicine proposed that gout was caused by one of the mysterious humors that circulated in the body and settled, drop by drop, in the affected joint.

Gout is a true form of arthritis because it involves the inflammation of a joint. However, gout is unlike many of the other arthritic diseases we've discussed because it primarily involves the body's metabolism, not the immune system. The inflammation is the result of an accumulation of crystals deposited within a joint. These crystals are composed of a chemical called monosodium urate.

People with gout have excessively high levels of uric acid, a waste product normally present in the blood. Uric acid results from the breakdown of purines, a group of chemicals derived from nucleic acids, the material involved in heredity. Purines are found in high concentrations in meat, especially organ meats, which are high in cell nuclei. Your body also produces purines on its own, which then get broken down into uric acid.

Excess amounts of uric acid are normally filtered out by the kidneys and excreted in the urine, but when your blood is supersaturated with uric acid, excess crystals may settle out, much the way sugar crystals do in a coffee cup. The sharp, needle-like crystals of monosodium urate can be deposited in your joints, where they sometimes cause inflammation and excruciating pain. Of course high uric acid levels do not always result in gout. Older people, many with kidney disease, many people on diuretics, and diabetics may have high uric acid levels and never develop gout. So some other factor must keep crystals from forming in certain people.

Who Gets Gout?

Gout is mainly a disease of men who are middle-aged and older. Factors that may increase the likelihood of gout include having high blood pressure, being overweight, and drinking excessive amounts of alcohol. Women are far less apt to get gout, probably because their blood uric acid levels are much lower than men's are up until menopause. After women go through menopause, their uric acid levels rise, but it takes approximately twenty years for their blood levels to catch up with those of men.

Signs and Symptoms

Gout usually strikes a single joint suddenly and violently (the medical name for such an attack is acute monarticular arthritis). The episode begins with the classic signs of inflammation—redness, heat, swelling, and pain. Less commonly, gout can develop more slowly and involve multiple joints in a pattern that resembles rheumatoid arthritis.

For some unknown reason, the big toe is commonly affected first. The pain in the big toe is very distinct and is called podagra. Other joints may also be involved, including the feet, knees, and elbows. Wrist or finger joints are less frequently involved in early attacks. It is unusual for the shoulders, hips, or the spine to be affected.

Most of the time gout begins rather dramatically, often in the middle of the night. Many of my patients say they go to sleep feeling absolutely fine, with no indication of inflammation, and then wake up at 2:00 or 3:00 A.M. in great pain. The joint with gout is so sensitive that even the lightest touch of a sheet or a breeze on it is excruciating. Patients say this is the worst pain they have ever felt. One patient told me that during an attack he noticed a housefly in the bedroom and couldn't take his eyes off that fly, terrified it would settle on his toe. Another worried that a piece of peeling paint from the ceiling was going to drop off onto his toe. Systemic symptoms of chills and fever are also common.

Gouty joints show just about the most florid signs of inflammation of any form of arthritis. The skin around the affected joint may be pulled tight and may look shiny and bright red or purple.

An initial attack of gout may last several days and then disappear, even without treatment. You may not have another attack again for weeks, months, or even years. In fact some people never have subsequent attacks.

During the period between attacks, you may be completely symptom-free. If the gout is left untreated, attacks sometimes recur with increasing frequency, last longer, and may affect more joints. In severe cases, repeated attacks over time may cause damage to the joints and loss of mobility. However, with today's good treatments, recurrent attacks can be avoided.

Gout attacks seem to occur more often under certain conditions. Acute attacks may be triggered by alcohol consumption, overeating, and physical stresses such as surgery and acute medical illness. If people take good care of themselves and stop drinking and eating to excess, attacks may not recur.

Sometimes when there are high amounts of sodium urate in the system, crystals can accumulate to form lumps under the skin. These lumps are called tophi. Tophi may not develop until many years after the onset of the disease. Not everyone develops tophi. When they do occur, these lumps are usually found around the affected joints, where they can cause joint damage, and at sites that involve irritation. Tophi are most commonly seen near the elbows, where you lean against a table; at the Achilles tendon, where shoes or boots rub; and in the cartilage on the outer ear. In some patients, if untreated, sodium urate deposits may also occur in the kidneys, where they can impair function.

Tophi can sometimes be confused with rheumatoid nodules, but a biopsy or examination of the fluid inside can help the doctor distinguish between the two. Sometimes the skin becomes ulcerated and breaks open and a white, chalky discharge composed of urate crystals can be seen.

What Causes Gout?

There are many portraits in art and literature of people with gout. The stereotypical image is that of a portly and prosperous middle-aged European man. He eats and drinks with reckless abandon, his bandaged leg propped on a chair. Historically, gout has been associated with gluttony and overindulgence. It was considered a disease of the rich and greedy. Today we know that such stereotypes do not tell the whole story and that people of any socioeconomic level can get gout. While diet and excessive drinking are linked to gout, the disease appears to be caused by a combination of factors, including a hereditary tendency that predisposes some people to elevated levels of blood uric acid.

When uric acid reaches a certain level in the blood (7 milligrams in each 100 milliliters) the blood cannot hold any more and is said to be saturated. When this saturation point is reached, the uric acid may precipitate out of the blood in the form of monosodium urate crystals, which may be deposited in the joints. When a person's uric acid levels are too high, he or she is said to have hyperuricemia. There are three basic reasons for having hyperuricemia: (1) You are eating too many purine-containing foods; (2) your body may have a metabolic defect that causes you to overproduce uric acid; or (3) your kidneys aren't doing an effective job of eliminating excess uric acid, and you aren't excreting enough of it. In many patients, a combination of these factors results in high levels of uric acid.

Dietary habits and alcohol consumption may trigger gout attacks among susceptible individuals. Many gout patients are overweight and many drink to excess. A diet rich in purines, frequently from organ meats, may raise the levels of uric acid in the blood; alcohol in turn affects kidney function and uric acid metabolism.

Several other environmental factors can also raise the uric acid concentration in your blood, including the use of certain drugs, such as diuretics, that can block the elimination of uric acid in the urine. Lead ingestion can also predispose a person to gout. In nineteenth-century England, when lead containers were used to store port, the incidence of kidney damage and gout increased. In the past, gout was found among patients who drank unbonded liquor or moonshine, which contains lead derived from automobile radiators. This is called saturnine gout.

Those with a high level of uric acid in the blood, however, do not automatically get gout. In fact most people with hyperuricemia never develop gout. Perhaps it's not the high level of uric acid itself that causes gout, but rather a rapid change in uric acid levels that may act to trigger an attack. For example, heavy drinking and the ingestion of a rich meal, classically associated with an attack of gout, are both accompanied by rapid rises in the level of uric acid in the blood, which may cause an attack.

Gout can occur in association with other diseases, such as diabetes and hypertension. Since women rarely suffer from gout before menopause, its occurrence may also be linked to hormonal changes.

What Happens Physiologically?

Crystals of monosodium urate form and are deposited in the body's connective tissues and joint spaces. Exactly why specific joints, such as the big toe, are prime targets is unclear. The crystals in the joint evoke intense inflammation in the joint space and cause the immune system to respond by sending in white blood cells. The result is swelling and inflammation. Sometimes crystals appear to be knocked out of the connective tissue and into the joint space as a result of metabolic changes or a physical injury. That's probably what happens to patients who report that a gout attack began late at night after they stubbed their toe in the dark on the way to the bathroom. If left untreated, the crystal deposits and joint inflammation can damage the cartilage and bone and lead to deformity and reduced mobility. If you get prompt treatment, however, the disease usually does not progress to this stage.

Diagnosis

A definitive diagnosis of gout can be made by examining a bit of joint fluid under a special type of microscope called a polarizing light microscope. Joint fluid is obtained by aspiration with a needle, also referred to as tapping the joint. Your doctor will sterilize and anesthetize the skin surrounding the affected joint, usually with a freezing solution, and then will withdraw some fluid for examination. When I tap a joint, I try to remove as much fluid as I can, not only so I can diagnose the condition properly but also because it helps to relieve the patient's painful swelling. The procedure may cause some discomfort. It is usually done on an outpatient basis.

Since the joint is severely inflamed, the joint fluid is loaded with white blood cells. In addition, it contains crystals, which can be seen under the polarizing light microscope as vividly colored needles.

Because not all offices or emergency rooms have light polarizing microscopes, a doctor sometimes has to base his or her diagnosis on the patient's symptoms and the physical examination. This is usually possible, especially with the unique and characteristic presentation of gout.

You may also have a blood test to assess your uric acid levels. But as I've already mentioned, hyperuricemia alone is not sufficient evidence for a diagnosis of gout; most patients with hyperuricemia do not have gout. Elevated uric acid levels indicate only that you may have a tendency toward this disease. In fact some patients with gout have normal blood uric acid levels.

X-rays are not usually necessary if a tapped joint shows evidence of crystals. However, in some cases when the diagnosis is less obvious, I may order an X-ray. For example, I recently saw in consultation a sixty-year-old patient with a presumptive diagnosis of rheumatoid arthritis who was not responding well to treatment. The lumps under the patient's skin could have been either rheumatoid nodules or tophi. X-rays were performed, and I was able to see evidence of the characteristic changes of gout. I then performed a joint aspiration and confirmed the diagnosis of gout by polarization microscopy.

A definite diagnosis of gout is key in view of the possible need for long-term preventive treatment. You do not have to be in the middle of an acute attack of gout to have crystals present in your joints. Gouty crystals can be withdrawn from joints even between attacks, after symptoms have subsided. I recommend, wherever possible, that patients have the joint fluid aspirated and examined for crystals, especially if the diagnosis of gout is uncertain.

Treatment

Treatment of gout varies, depending on whether you are dealing with the initial acute attack or the chronic phase of the disease.

The initial attack is self-limited and goes away by itself in a few days, with or without treatment. Exactly why these painful flare-ups subside by themselves is unclear. It's possible that the irritating crystals dissolve in the joint space, and because the immune system is no longer stimulated, the swelling goes down.

Acute attacks of gout are extremely painful, and there is no reason to let them run their natural course. Excellent treatments are available that can bring prompt relief.

Colchicine is an effective drug that is derived from a European plant, *Colchicum autumnale,* or autumn crocus. The roots and seeds of this plant have been used to treat gout since at least the fifth or sixth century A.D. Colchicine, the active ingredient in the plant, was chemically isolated in the nineteenth century.

Colchicine is believed to work by slowing down the migration of white blood cells and their release of inflammatory mediators that can cause pain. Treatment with colchicine has to be started within the first two days of the gout attack. After forty-eight hours, it tends to be less effective.

One of the advantages of colchicine is that it can be used to establish a definite diagnosis of gout. Colchicine is not very effective for other forms of arthritis, so if a patient feels relief from pain after receiving this drug, the pain was probably caused by gout. The main drawback of colchicine is the gastrointestinal side effects. Colchicine can cause nausea, vomiting, abdominal cramping, and diarrhea.

To help prevent side effects, colchicine is given in small, frequent doses over the course of a day, usually no more than 6 to 8 milligrams in twenty-four hours. Individual doses are tailored to body size, and during an acute attack, you can take colchicine tablets hourly until either the pain is gone or you develop gastrointestinal side effects—whichever occurs first.

Colchicine is excreted slowly from the body and excess accumulations can sometimes lead to serious blood problems, especially if there is kidney dysfunction; so another dose should not be given for at least a week after the patient completes the full initial treatment. This drug can also be injected into a vein or given intravenously in the hospital when necessary. You wouldn't normally need to have the drug delivered intravenously unless, for example, you have recently had surgery and are not allowed to take anything by mouth. When colchicine is given intravenously, many of the gastrointestinal side effects are avoided, and for some patients, this may be of special benefit. The drug is more commonly administered in tablet form, on an outpatient basis.

Great care has to be used when prescribing colchicine for people with blood, kidney, or liver problems and for the elderly, who may have reduced kidney function.

Nonsteroidal anti-inflammatory drugs (NSAIDs) are highly satisfactory alternatives to colchicine therapy, indomethacin being the most commonly prescribed. Therapy with NSAIDs is usually begun at the maximum dosage, which is cut down gradually as you begin to respond to treatment, usually within a few hours.

NSAIDs can be effective drugs even when treatment has been delayed by a few days. However, NSAIDs have some common side effects. They may affect kidney functioning, and since gout is sometimes associated with reduced kidney function, this can be a problem. Also, gout often occurs in older people, mainly those who have had previous kidney or heart problems, which are associated with fluid accumulation. People with a history of heart failure should also avoid NSAIDs.

Aspirin, though classified as an NSAID, is not used for acute attacks of gout because it takes too long to work; in addition, low doses of aspirin can elevate uric acid levels by blocking kidney excretion.

Occasionally, when a patient fails to respond to colchicine or NSAIDs, the doctor may try a corticosteroid. Such drugs may be injected directly into the affected joint or given systemically to bring the inflammation down.

Sometimes just tapping a joint is the only treatment necessary. If a person is sick or has had heart or kidney failure or a recent operation, and you don't want to give him or her additional medications, withdrawal of fluid from the joint may sufficiently relieve the pain.

Treatment of Chronic Gout

Once you've had a gout attack, you know you have a predisposition to the disease. Will you ever have another attack? How often will subsequent attacks occur? Unfortunately, we do not have answers to these questions. You may not have another attack for months or even years after the first episode. Some patients seem to have frequent attacks, especially when they slip back into former eating and drinking patterns. For example, Fred, a gas station attendant, has had four attacks within the last two years. Harry, a sixty-year-old patient, on the other hand, had one isolated attack when he was admitted here at the hospital for gallbladder surgery. Three days after the operation his big toe became red, very painful, and swollen, and I was called in for consultation. His toe was tapped, and he was treated with colchicine. It's been several years since this attack, and the gout has never recurred.

There's no way to know how an individual will react; therefore, I like to observe my patients for some time before making a recommendation about potentially lifelong therapy.

Fairly simple alterations in lifestyle can help reduce your risk of subsequent gout attacks, and it makes sense to begin with these. Since there is a link between gout and obesity, if you're overweight you should consult your doctor about a sensible weight reduction plan. Weight control is really very important, and it's an area in which you can really take charge of your own health. However, I would caution against quick-loss fad or crash diets, as fasting can increase the levels of uric acid in your blood and bring on another gout attack. Instead, wait until your condition stabilizes after a gout attack and then begin a gradual weight-loss program.

I recommend you go on a low-fat diet and eliminate purine-rich foods. Foods to avoid include fatty meats, especially organ meats. The following foods contain an especially high level of purines: liver, sweetbreads, fish roe, mussels, anchovies, and sardines.

Drink at least eight glasses of fluids each day. However, note that caffeine-containing beverages such as coffee can actually make you more dehydrated. Also, avoid excess alcohol consumption. One to two drinks per day is considered moderate; however, alcohol can raise uric acid levels in your blood and precipitate an attack. If you have gout, you should probably avoid alcohol altogether.

Weight control and sensible eating and drinking habits can not only reduce your chances of another gout attack but also provide other health benefits as well. However, if gout attacks recur despite your efforts, then preventive treatment for long-term control may be necessary.

The first approach is usually low-dose treatment with colchicine, one or two tablets—0.6 to 1.2 milligrams—a day. This dosage will usually be reduced even further if you have a history of kidney problems. You may have to take colchicine for a few months, but your doctor will probably discontinue it once your levels of uric acid are down. If those levels don't respond, however, your doctor may extend the treatment.

Overproducers versus Underexcretors

The next step in treatment depends upon what's causing the high uric acid levels in your blood. Gout patients are subdivided into two groups: overproducers of uric acid or underexcretors. In other words, patients either produce too much uric acid or excrete too little in their urine.

In order to assure that you are placed on the correct treatment regimen, your physician will measure the total amount of uric acid in your urine over a twenty-four-hour period. You simply collect in a jar all of the urine you produce in one day. An analysis of the uric acid in this sample helps your doctor classify you as either an underexcretor or an overproducer. I advise my patients to go on a low-purine diet for at least a few days before the urine collection; otherwise, your doctor may get confused and identify you as an overproducer when you've simply eaten a purine-rich diet.

If you are an underexcretor, you will probably be treated with a uricosuric drug—i.e., drugs that work by dissolving crystals and increasing the excretion of uric acid in your urine. Two commonly prescribed uricosuric drugs are probenecid (Benemid) and sulfinpyrazone (Anturane). Benemid has fewer side effects than Anturane and is a relatively safe drug that has been used for many years. A popular preparation, Col-BENEMID, is a combination of colchicine and probenecid.

By increasing the amount of uric acid in the urine, uricosuric drugs may increase the risk of kidney stone formation. To avoid such a risk, you must dilute your urine by drinking plenty of fluids every day. Benemid should be used only by people with normal kidney function who do not have a history of kidney stones.

If you are an overproducer of uric acid, then you may be prescribed the drug allopurinol (Zyloprim). This drug blocks the enzyme necessary for the formation of uric acid. Allopurinol is one of the most specific biochemical interventions for the control of disease in all of medicine and is a triumph of modern pharmacology.

The development of this drug can be traced in part to Duke University, which has historically been a place for the study of purine metabolism. Duke was one of the institutions that originally participated in studies on the effects of allopurinol. The drug was developed as a way to make chemotherapy more effective for cancer patients by preventing the breakdown of other drugs used to kill tumor cells. When allopurinol was used to treat malignancies, it was observed that patients' uric acid levels were also being lowered. Consequently, researchers thought this drug could be useful in lowering uric acid levels in gout patients. So a drug used by hematologists and oncologists ended up being useful for arthritis.

Though allopurinol is a generally safe drug, its dosage must be adjusted if you have any problems in kidney function. Possible side effects include gastrointestinal upsets and a severe skin rash.

Because allopurinol is so effective and can generally be tolerated well, some physicians prefer to use it for all gout patients. It is not always easy to distinguish between underexcretors and overproducers, so the use of a single agent is attractive.

Drugs used to treat chronic gout may at first cause rapid changes in your uric acid levels. When such therapy is initiated, it may trigger an acute attack of gout. Therefore, when drug therapy is first started, gout attacks may become more frequent. The attacks will subside once the drug takes effect and the levels of uric acid stabilize at a normal point. In order to minimize the possibility of attacks, doctors usually start uric-acid-lowering drugs along with colchicine. This combination works very well.

Many doctors recommend that you always have a supply of colchicine or an NSAID on hand, even when you are being treated with drugs to lower uric acid. I usually give my patients 50-milligram tablets of Indocin in case they forget to take their medications and experience an attack. A full-blown crisis can often be averted when NSAIDs or colchicine are started as soon as you notice the initial symptoms of an attack.

Drug Interactions

Gout medications can interact with other drugs and produce undesirable results. You must discuss with your physician any drugs that you may be taking, including over-the-counter medications. Aspirin, for example, can affect the normal excretion of uric acid and alter actions of other drugs. Thiazide diuretics, used to treat hypertension, can also prevent the normal excretion of uric acid, and your physician may consider switching you to another medication (e.g., beta-blockers or calcium channel blockers) to control your high blood pressure. Gout medications may also affect the actions of antibiotics, decongestants, and insulin, among others.

Preventive Therapy

Should people with high levels of uric acid be treated prophylactically so that they do not develop gout?

Many people with high uric acid levels have kidney disease, and it was long thought that gout was the cause of kidney disease. Given the serious problems associated with kidney failure, drugs to lower the levels of uric acid and prevent gout seemed to make sense.

Studies have since suggested the cause of kidney disease in people with hyperuricemia is not the high uric acid levels, but hypertension. Hypertension is the condition that needs to be treated, not high levels of uric acid. Furthermore, we know that many people with high uric acid levels never develop gout. So high levels of uric acid alone, without any symptoms, are not an indication for treatment.

Today we do not give allopurinol or other uric-acid-lowering drugs to prevent gout in patients who have elevated uric acid levels but who have never experienced a gout attack. Instead, we emphasize prevention of kidney disease by dietary measures and treatment of hypertension.

Long-term Therapy

What about those patients who have already had an initial attack of gout? Should they be placed on long-term therapy to bring their uric acid levels down to normal? This issue is of special concern for patients whose disease begins when they are young and who might have to use these agents for thirty to forty years. The long-term safety of these drugs is not known; moreover, they are expensive.

The long-term use of therapy to lower uric acid levels has to be measured against the frequency and severity of gout attacks. If someone has had one attack and then feels perfectly fine, he or she may be unwilling or financially unable to continue an indefinite course of daily medication. Some patients are willing to bet that the next attack of gout won't happen soon, if ever, or that if an attack does occur, a quick course of an NSAID or colchicine would halt it quickly.

My own approach is to wait for the second attack of gout before considering long-term therapy. Sometimes gout can be triggered by something—an unusual stress or surgery, for example—that is unlikely to recur. Limited treatment with colchicine or NSAIDs may control the acute attack, but it is hard to justify unlimited therapy for a single event, no matter how painful. Once the disease recurs, however, the decision is much more obvious and lifelong therapy more justifiable.

Prognosis

The prognosis for this disease is very good. Early attacks do not normally damage joints or leave any long-term effects. So if therapy is instituted for recurrent episodes of disease and conscientiously followed, future attacks can be prevented. Gout is a very well understood and easily controlled disease that should have little effect on your normal daily life.

Pseudogout

In the early sixties, physicians examining joint fluid of patients thought to have gout discovered that some of the crystals had unusual shapes and were bending the microscope's polarizing light in uncharacteristic directions. Gout crystals are normally needle-shaped, but these crystals were rhomboidal. Chemical analysis showed that the new crystals were composed of a salt called calcium pyrophosphate dihydrate (CPPD). The symptoms caused by the deposition of these crystals were similar to those caused by the monosodium urate crystals in gout. As a result of the resemblance, scientists named the new disease pseudogout. The crystal-induced disease is also called calcium pyrophosphate dihydrate deposition disease, or CPPD disease.

Pseudogout is only one form of CPPD disease. Some forms of CPPD disease resemble osteoarthritis, and some forms look like rheumatoid arthritis. When CPPD crystals are deposited in the cartilage, the condition is called chondrocalcinosis (meaning calcium in the cartilage).

What Causes Pseudogout?

Like gout, pseudogout is caused by the formation of crystals in the joints. We don't know why these crystals form, but their presence in the joint stimulates the immune system to send white blood cells to the area, and the joint becomes painful and inflamed. It is not clear whether the crystals are the cause of the problem or the result of some sort of joint damage.

Pseudogout may be triggered by surgery and severe medical illness. Sometimes it is a sign of an underlying medical condition. CPPD disease may be caused by a hormonal or metabolic disturbance—for example, a problem with iron or calcium metabolism, or an overproduction of growth hormone.

Who Gets Pseudogout?

Pseudogout affects mainly older people, most commonly those over sixty. Men and women are equally likely to get this disease. Often this disease develops in the hospital after surgery, as it did for a sixty-seven-year-old man who recently came in for a hernia repair. Three days after the operation, his knee became severely painful and swollen. We tapped it and the pseudogout resolved itself.

Signs and Symptoms

The pattern of attack may vary from individual to individual. Pseudogout generally resembles gout. In the acute form, the pain may come on suddenly, and your joint may become red, painful, and swollen. While the big toe may be involved, it is usually not the joint that's affected. Sudden acute attacks of pseudogout are more likely to affect the knees. Symptoms may last several days and then disappear.

In the more chronic forms of CPPD disease, symptoms may come and go, much like the pattern of rheumatoid arthritis. Chronic attacks are usually less painful than gout and are likely to affect several joints at once, most commonly wrists, fingers, and knees.

Diagnosis

As in the case of gout, an analysis of the joint fluid will give a definitive diagnosis. An X-ray may show cartilage changes due to crystal deposition. By the time we reach eighty years of age, most of us will have evidence of calcium in the cartilage layer of our joints. This can be an essentially normal degenerative change and may not produce symptoms.

Treatment

There is no medication available that can dissolve CPPD crystals or prevent their formation. Therapy is directed toward alleviating painful inflammation. When the attack is sudden and very painful, treatment usually involves NSAIDs and the aspiration of fluid from the joint. Aspiration serves two purposes: It removes the fluid containing the CPPD crystals, and so reduces pain and inflammation; and it also provides a fluid sample for microscopic analysis. Sometimes just tapping the joint is treatment enough, especially for elderly people who are in poor health and who may want to avoid taking NSAIDs.

NSAIDs are usually taken for from three to ten days at mealtimes to reduce the chances of gastrointestinal upset. During a painful acute attack, your physician may inject corticosteroids into the joint to quickly reduce inflammation.

If the disease is chronic, you may have to continue taking NSAIDs on a long-term basis in order to avoid recurring attacks.

Prognosis

Most people with pseudogout live normal lives and are unhampered by their disease. While there is no cure, symptoms can be controlled well through medication.

GOUT

Joint inflammation caused by deposits of crystals of monosodium urate within the body's connective tissues and joint spaces.

WHO GETS IT? Mainly middle-aged and older men. High blood pressure, overweight, excessive alcohol consumption, and a diet high in organ meats add to the risk

SIGNS AND SYMPTOMS: Usually strikes a single joint, most commonly the big toe, with sudden, violent swelling and pain. Initial attack disappears in several days; subsequent attacks may occur more frequently, last longer, and affect more joints.

CAUSE: A hereditary tendency predisposes some people to elevated levels of uric acid in the blood. Also linked to a diet high in purines, obesity, excessive drinking, lead ingestion; may be associated with other diseases such as diabetes and hypertension.

DIAGNOSIS: Microscopic examination of joint fluid derived from needle aspiration reveals characteristic crystals.

TREATMENT: Initial treatment with colchicine or NSAIDs to bring down inflammation. Weight reduction, decreased alcohol consump-

(continued)

tion and purine-free diets are advised. In chronic cases, uric acid underexcretors are placed on uricosuric drugs to promote excretion of uric acid in urine; overproducers may be placed on allopurinol, which blocks uric acid formation.

PROGNOSIS: A well-understood and -controlled disease that should have little effect on your normal daily life.

PSEUDOGOUT

Similar to gout, except crystals are composed of calcium pyrophosphate dihydrate (CPPD). Is part of a larger group of crystal-related diseases called CPPD disease.

CAUSE: Crystals in joint spaces and connective tissues cause inflammation. May be related to a hormonal or metabolic tendency to crystal formation.

WHO GETS IT? Mainly older men and women over age sixty.

SIGNS AND SYMPTOMS: Attacks may be sudden. May affect several joints, especially the knee.

DIAGNOSIS: Joint fluid analysis reveals crystals. X-rays can show calcium deposits in cartilage.

TREATMENT: Aspiration of joint fluid and NSAIDs.

PROGNOSIS: Symptoms can be controlled well through medication.

10

Muscle Pain: Polymyositis/ Polymyalgia Rheumatica/ Fibrositis

A forty-five-year-old man I know, a sedentary hospital administrator, recently went off on a Boy Scout wilderness campout with his son's troop. Although he had fond memories of his own days as a Boy Scout, he hadn't been very physically active since he graduated from college. After three days of canoeing, hiking, and setting up camp, he felt so sore that he could hardly pack his gear and load it into his van. When he got home, he took a warm bath and dove into bed. "I feel muscles where I didn't know I had them," he groaned miserably to me the next day over lunch at the hospital cafeteria. I assured him he'd feel just fine within a few days.

If you've ever performed a physical chore or played a sport that requires motions you don't ordinarily do, you may well wake up the next day with stiff, painful muscles. During a bout with the flu, you may have a weak, achy-all-over feeling in your muscles. Routinely, you would not need to consult a physician for these problems.

But sometimes muscle soreness and weakness occur for no reason and grow worse with time, rather than get better.

When muscle problems persist, you should consult a doctor. Muscle aches can signal a variety of hereditary, inflammatory, metabolic, and neurological problems, and may be treated by any number of specialists. In this chapter I will concentrate on the muscle problems most commonly treated by rheumatologists. These include polymyositis, polymyalgia rheumatica, and fibrositis. I group these together because they all involve either weakness or pain in the muscles. Though their names sound similar, as you will see, they have very different causes.

Polymyositis

Elsie is a fastidious fifty-seven-year-old who prides herself on being fit and trim. She bikes and swims regularly, and keeps an immaculate home. One of her hobbies is gardening, and Elsie spends many hours each week pruning, weeding, and tending her shrubs and flowers. This year she hired someone to rototill a corner of her garden so she could have a vegetable patch. She was looking forward to planting and harvesting her own produce.

She doesn't know exactly when it started, but over the course of several weeks, Elsie began to feel quite weak and easily fatigued. Not one to complain, she pushed herself through the days with increasing difficulty. Anyone who knew Elsie well could sense that something was wrong: The dust began to collect in her house, and the garden went untended. She could neither climb stairs nor push a vacuum; she couldn't bend or stoop to weed. The new vegetable patch never got planted, the housework was neglected, and finally she could hardly even get herself out of bed in the morning or lift her arms high enough to comb her hair.

When her daughter Karen visited, she was shocked by her mother's condition and took her to the doctor. After Elsie's doctor examined her and found that she had a significant decrease in her muscle strength, he recommended immediate hospitalization. Three days later, after a few carefully selected tests were done to determine the cause of the muscle weakness, a diagnosis of polymyositis was made and Elsie was put on prednisone. After two days on prednisone, she felt much better. She could get out of bed unassisted and could comb her hair. After a week, the weakness had all but disappeared.

Over the next year, Elsie's doctor tried to slowly decrease her dosage of prednisone. As she took less and less of the drug, she experienced some ups and downs, with some recurrence of her muscle weakness. Eventually Elsie was able to remain on a very low dose of prednisone and is doing very well. She has even been able to do some gardening and swimming again.

What Is Polymyositis?

Polymyositis is a disease of generalized weakness resulting from inflammation of the muscle tissues. In fact its name, derived from the Greek, means inflammation of many muscles. (*Poly* means many; *myo* means muscles; and *itis* means inflammation.)

The main muscles affected are the proximal muscles—the larger muscles close to the body, such as the shoulders, upper arms, thighs, and hips. Sometimes the neck muscles and the muscles that control swallowing and breathing are also involved.

Sometimes this condition is accompanied by a rash. In such cases, when both skin and muscles are inflamed, the condition is known as dermatomyositis. Because they are so closely related, we will consider dermatomyositis and polymyositis together, using only one name for convenience.

Who Gets Polymyositis?

Polymyositis is a relatively rare disease. The Arthritis Foundation estimates that only five out of every million people contract the disease annually. Women are more likely to have polymyositis than men. And while people of any age can get it, it most commonly affects those between the ages of thirty and sixty. Children have also been known to have polymyositis. This disease does not appear to be inherited. Other patients have what is called an overlap syndrome or mixed connective tissue disease characterized by features of several rheumatic conditions, including polymyositis.

Signs and Symptoms

Symptoms may vary a great deal from one person to another. The disease frequently comes on gradually, over a period of weeks, months, or years; but it may also happen quite suddenly. To illustrate, a fifty-five-year-old colleague of mine at the hospital, usually quite active, began over a two-year-period to feel generally sluggish. He knew he didn't feel quite right. He tired more easily on the tennis court, and his shots were not as good. He noticed occasional fevers and joint pains, but had no idea that this was the beginning of a potentially serious illness. On the other hand, some of my patients are bedridden immediately. They may have trouble breathing and may have to be monitored carefully for signs of respiratory failure.

Muscle weakness is usually the first sign of polymyositis, often initially affecting muscles in the hips and shoulders. You may or may not feel any muscle pain. Patients report difficulty lifting heavy objects, such as groceries; climbing the stairs; or lifting their arms to comb their hair or put on a coat. The weakness can progress to the point at which it becomes increasingly difficult to rise from a chair, get out of the tub, or roll out of bed in the morning.

If the neck muscles are involved, you may find it hard to lift your head when you're lying down. Less commonly, throat muscles may be affected, making it hard for you to swallow and possibly affecting your voice. Should the chest muscles be affected, you may have difficulty breathing.

You may also have joint pain. Some of my patients experience arthritis as a first symptom of polymyositis.

When the skin is affected, patients have a characteristic violet-colored rash and puffy skin around the eyes. They may also have a patchy red rash on the face, upper chest, and neck, and possibly on fingers, forearms, knees, shoulders, and upper back. These rashes may occur before, during, or after the period in which muscle weakness develops.

Polymyositis is a systemic disease, as are rheumatoid arthritis and lupus; symptoms may crop up throughout the body. You may have fever, weight loss, general malaise, and Raynaud's phenomenon (an extreme sensitivity to cold, especially in your fingers).

What Causes Polymyositis?

The cause of this disease is unclear. There is no known genetic link. Some suspect that a malfunction in the immune system may cause the body itself to attack healthy muscle tissue. People with polymyositis often have antinuclear antibodies in their blood, as do many patients with lupus and RA. No one knows why these antibodies are present, but they indicate an immune system problem.

Other theories hold that an infectious agent, such as a virus, may attack muscles directly. In laboratory animals, muscle disease has been shown to follow certain viral infections, but it's not clear if a similar scenario holds true for humans.

An interesting association, the significance of which has yet to be evaluated, is found between cancer and polymyositis. Some patients are found to have both conditions at once. Often, muscle weakness is so closely related to the time at which cancer is diagnosed that it seems unlikely to be coincidental. In addition, weakness in some patients has been reported to improve after surgical removal of a cancer. The incidence of malignancy associated with polymyositis is highest in older men. However, only a small percentage of people with polymyositis have cancer, perhaps 10 percent or less.

Toxins, most commonly alcohol, can also cause muscle disease. Doctors advise patients with this condition not to drink alcoholic beverages.

Diagnosis

When patients complain of muscle weakness, I ask some specific questions during the medical history and make certain observations during the physical exam to check for polymyositis. During the physical examination, I'll examine every muscle group to assess a person's strength. Muscles are rated on a numerical scale from 0 to 5, with 5 being the normal range.

Normal muscle strength is relative: it depends upon whether you are a man or a woman and on how old you are. One of my patients is a big, strapping lumberjack whose job consisted of chopping trees and hauling logs. He came to my office because he couldn't do his job. Yet when I tested his muscle strength, he rated a 5. The amount of muscle strength required by this man for his work was far above the norm. Even though I rated his muscle strength a 5, it was below the power he normally needed to perform his job.

Most people today are more aware of the value of exercise and keep themselves in better shape than those of the previous generation did. As a result, our norms for muscle strength have changed. What would have been sufficient strength for women of a generation ago to get a 5 has since been revised.

I can make a good determination of muscle strength by asking my patients to grip my hands, make a muscle, push me away with their arms, and hold their arms up to see if they can prevent me from pushing their shoulders down. I also test muscle strength by asking patients to move their necks, lift their hips, flex their knees, and push down and then lift up with each foot.

I try to assess whether there is tenderness in their muscles. And I'll look for signs of joint swelling, pain, or tenderness, to ascertain whether they have any arthritis. I'll also concentrate on skin disease and look around the nail beds for telangiectasias, small red marks caused by dilated blood vessels.

In addition, I'll perform a blood test to assess levels of creatine phosphokinase, or CPK. CPK is an enzyme found mainly in muscles. When muscles are damaged, it leaks out into the bloodstream, causing CPK levels in the blood to rise. In general, the greater the muscle damage, the higher the level of this enzyme in your blood. Conversely, when CPK levels fall, this indicates that your condition is improving. For this reason, I may take blood tests for CPK repeatedly throughout the course of a patient's treatment, to monitor the progress of the disease.

Other standard blood and lab tests will be performed to exclude other conditions, such as lupus, rheumatoid arthritis, and scleroderma. Thyroid and nerve disease can also cause muscle problems, and appropriate tests will be performed. Since polymyositis is sometimes associated with malignancy, especially in older patients and in men, many physicians do routine basic studies—a chest X-ray, tests for blood in the stool, and a pap smear or breast examination—to rule out this possibility.

If the medical history, physical exam, and CPK tests indicate polymyositis, I usually admit the patient to the hospital to complete the diagnostic workup. I also admit patients to the hospital when their weakness is progressive and they are unable to care for themselves. I'm especially concerned when their breathing muscles are involved, because a rapid deterioration of these muscles can lead to respiratory failure.

When muscle disease is rapidly progressive and shortness of breath is present, I'll immediately order a pulmonary function test. I'll ask a patient to take a deep breath and blow into a machine that records how well and efficiently the lungs and chest muscle are working. I'll also perform a blood gas test to get a measure of the amount of oxygen and carbon dioxide in the blood.

Once patients are in the hospital, I have them undergo an electromyogram (EMG) test. This test is similar to an electrocardiogram, but it measures the electrical activity of muscle. An EMG involves the insertion of needle-like electrodes into muscles to stimulate and record their activity. The test can distinguish between muscle weakness caused by nerve damage and that caused by muscle fiber damage. Some patients complain that the test produces some discomfort.

In addition, I'll perform a muscle biopsy to confirm the diagnosis prior to putting someone on long-term therapy. We usually biopsy muscles that are exhibiting symptoms. This may require a surgical incision under a local anesthetic, although we may be able to avoid an incision and obtain the sample with a needle. The biopsy is usually done in the hospital while patients are getting a general workup for polymyositis. It is not a major surgical procedure. Muscles affected by polymyositis may show microscopic signs of inflammation or of its consequences (dying muscle cells).

What Happens Physiologically?

The physiologic changes in this disease are not clearly understood. We don't know exactly why the muscles are impaired. The muscles become inflamed—either because of an irritating substance produced at the site or because of antibodies that attack the muscle tissue—and the muscle fibers may become damaged.

Treatment

Treatment with corticosteroids, a class of drugs related to the hormone cortisone, frequently reduces inflammation and restores muscle strength. However, some patients may be on corticosteroids for months, yet show little improvement.

Prednisone, the corticosteroid of choice, is usually started orally, in pill form, at high levels (1 milligram per kilogram per day) in divided doses. If a patient is extremely ill, I may start him or her on an intravenous preparation of methylprednisolone, a related corticosteroid.

Improvement in muscle strength can be dramatic. For example, Joan, a sixty-year-old patient, was bedridden when she first came to my office. Her husband had to help her eat and dress. After being on prednisone for a week, she was able to get up and walk around by herself. After several weeks, she felt entirely herself.

There is great variability in patients' responses to corticosteroids. I've seen people bedridden one day and completely better the next. However, I've also seen patients go for weeks, months, or even years before they experience any significant improvement.

Sometimes patients don't respond well to corticosteroids and may require a higher dose, or the addition of an immunosuppressive drug such as methotrexate or Imuran. Currently, the new drug, cyclosporine—a powerful immunosuppressive used to prevent organ transplant rejection—is being tried.

Prednisone is a potent drug with potentially serious side effects, including puffiness of the face, easy bruising, high blood pressure, thinning of bones, depression, cataracts, and diabetes.

Another possible side effect of long-term high-dose prednisone is a muscle problem called steroid myopathy. Like polymyositis, this condition also causes muscle weakness, and a doctor may suspect this problem when a patient has been on high doses of prednisone for a long time without any apparent improvement. Steroid myopathy is not caused by inflammation, and can be distinguished from the muscle damage of polymyositis by an EMG. Sometimes a rebiopsy of the muscle may be necessary for diagnosis. If we lower the dosage of prednisone and the patient gets better, we strongly suspect that the medication may be the cause of the problem.

To avoid side effects, corticosteroids are given in the lowest dose possible and the dosage is gradually reduced as muscle strength increases. Repeated CPK tests help your doctor assess the effectiveness of your treatment and adjust drug dosages slowly downward when indicated. It can take weeks or months until you are brought down to a low-dose maintenance level of prednisone. Some people are eventually able to go off prednisone altogether; others may have a more protracted illness, requiring therapy for years or even indefinitely.

Your doctor will carefully monitor the status of your disease and advise if and when you should change your prednisone dosage. Once you have been treated with high dose corticosteroids for any length of time, your body must readjust gradually to lowered dosages. Going off these drugs cold turkey can have serious side effects. Your doctor may instruct you to lower the dosages bit by bit over the course of weeks or months.

Prolonged periods of inactivity can cause muscles to become weak and reduce their range of motion, so a medically supervised exercise program should also be part of your recovery plan. You should start these exercises only after your condition has been brought under good control and under the supervision of your doctor or physical therapist. Exercises begun during a flare or too soon after recovery can actually damage delicate muscle fibers.

I advise my patients not to drink alcohol, partly because it interacts with many medications but also because alcohol itself can damage muscles.

Prognosis

In most instances, the prognosis for polymyositis is good. Treatment with prednisone is usually quite effective and helps restore muscle strength.

Most patients are able to get the disease under control, and while some will continue to have chronic symptoms, many go on to lead relatively normal, active lives.

Polymyalgia Rheumatica

Anne and her husband George are both retired schoolteachers who enjoy square dancing once a month at their local church. Last week, on the morning after the dance, Anne awoke with an uncomfortable ache in her hips and shoulders. She was surprised at these sensations. She and George had often danced strenuously for hours, and she had never been affected by it. She assumed that maybe this time she had overdone it, so she stayed in bed most of the day and took a hot bath in the evening. But the next morning she felt even worse. She awoke stiff and sore and had a slight fever; she didn't feel like eating. She took some aspirin and continued resting, thinking she must have the flu. Three more days passed and the symptoms persisted, convincing Anne that she should go see her doctor.

Though Anne told the doctor her muscles ached, he could find no evidence of muscle tenderness or arthritis. Initial lab tests did not show rheumatoid factor, but did show a high sed rate, a sign that there might be inflammation involved. The doctor wanted Anne to return in two weeks for some additional testing before he could confirm the diagnosis. In the meantime, he sent Anne home with instructions to take twelve aspirin a day.

The next few days went very badly. Anne ached, her appetite was poor, and she lost three pounds. She had fever on and off and spent most of her time in bed. Two weeks later, she returned to her doctor, who repeated the laboratory tests. Her sed rate was still elevated, but there was no other evidence of arthritis. So the doctor sent Anne to Duke's rheumatology clinic, where a complete medical history, a physical exam, and a series of laboratory tests pointed to a disease called polymyalgia rheumatica. Anne was started on a therapeutic trial of two 5-milligram prednisone tablets a day.

The day after starting the prednisone, Anne felt much better. The aching in her shoulders and hips subsided. Two days later, she was up and about, able to take a long walk with her husband. Within a year, the disease cleared up and Anne was able to reduce her medication.

What Is Polymyalgia Rheumatica?

As its name implies, polymyalgia rheumatica, or PMR, means pain in many muscles (*poly* = many; *myo* = muscles; *algia* = pain). The disease causes severe muscle pain and stiffness in the neck, shoulders, and hips. Unlike other arthritic diseases, the symptoms may be self-limiting. That is, the disease eventually subsides, and symptoms may disappear completely. We have good treatments that can effectively reduce or eliminate pain during the active phase.

Who Gets PMR?

PMR rarely occurs in people under fifty, and its incidence increases with age. The disease affects more women than men and is more common among whites than in other racial groups. The Arthritis Foundation estimates that five out of a million Americans develop this disease annually.

Signs and Symptoms

The main symptom of PMR is a constant aching in the muscles of the hips, neck, shoulders, upper arms, thighs, buttocks, and lower back. Most of the time the onset of the disease is sudden, with no apparent cause. It's not unusual for a patient to go to bed feeling perfectly fine, then awaken the next day feeling stiff and sore, as if she had done some strenuous physical activity. Typically I'll ask a patient, "When did it first start?" And he'll tell me, "Oh, I know exactly when. It was May 12. Everything was perfectly fine, and then I woke up that day and never felt so bad in my life." Less commonly, PMR can come on more gradually.

If you have PMR, you will likely find that your muscles are stiff when you awaken in the morning, but loosen up as you become more physically active. Muscles may also stiffen up when you stay in one position for too long.

Patients may report painful sensations that seem to resemble the symptoms of rheumatoid arthritis. Yet when we examine the joints, we can find no evidence of an active arthritis. So the pain seems out of proportion to the visible signs. If there is any inflammation of the joints, it is usually much milder than that of rheumatoid arthritis.

As in other forms of inflammatory arthritis, you may experience systemic symptoms, including fever, weight loss, fatigue, and a general achiness and feeling of malaise.

What Causes PMR?

We do not know the exact cause or the origin of the pain of polymyalgia rheumatica. The muscles themselves are not inflamed, as they are in polymyositis. The synovial membrane that lines the joints may show some evidence of inflammation, but never to the same extent as in rheumatoid arthritis.

Diagnosis

PMR is a diagnosis of exclusion—that is, doctors have to rule out other forms of disease, because we have no specific tests for PMR itself. PMR mimics several other arthritic diseases; for example, patients with rheumatoid arthritis or lupus can have similar pains in and around the shoulders and hips. They too may experience fever, weight loss, loss of appetite, and general malaise.

The medical history and physical exam will give your doctor some clues that will help him or her distinguish PMR from other diseases. Age at onset may be one indication: PMR usually begins in people over age fifty, while other connective tissue diseases, such as ankylosing spondylitis or rheumatoid arthritis, more typically affect the young.

Lack of signs of joint inflammation may offer a second clue. With rheumatoid arthritis, affected joints are obviously inflamed—with signs of redness, warmth, swelling, and pain. With PMR you may report a lot of pain around your joints, but an examination will reveal no overt signs of inflammation.

You will need to have routine blood and laboratory studies performed (see chapter 3 for a complete discussion of these). Patients with PMR may show a low red blood cell count, which indicates that they are anemic. They may also have a high sedimentation rate—a measurement of how fast red blood cells fall to the bottom of a glass tube—which indicates the presence of an inflammation and is found also in patients with lupus and rheumatoid arthritis. Other lab tests will therefore be done to rule out rheumatoid arthritis and lupus (see chapters 4 and 6).

A final way to diagnose PMR is to observe a patient's response to low levels of corticosteroids, usually prednisone. You may be given a low-dose therapeutic trial of the drug (usually 10 to 15 milligrams a day). PMR patients respond promptly to such low doses, with dramatic relief of symptoms. If the initial trial dose is high, however, it will not help the doctor distinguish between PMR and other diseases. Several other arthritic conditions can also improve with high doses of prednisone.

Treatment

Polymyalgia rheumatica is considered a self-limited disease. In other words, it will frequently run its natural course and subside within two or three years or less. Treatment involves corticosteroids, at dosages as low as possible, to keep symptoms under control and the sedimentation rate normal. There is some concern about the side effects of prednisone in older patients, especially since prednisone can worsen osteoporosis and lead to bone fractures. Many people are able to decrease their dosage of steroids significantly after a year; however, others may require more prolonged treatment.

To avoid possible complications, some physicians treat PMR with nonsteroidal anti-inflammatory drugs (NSAIDs) alone or in combination with lower doses of prednisone. NSAIDs take longer to relieve symptoms. A patient on NSAIDs may have to wait a few weeks before he or she feels relief; on prednisone, symptoms may be controlled in only a few days.

Polymyalgia Rheumatica and Giant Cell Arteritis

Some people with PMR may also have a condition known as giant cell arteritis (GCA). In GCA, the walls of certain arteries become inflamed. When the arteries leading to the temples in the head are involved, the condition is also called temporal arteritis, or cranial arteritis. Unless you do a biopsy on all patients with PMR, it's difficult to say what percentage of them will have giant cell arteritis. However, I would estimate that as many as half of all people with PMR have this condition.

Inflammation in the arteries can cause the blood vessels to become narrowed, so they are unable to supply enough blood and oxygen to the tissues they serve. Without adequate blood, a tissue is said to be ischemic (*ischemia* means lack of blood) and it hurts. Unless blood flow is restored, the tissue may die.

Giant cell arteritis most commonly affects the arteries in the head and neck. Blood vessels supplying the eyes, tongue, and scalp may be involved.

Symptoms caused by a lack of blood flow to the tissue include headache; pain in the scalp, tongue, and jaw; and visual problems, such as blurring, seeing double, intermittent darkening, or loss of vision. Since GCA involves inflammation, it may also produce symptoms such as fatigue, anemia, weight loss, and general malaise.

The most dreaded complication of GCA is blindness, resulting from a blockage of the blood vessel that nourishes the optic nerve, which carries nerve impulses from the eye to the brain. Today, with better recognition of GCA and the often-connected polymyalgia rheumatica, aggressive treatment can be instituted earlier and loss of vision occurs far less frequently.

No one knows the exact cause of this disease. There does appear to be a genetic link, however, and the disease occurs mostly in whites.

If GCA is suspected, your doctor will try to establish a diagnosis by removing a piece of tissue from one or both temporal arteries. In order to determine which artery to biopsy, I usually palpate the area and look for signs of tenderness and little nodules or bumps in the artery that result from inflammation. Sometimes these changes can be felt on both sides of the temple. The biopsy is done under a local anesthetic through a small incision in the scalp. This is a relatively minor procedure and does not require hospitalization. These biopsies are safe, as the blood supply of the scalp is so rich that the removal of a small piece of blood vessel will not deprive the area noticeably of blood. When examined under a microscope, the arterial wall shows inflammation and tissue damage; in fact, giant cell arteritis got its name because some of the cells in the inflamed walls enlarge to great size and are distinctive under a microscope. The results of the biopsy are important to be certain of the diagnosis and to determine the course of treatment and the need for high-dose corticosteroids.

The relationship between PMR and GCA is unclear. Not everyone with polymyalgia rheumatica will develop GCA. Should temporal artery biopsies be done routinely in patients with PMR? Certainly the patient who is having serious headaches and blurred or distorted vision should have such a biopsy; early diagnosis and treatment may prevent blindness. But what of patients who have no obvious symptoms?

If you meet the criteria for PMR, are responding well to therapy, and show no signs of cranial circulation problems, I believe that you need not undergo a temporal artery biopsy.

Treatment for GCA involves regular monitoring and high doses of corticosteroids, usually prednisone. You take a higher dosage of prednisone than you would were you being treated for PMR alone. As in the case of PMR, you will receive the lowest dose of prednisone necessary to control your symptoms and lower your sedimentation rate.

Prompt treatment with cortiscosteroids is highly effective in reducing inflammation and in preventing blindness and other complications. Like polymyalgia rheumatica, GCA can be self-limited and may eventually run its course. However, if you suffer serious vision loss from GCA, this usually cannot be undone, even if therapy with prednisone is begun immediately. You must be aware of the symptoms of GCA. If you think you have arthritis and are having vision problems, such as blurring or transient vision loss, you may actually have temporal arteritis and should see a doctor at once.

Prognosis for PMR and GCA

People who have PMR and GCA usually do well, though some may continue to have symptoms. If such symptoms are severe, you may need a prolonged course of steroids, and this may cause some problems, especially if you're an older person. With proper medication, we can effectively relieve the symptoms and prevent potentially serious complications. Many people are able to lead normal lives and go on with their usual daily activities.

Fibrositis

Betty is a forty-year-old businesswomen with three children and a full-time administrative job at a bank. After a great deal of soul-searching, her husband, Mark, decided to accept a very promising job with an international investment firm that requires a great deal of foreign travel. With her husband gone for weeks at a time, Betty was finding it increasingly difficult to juggle her job and the needs of her children, ages five, eight, and twelve. Her co-workers at the bank had no idea how strained Betty had been feeling lately; she worked hard to appear neat, efficient, and unruffled at work. She also pushed herself to the limit at home, keeping an immaculate house and trying to keep up with her children's school activities.

Over the past few months, Betty had been experiencing aches and pains, as well as stiffness around several joints and muscles. She also tired more easily than normal and was having problems sleeping. She took hot showers and applied warm compresses to alleviate the pain, but it always seemed to return.

Betty thought she had arthritis and consulted a doctor; however, her physical exam and laboratory tests showed no evidence of arthritis. The doctor told her to rest more and to take aspirin for her pains. This advice did not prove helpful. The muscle pain persisted, and Betty was miserable. She subsequently consulted several more physicians before one of them made the diagnosis of fibrositis.

The diagnosing physician explained to Betty that this disease did not cause any disability or deformity, and that it was most probably linked to her stressful lifestyle. He prescribed some medication to help her sleep, but explained that Betty might have to change her lifestyle, too, to help herself get well.

Betty followed the doctor's advice and pared down her hectic work schedule; she also tries to incorporate some time into each day during which she can totally relax—reading, taking a long, brisk walk, or just soaking in a warm bath. The aches and pains seem to be greatly reduced, and she has much more energy than before.

What Is Fibrositis?

Fibrositis is a disease involving muscle pain. The name fibrositis is misleading: It means an inflammation (*itis*) of the fibrous tissue. Yet this condition involves neither inflammation nor fibrous tissue, though to the patient it may feel as if it does. The disease has also been called fibromyalgia, meaning pain (*algia*) in the muscles and soft tissues. Fibrositis is pain in the muscles around the joints that is apparently caused by an interplay of physical and psychological factors.

By the time I see a patient with this disease, he or she has probably already been to several doctors and has tried several treatment regimens with no apparent success. This disease can be difficult to diagnose with precision and may be linked to certain personality types. Experienced rheumatologists who have seen many of these patients have more success in diagnosing and treating this disease.

Who Gets It?

This is a disease mostly of women. It begins most often in the middle years, but can happen at any age. The disease appears to be linked with high-stress situations. Hard-driving, perfectionistic, and compulsive types of people seem more susceptible. Also, certain other physical ailments are associated with fibrositis, including irritable bowel syndrome, irritable bladder, tension headaches, migraines, and painful menstruation.

Signs and Symptoms

The major symptom of fibrositis is pain in the muscles in various parts of the body. The location and severity of pain can vary from person to person. The pain may affect many areas in the body and may come and go, varying in intensity. Some of my patients have described the pain as "a pain in my flesh" or "in my tissues." They speak of their pain in very graphic terms. Many say they hurt all over, not just around the joints, and that the pain is "burning" or "searing." While patients often complain that the tissues around their joints feel tender and swollen, no sign of inflammation can be detected during an examination. Nor do they have any other signs of inflammation, such as fever and weight loss.

Often, muscle stiffness is worse in the morning, but eases up as the person begins to move around. For some people, however, the stiffness may persist throughout the day.

Sleep disturbances are common. I'll see patients at the clinic who'll say, "I haven't had a good night's sleep in five years." If you ask how they feel, they often tell you that they wake up feeling fatigued and feel tired all day long, or that they just don't feel well in general. They may have trouble getting through a normal day with their usual stamina.

Some patients say they notice that their symptoms grow worse during cold, damp spells or in highly stressful situations.

The disease frequently lingers, especially if not treated appropriately. As I mentioned earlier, patients often get many workups and move from doctor to doctor. It may take weeks, months, or possibly years to alleviate their symptoms. However, this disease does not cause any physical damage or deformities.

What Causes Fibrositis?

The exact cause of fibrositis is unknown, although there does appear to be some interaction between physical, environmental, and emotional factors that may result in muscle pain.

Chronic stress is associated with a number of physical reactions. Some people respond to life's stresses with headaches or gastrointestinal upsets. For the fibrositis patient, stress may be translated into muscle tension and pain.

Often it's not so much the situation that generates stress; it's the individual's response to stressful situations. One person may find his or her job stressful, while another in the same situation copes quite well. In one study, an increased prevalence of fibrositis was found among men who were laid off from their factory jobs.

The pain of fibrositis has been compared to the pain of a headache. Although your head may throb with pain, an X-ray usually doesn't show any changes that could cause your headache. Similarly, with fibrositis, you feel a very real pain, but no physical basis for it will show up on X-rays or examination. Stress and tension can cause and exacerbate a headache just as it may trigger the muscle pain of fibrositis.

Since there is no easily identifiable source of pain, many patients want to know if the pain is "all in my head." Technically speaking, pain is *always* in the head, because that is the place where all of our feelings and senses get integrated. Whether the source of pain is a joint, a muscle, or some other site in the body, the result is the same—pain that must be relieved. The pain of fibrositis is very real and requires appropriate treatment.

There may also be a relationship between muscle pains, fatigue, and the sleep disturbances that people with fibrositis so commonly experience. Fibrositis patients do not seem to enter the deeper, more refreshing stages of sleep. They toss and turn and wake up feeling tired. In experiments, normal people deprived of sleep also develop muscle pain and soreness. As a doctor, I can remember that during my training, when I had to stay up all night treating patients, I felt miserable the next day. And anyone who has ever gone on an overseas airline trip and stayed up all night will probably hurt the next day because he or she didn't sleep well. So it seems a reasonable conclusion that sleep difficulties probably contribute to the physical symptoms of fibrositis. Conversely, muscle aches and pains may also be the cause of sleep difficulties. People with other forms of arthritis also find that painful joints may prevent them from sleeping well, and this in turn may add to their general discomfort.

Diagnosis

Since people with this disease are often involved in stressful situations, either at home or at work, some key questions asked during the medical history can provide me with some valuable insight. The patients themselves may not perceive their situations as stressful, but their symptoms indicate that stress may be a problem.

You need to find a doctor who will take the time to sit down and talk with you. At Duke, we understand that this disease involves a person's whole life. If I ask a patient what she does, and she says she's a homemaker, I then ask her to tell me about her home. What's it like? Does she like to keep a clean house? How much time does she spend cleaning? How does she feel if someone messes the house up? If someone says she's an account executive at an advertising agency, I might then ask what aspect of her work she likes best or what she does when she makes a mistake. I want to get a sense of what this patient is like as a person and of how she feels about her life and work. I also want to know how well my patients sleep at night. These aren't always routine questions in a medical history; they require some extra care and persistence.

Though you may report persistent pain, your doctor will usually find no physical evidence of swelling in your joints or muscles. Furthermore, there are no tests that can confirm the presence of this disease. The results of any laboratory studies will be normal, and while lab studies help your doctor rule out other types of arthritis, they cannot confirm the presence of fibrositis.

The physical exam does, however, reveal the existence of certain trigger or tender points. When the physician firmly palpates certain muscle groups, the patient with fibrositis reacts with heightened sensitivity, especially in areas around the neck, shoulders, elbows, hips, groin, knees, and ankles. Sometimes the pain travels along your nerves and you'll feel it elsewhere in your body. This is known as referred pain. While arthritis patients may hurt in their joints and nowhere else, fibrositis patients seem to hurt all over.

Treatment

Nonsteroidal anti-inflammatory drugs, such as aspirin, are often recommended to relieve the pain of fibrositis. However, these drugs do not work for every patient.

Doctors currently prefer to treat fibrositis with a group of drugs called tricyclic antidepressants. This does not mean that people with fibrositis are depressed or have a psychiatric problem. In fact, patients with fibrositis are usually not depressed. Doctors prescribe antidepressants because they help improve sleep and so eliminate some of the problems that poor

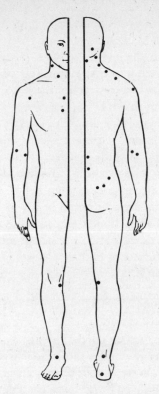

**FIBROSITIS
(TENDER POINTS)**

sleep patterns may cause. These drugs also appear to relieve pain. I commonly use Elavil (amitriptyline), but many others are available. Doses are started at 50 milligrams and increased up to 150 milligrams as needed. Some patients say they feel drowsy or doped up on antidepressants, but this feeling usually subsides after a few days. The major side effects of Elavil are dry mouth and trouble emptying the bladder. Since it can cause urinary problems, this drug should be used with caution in patients with prostate conditions.

You may also find that applying heat to an area will bring temporary relief of symptoms. Your muscles may feel less sore after you take a warm shower, soak in a warm tub, or apply warm compresses to affected areas. A firm mattress may foster good sleep.

Your doctor may also recommend that you try to change your attitudes or modify the situations that cause you stress. A busy business executive and workaholic, for example, may have to learn to take some time out each day for relaxation. On the other hand, an unemployed person may need help finding a new job, being retrained for another job, or looking for financial assistance. A perfectionist may have to learn to loosen up a little, to relax his or her standards.

Exercise can be an excellent stress reducer, especially if it is an aerobic activity, such as fast walking or bike riding. There is some evidence that intense aerobic activity causes your body to secrete endorphins, morphine-like substances that relieve pain and promote a feeling of well-being. Exercise also increases the amount of oxygen getting to your brain and promotes deeper, more refreshing sleep—further increasing your sense of well-being. You should, however, consult your doctor before embarking on a new exercise program. The rule of thumb here is to start gradually and work your exercise level up slowly.

If you're experiencing stress at home or at work, you might want to attend a class in stress reduction, yoga, meditation, or biofeedback to learn how to relax consciously. Such workshops are often offered at local American Red Cross branches and in many YMCAs and community centers across the country.

Prognosis

The prognosis for fibrositis is good. Finding a sympathetic doctor is essential, because you may not get satisfactory treatment if your doctor doesn't understand the nature of your illness. This is not the kind of illness that you can treat by reading a book. It is a nagging kind of condition that often takes hard work on the part of both you and your doctor. This disease does not result in any long-term deformities or disabilities, but it can affect your lifestyle and happiness. Through a combination of medication, exercise, and stress-reduction measures, you can usually expect to lead a normal life.

MUSCLE PAIN

The following three diseases are grouped together because they all involve muscle problems—either weakness or pain.

POLYMYOSITIS: A disease of muscle weakness that results from inflammation of muscle tissues.

CAUSE: Unknown. May be a direct effect of a virus or of immune system malfunctioning.

SYMPTOMS: Progressive muscle weakness, skin rash, fever, weight loss, general malaise, and Raynaud's phenomenon. Sometimes difficulty breathing.

WHO GETS IT? Relatively rare. More women get it than men. Most common in people between thirty and sixty years old. Not hereditary.

DIAGNOSIS: Evidence of muscle weakness and skin changes. Tests include CPK test, electromyogram, muscle biopsy, pulmonary function tests, and blood gas test.

TREATMENT: Corticosteroids, usually prednisone, in high doses initially and then tapering down to the lowest possible dose to keep symptoms under control; also, medically supervised exercises.

PROGNOSIS: In many instances, good. Disease can be controlled, allowing a relatively normal life; some may remain symptomatic.

POLYMYALGIA RHEUMATICA (PMR): Severe muscle pain and stiffness in neck, shoulders, and hips. Usually self-limiting. May be accompanied by an inflammation of arteries called giant cell arteritis (GCA).

CAUSE: Unknown. Despite reported joint pains, there are no physical signs of inflammation.

SYMPTOMS: Aching muscles of hips, neck, shoulders, upper arms, thighs, buttocks, and lower back. Muscles usually most stiff on awakening but improve over day. May be fever, weight loss, fatigue, and general achiness.

WHO GETS IT? People over fifty. More women get it than men. More common among whites.

DIAGNOSIS: No specific diagnostic test. Diagnosis is based on medical history, physical exam, high sed rate, negative results of tests for

(continued)

other diseases. Improvement after a clinical dose of corticosteroids is suggestive of PMR. If GCA is suspected, a temporal artery biopsy is performed.

TREATMENT: Is frequently self-limiting. Low-dose corticosteroids keep symptoms controlled. NSAIDs may also be used, but take longer to act. If GCA is also present, higher doses of corticosteroids are used.

PROGNOSIS: Generally good for both PMR and GCA.

FIBROSITIS: Muscle pain around the joints with no sign of underlying connective tissue disease.

CAUSE: Unknown, but some interaction between physical and psychological factors.

SYMPTOMS: Pain in muscles, tendons, and ligaments throughout body, described as burning, searing, and persistent. Also, sleep disturbances and fatigue.

WHO GETS IT? Mostly women in the middle years. Linked to stress and hard-driving, perfectionistic, and compulsive personalities.

DIAGNOSIS: Based on medical history, lack of physical evidence of swelling, normal lab studies, and presence of tender points.

TREATMENT: NSAIDs and sleep-promoting drugs, lifestyle modification, exercise, and relaxation techniques.

PROGNOSIS: Can be good, but pain may linger. Does not result in deformities or disabilities.

11

Infection and Arthritis

Each of the previous chapters has focused on an individual form of arthritis. Here, however, I am going to discuss a wide array of conditions that are very different from one another in terms of cause, symptoms, treatment, and prognosis. The common thread that binds them is that all are caused either directly or indirectly by some infectious agent, either a bacterium, a virus, or a fungus.

Some of the diseases discussed in this chapter are so rare that most people do not have to worry about acquiring them. On the other hand, some are quite common, and your risk of contracting them may vary, depending upon where you live and on your age and lifestyle. If you live in the northeastern United States, where the deer tick that carries the bacterium for Lyme disease is most prevalent, for example, you may have an increased risk of contracting Lyme arthritis. A sexually active young adult may be at higher risk for gonococcal arthritis, because gonococci are transmitted through sexual contact.

Reiter's syndrome is a somewhat special case. It is included in this chapter because it often follows a bowel or urinary tract infection; however, some people get Reiter's syndrome without any evidence of a prior infection. Reiter's is also classified as a spondyloarthropathy, and you may want to refer to chapter 8 for a more complete overview of that category of diseases.

What's key about all these diseases is that there is a strong interaction between the host and the infection. In other words, not everyone who is exposed to the initial infection will develop symptoms of arthritis. For example, some people exposed to the spirochete bacteria that cause Lyme disease will go on to develop progressive arthritis, but many will not. Similarly, only a fraction of those who come down with a strep throat will develop rheumatic fever and arthritis. Your chances of developing arthritis from any of these diseases is a result of many factors, possibly including your particular genetic makeup and your overall health.

How Infections Cause Arthritis

Before we focus on individual diseases, let's look at the way infections in general may cause arthritis. In most instances, the infection begins in another part of the body and then travels via the bloodstream to a joint. However, an infectious agent may also enter the joint directly—through, for example, a surgical incision, wound, or needle puncture. Once in a small, enclosed joint space, the invading organism reproduces rapidly. Its presence signals your white blood cells to rush to the area in defense of your body. The joint space soon fills with pus and the joint becomes red, swollen, and painful.

Some types of infection result in a sudden, rapid, painful swelling in one joint. This is called septic arthritis. The person with septic arthritis is very sick, with chills and fever, and requires hospitalization and intravenous antibiotics. Other types of infection take a slower course and require different treatment approaches. As you will see, the cause, symptoms, and treatment of infection and arthritis vary, depending on the microorganism responsible for the infection. Since it is impossible, within the scope of one chapter, to fully explore every type of infection-related arthritis, let me emphasize the most common diseases.

Lyme Disease

Tom, a nineteen-year-old college student, spent the summer of his junior year working on Cape Cod as a counterboy in a fast-food restaurant. He worked long hours, but still found the time to do some hiking and camping. The combination of hard work and beach life seemed to agree with Tom, and except for a bout with a brief, flu-like illness in the middle of the summer, he thoroughly enjoyed himself.

But two weeks after he returned to college, Tom noticed some unusual symptoms. His right knee became tender and swollen and hot to the touch. He had trouble walking and occasionally felt sharp, shooting pains in his other joints. Although he had always played football and other vigorous sports, he had never had any joint problems before, nor could he recall any recent injury that could be causing his current problems.

The swelling in Tom's knee persisted, and he visited the student health clinic, where he was told he had a severely sprained knee. The doctor prescribed a knee immobilizer and medication to reduce the inflammation. These measures failed to bring any relief. So the health clinic referred Tom to an orthopedic surgeon. The surgeon could not find any signs of mechanical injury to the knee, although it was obviously swollen. He in turn sent Tom to a rheumatologist.

Tom's initial symptoms made rheumatoid arthritis seem unlikely. Since Tom was a healthy young man, the doctor wanted to rule out gonorrhea, so he asked Tom some questions about his sexual activities. He also asked Tom about what he had done during the summer: Had he spent his time near the seashore, or did he also go into the marshes and woods? Had he been near any animals? Had he been bitten by a tick? Did he recall having a rash? Tom did not remember having been bitten by a tick or having had a rash, but he had been around his friend's two dogs all summer, and he had also camped out several times in the woods.

The rheumatologist ordered some routine laboratory tests and a test for Lyme disease. The Lyme test returned positive, and a diagnosis of Lyme arthritis was made. Tom was immediately placed on a course of intravenous antibiotics. Within a few weeks his arthritis subsided, and Tom was able to return to his normal activities without any further problems.

What Is It?

Lyme arthritis is a joint condition caused by infection with a bacterial organism transmitted by a tick that feeds on deer.

This disease was first recognized in the early 1970s in the town of Lyme, on the southern shore of Connecticut. Around that time there was a curious cluster of arthritis cases, all found in the area surrounding this town. Sometimes entire families—mother, father, and children—were diagnosed with arthritis. The pattern of symptoms exhibited by patients with this particular form of arthritis did not match any textbook description. Patients with this disease underwent repeated batteries of tests and received a variety of diagnoses, including rheumatoid arthritis, viral meningitis, juvenile rheumatoid arthritis, and even neurosis.

The breakthrough in the understanding of this disease was based on keen observation—some of it by the patients and their families—and astute clinical detective work performed over the next decade by medical epidemiologists at Yale University.

The most striking feature of this outbreak of Lyme disease was the restricted area it occurred in. In fact, many cases cropped up in the same neighborhood. Furthermore, many of the original patients were children, and the clustering of several cases of juvenile rheumatoid arthritis in the same area by simple chance was more than statistically unlikely: it defied credibility. It seemed more likely that this disease was acquired from one common source that had to be located and identified.

Certain facets of the illness provided clues to its origin. The peak incidence of disease was in the summer months (this is the time that insects are most active); the area was heavily wooded and inhabited by domestic as well as wild animals; and, most important, many patients said they had had a rash during the course of the illness. These features seemed to point to an insect-borne disease. Since the rash was similar to a rash associated with tick bites in Europe, the animals in the area were searched for ticks.

Indeed, ticks were found on the local deer, providing evidence of a carrier. Scientists were able to isolate bacteria called spirochetes from these ticks. This proved a valuable discovery, since spirochetes have long been known to cause disease in humans, particularly syphilis.

The next steps were to isolate these spirochetes from affected patients and to show that these patients were producing antibodies to the spirochete and that the production of these antibodies increased during the course of their illness. This too was accomplished.

Perhaps most important, it was shown that treatment with antibiotics known to affect spirochetes could prevent or eliminate the arthritis.

Lyme disease is now recognized as the most common tick-borne disease in America. Although the disease was originally identified in Connecticut, cases have been reported in other areas of the Northeast and throughout the United States. To date, cases of Lyme disease have been found in thirty-two states as well as in eighteen other countries. Many of the cases have been associated with wooded areas, but it appears that the ticks are spreading to suburban areas, including the counties surrounding New York City.

Who Gets It?

Anyone bitten by the tick that carries this disease can get Lyme arthritis. Children who spend a lot of time outdoors playing in areas likely inhabited by ticks are frequently affected.

What Causes It?

The disease is caused by spirochete-bearing ticks that can live on a variety of animals, including mice, deer, and dogs and other domestic animals.

Symptoms

Symptoms occur following a tick bite and progress in three stages. The first stage includes fever, malaise, headache, and flu-like symptoms as well as a characteristic rash, called erythema chronicum migrans, at the site of the tick bite. The rash is circular with a bright-red outer border and may be hot, painful, or itchy. It then disappears, leading to the next phase of disease.

The second stage may include signs of inflammation of the heart (usually abnormal heart rhythm) and nervous system, severe headache, neck pain and stiffness, meningitis, and paralysis of the muscles of the face. In addition, joint and muscle pains may come and go.

The third stage is marked by arthritis, which frequently affects the knees but can involve other joints such as the shoulders, elbows, jaw, ankle, wrists, or finger joints. The affected joints may be painful and swollen.

Without treatment, the arthritis of Lyme disease may come and go for months or years. Some people develop a condition similar to rheumatoid arthritis and may have some joint damage.

Diagnosis

A doctor should suspect Lyme disease when the patient has the characteristic disease pattern mentioned above and lives in an area in which the tick is endemic. The tick is very small, and many individuals with Lyme disease can't recall having been bitten by a tick or having seen the characteristic rash. So a physician must suspect the disease when patients report intermittent swelling of their joints, especially of the knee joints. The diagnosis can be confirmed with a blood test that reveals antibodies against Lyme disease spirochetes.

Treatment

The timing of treatment is key here. Prompt treatment with oral antibiotics can get rid of the rash more quickly and prevent the occurrence of arthritis. You must watch for the typical skin rash and other early symptoms and report them at once to your physician, who can begin treatment with oral antibiotics and arrest the disease. If you wait until the disease has progressed to a later stage, your physician may still try to treat you with oral antibiotics. If these do not work, however, you may need two to three weeks of antibiotics administered intravenously. Penicillin is the antibiotic of choice, although other antibiotics are being evaluated as alternatives. You may not respond to treatment with antibiotics for weeks or months and may need to continue taking them longer. The fact that antibiotics can be successful in preventing the arthritis, even at later stages of disease, indicates that the arthritis is caused by the persistence of the spirochete, which invades and remains in affected tissues throughout the illness.

Those who live in affected areas can take some simple precautions during the summer months to reduce the chances of infection. Use insect repellent when going into wooded areas; wear protective clothing, such as long-sleeved shirts and long pants tucked into high socks. Check your children and yourself carefully for ticks. If you find a tick, remove it carefully, making sure you remove the head and body; use tweezers if possible. Dogs and cats in tick-infested areas should wear flea and tick collars, since they can carry the tick into the home.

Prognosis

Recognition of this disease has increased enormously, so most people in affected areas have become alert to early symptoms and seek treatment before arthritis develops. With prompt treatment, the prognosis is good and there is no permanent joint damage.

Gonococcal Arthritis

Matt, a twenty-two-year-old man, came to the clinic with a painful, swollen knee. He said that he had fever and chills, but when I asked him specific questions about his sexual activities and the possibility that he had venereal disease, he at first denied it. His medical history and physical symptoms, however, made gonococcal arthritis a likely cause. So I explained to Matt that he had to give me honest answers about his sexual activity because those answers would help me make decisions about how to treat him; if he did have gonorrhea, it was also important to inform those he'd had sexual contact with so that they too could be treated. With some embarrassment, Matt confided that he occasionally visited prostitutes. Because of his age, his sexual activity, and evidence of a genital discharge, I placed Matt on a trial of antibiotics. A culture of his body fluids confirmed the diagnosis; his prompt response to the penicillin further indicated that this was an arthritis related to the gonorrhea.

What Is It?

This is the most common form of infectious arthritis. It is caused by the gonococcus that causes gonorrhea, a sexually transmitted disease. The bacteria spread from the genitals through the bloodstream to the joints.

Who Gets It?

Gonococcal arthritis is most common among young, healthy people who are sexually active. Women are more likely than men to have gonococcal arthritis, because men have more overt symptoms of gonorrhea, including painful urination and discharge of pus from the penis. They're therefore more likely to seek prompt treatment of their venereal disease before it can spread to the joints. Women, on the other hand, tend to have fewer obvious symptoms during the initial stages of the disease, giving the bacteria a lot more time to spread elsewhere.

Symptoms

The onset of gonococcal arthritis is usually sudden, and in women is often accompanied by fever and abdominal pain. As mentioned above, men usually have a warning in the form of a penile discharge. Joint pain appears to move from one part of the body to another, affecting both upper and lower extremities. Another symptom is tenosynovitis, a swelling of the tendons and tendon sheaths. Little skin blisters may appear on various parts of the body—an indication that the gonorrhea has spread.

Diagnosis

The physical exam and medical history often give strong clues to the diagnosis. I would suspect gonococcal arthritis if a person is young and sexually active and has evidence of a genital discharge or other symptoms of venereal disease. Other signs are red streaks along the tendons in the hand and small, pus-filled blisters. Various body fluids can be cultured to isolate the gonococcal organism and make the diagnosis firm. These cultures are obtained from genital discharges or from the rectum or mouth, which can be infected. It is difficult to grow an organism from the fluid in the joint itself, so the joint is seldom tapped for this purpose when the diagnosis appears likely.

Venereal disease is a very sensitive issue, and as a physician, I have encountered situations that can be very embarrassing for the patient, especially if he or she is married. I'll often ask about the sexual history in private, without the spouse being present.

Sometimes the patient has Reiter's disease and not gonococcal arthritis. It is sometimes tricky to distinguish between these two diseases, because their symptoms can be so similar. It's important to make this distinction, however, especially when you take into consideration the potential effect a diagnosis of gonorrhea can have on a patient's personal relationships. A prompt response to antibiotics indicates the presence of gonorrhea, and is almost diagnostic in itself.

Treatment

Treatment usually involves the administration of penicillin, and you may be hospitalized during the first few days so that the penicillin can be administered intravenously; this may be followed by ten days to two weeks of oral antibiotics. Penicillin usually acts very promptly, bringing relief within a few days. Depending on the severity of the symptoms, the disease may completely clear up within several weeks of therapy. Other antibiotics may also be used if you are allergic to penicillin.

Prognosis

The prognosis for this disease is very good. Gonococcal arthritis responds very well to penicillin and symptoms usually disappear completely, without any lasting damage to the joints.

Nongonococcal Infectious Arthritis

Stephen, a fifty-five-year-old businessman, had had rheumatoid arthritis for many years and was doing quite well. Recently he had developed a mild cough and was bringing up phlegm; ten days after that, he developed a fever and sweats, and his right knee became red, swollen, and painful. He'd had flares of his rheumatoid arthritis in the past, but this pain was different. It was so excruciating he couldn't move his leg. He called his doctor, who told him to come right in to the office. The doctor tapped the painful joint and found pus. He performed a Gram's stain on the fluid from the joint and discovered the presence of bacteria there. This was a nongonococcal infection, and Stephen was immediately placed in the hospital and treated with high doses of intravenous antibiotics.

What Is It?

Many types of bacteria other than the gonococcus can cause joint space infections; the most common are staphylococcus, or staph, and pneumococcus. Some strains of staphylococcus are virulent and can seriously damage joints—even within a day or two—if not treated promptly. Other strains are weaker and much slower acting. As a group, these diseases are denoted as nongonococcal infectious arthritis or septic arthritis.

Who Gets It?

This type of arthritis is rare, and normal, healthy people do not usually develop it. When they do occur, joint infections are most likely in people who have already weakened or damaged joints—for example, those who have had previous joint injuries or joint diseases, such as rheumatoid arthritis.

There are certain conditions that can lower a person's resistance to infection and increase the risk for this disease. These include diabetes, kidney disease, and certain types of cancer. Others at higher risk for nongonococcal joint infections include alcoholics and drug addicts. The use of certain medications, such as corticosteroids and cytotoxic drugs, may alter the body's immune system and increase the chances for joint infection.

Cause

A nongonococcal joint infection is usually caused by a bacterial infection in another part of the body that spreads to the joints through the bloodstream.

Symptoms

This form of arthritis usually begins with a very painful, swollen, red-hot joint. The swelling often comes on quite suddenly, within hours or days of the infection. Usually, only one joint is affected, commonly the knee; but the disease occasionally begins with other joints, including wrists, shoulders, hips, and elbows. Small joints are rarely affected. Other signs of septic arthritis (or joint infection) include fever, chills, and a feeling of being sick all over.

Diagnosis

When a patient has a single hot, red, and painful joint, it is most commonly an indication of gout or pseudogout, which are caused by crystals in the joint space. Third on the list of possibilities is a bacterial infection. Patients with a septic joint are very sick. Their joints are red, hot, swollen, tender, and painful to touch or move. They usually have fever, and their white blood cell counts and sedimentation rates are elevated. The diagnosis is confirmed by removing fluid from the joint by needle aspiration and examining it under the microscope for signs of white blood cells and bacteria. The joint fluid will also be sent to a lab to be cultured so that the bacteria can be positively identified.

Treatment

A bacterial infection is usually a medical emergency; it can cause joint destruction and therefore requires prompt medical treatment with high doses of antibiotics. I always admit such patients into the hospital so that I can start them on an antibiotic intravenously. Afterwards, I may follow up this treatment with several more weeks of oral antibiotics.

In addition, I will drain the joint of excess fluid daily, in part to relieve the swelling, but also to see if the condition is clearing up and if the white blood cell count is going down. A septic joint is like an abscess; it needs to be opened and drained to promote healing and allow removal of bacteria and toxic products in the pus. I may be able to drain the joint using a needle to withdraw fluid; but if I can't, I'll call in the orthopedist to do this surgically. If your hip is infected, it will have to be drained immediately because of possible damage to the top of the femur, or thigh bone. Since hips are harder to get to, they have to be drained surgically. Surgical drainage of a joint is a major procedure and requires general anesthesia; however, arthroscopy is being used increasingly for this purpose and may simplify the procedure. After surgery, a drain will be left in, and you will be hospitalized, usually for several weeks. The drain will be removed when the infection clears. After that, I usually recommend physical therapy to rebuild muscle strength and restore mobility to the joint.

Prognosis

People who have this condition usually have damaged joints to begin with and are apt to have some residual problems, including some loss of joint function after the infection has cleared up. If left untreated, the infection can destroy a joint and eventually spread to other parts of the body and cause some very serious problems.

Rheumatic Fever

What Is It?

The medical community has been so effective in preventing rheumatic fever in this country that it's rare to come across a patient who has this disease. In fact, I have never actually seen a case of arthritis due to rheumatic fever at Duke.

Rheumatic fever usually follows a streptococcal infection. This disease is now rare in the developed world. General improvement in living conditions and the availability of antibiotics have contributed to its decline in the United States. In less developed countries, however, rheumatic fever remains a major cause of serious joint and heart disease.

Who Gets It?

Rheumatic fever occurs primarily in children between three and fifteen, although adults are occasionally affected. Only a few individuals with streptococcal infection will develop rheumatic fever. Some of the factors that determine whether a person will develop the disease include prior exposure to streptococcus; previous attacks of rheumatic fever (some people are more prone to multiple attacks); and genetic makeup (there is a genetic marker on the B cells of susceptible individuals).

Symptoms

This disease is a complication of a throat infection caused by streptococcus, a so-called strep throat. Two or three weeks after the initial infection, patients develop severe flu-like symptoms and a type of migratory arthritis that moves from one joint to another. These joints may be swollen, red, and extremely painful, or they may just ache. Their movement may become limited. In addition to the arthritis, rheumatic fever may also cause a red skin rash; nodules in the skin; uncontrolled movements of the extremities; and inflammation of the heart. If rheumatic fever is left untreated, the most serious complication that can result is damage to the heart, including possibly permanent scarring of the heart valves and disruption of their operation.

Cause

Certain types of streptococci seem to cause the body's immune system to malfunction. The immune system produces antibodies that attack not only the bacteria but the normal tissue of the heart and joints as well. This is known as an autoimmune response. It is well established that rheumatic fever is preventable. This infection can be avoided through good hygiene and less crowded living conditions.

Diagnosis

The physical exam and medical history will help your doctor to diagnose rheumatic fever, especially if you show evidence of a recent streptococcal infection. Although you may not remember having had a sore throat, blood tests can identify elevated antibodies to strep and document the infection.

Treatment

The joint inflammation of rheumatic fever is usually treated with non-steroidal anti-inflammatory drugs, most commonly aspirin. More severe cases may require corticosteroids.

Prompt recognition of strep throat and treatment with antibiotics (usually penicillin) can effectively prevent rheumatic fever. Throat cultures to identify the streptococcal bacteria can be simply taken in your doctor's office, and are certainly worthwhile for children who have sore throats and fevers. Some physicians treat a sore throat and fever with antibiotics immediately, just to "play it safe"; other physicians prefer to wait the day or two for the results of the culture before instituting antibiotic treatment. Not every strep throat will lead to rheumatic fever, and not every person is susceptible to this disease.

If you've already had rheumatic fever, your doctor may ask you to stay on antibiotics for several months, or sometimes indefinitely, especially if you have evidence of heart disease. This long-term antibiotic therapy can help prevent a recurrence of the disease.

If your heart valves do become damaged because of rheumatic fever, you should receive antibiotics during dental and medical procedures that could damage tissues and release bacteria into the bloodstream. While normal body mechanisms usually clear these bacteria out of the bloodstream easily and quickly, people with already damaged valves are more susceptible to infection and so require special precautions.

Prognosis

When this disease is prevented or treated promptly, the chances for a full recovery without any long-term joint disease are good.

Reiter's Syndrome/Reactive Arthritis

After basic training, Arthur, a twenty-one-year-old, developed a mild burning on urination and a slight genital discharge. He went to his doctor, who performed cultures and Gram's stains for gonococcus, thinking this might be a sign of gonorrhea. He treated the young man briefly with the antibiotic tetracycline. But lab results showed no evidence of gonococcus, and the initial signs of urethritis went away. Several weeks later, Arthur returned with a very swollen knee. The doctor drained the fluid for analysis, but tests showed no evidence of infection. He placed Arthur on the nonsteroidal anti-inflammatory drug indomethacin, and his knee gradually improved. Given the response to indomethacin and the history of urethritis, the doctor thought this might be Reiter's syndrome. He decided to do a back X-ray, and found evidence of sacroiliitis. A diagnosis of Reiter's syndrome was made.

What Is It?

Reiter's syndrome was originally described during World War I by a physician named Hans Reiter. He identified the condition in a German soldier who had a previous bout of dysentery. In its original classic definition, Reiter's was thought to be a disease that affected men only and followed a bowel or venereal infection. Since then the definition has been broadened. We now know that Reiter's affects women as well as men; and while it often follows either severe diarrhea or dysentery, or a genital/urinary tract infection—urethritis in men and cystitis in women—many people with Reiter's don't have a history of previous infection. They may just have isolated arthritis.

The major symptom of Reiter's syndrome is an inflammation of the joints and their surrounding structures. This type of arthritis is called a reactive arthritis because the joint inflammation is a reaction to an infection elsewhere in the body. The infectious organisms do not appear to travel to the affected joint.

Who Gets It?

Reiter's syndrome occurs most frequently in individuals with a history of an infection in the intestinal or genital/urinary tract. It most often affects young men in their twenties. However, many cases in women may go undiagnosed because it's harder to detect genital/urinary tract infections in women. The disease is more prevalent among whites than among blacks.

Heredity plays a part in susceptibility to this disease. A majority of people with Reiter's syndrome have the genetic marker HLA-B27 (this is the same gene associated with ankylosing spondylitis—see page 125). Just because you have this marker, however, does not mean you will develop Reiter's syndrome. While approximately 8 percent of the population has HLA-B27, only about 20 percent will develop some form of arthritis, including Reiter's syndrome.

Symptoms

The classic form of Reiter's syndrome consists of three main components: arthritis; conjunctivitis, an eye inflammation commonly known as pinkeye; and urethritis, an inflammation of the urethra, the small tube through which urine passes on its way out of the body. You can have only one or two of these symptoms, however, and still have Reiter's syndrome. In fact, you may have Reiter's syndrome without any evidence of a previous infection. When only one or two symptoms of Reiter's are present, the disease is sometimes called incomplete Reiter's syndrome.

You may not notice any symptoms of arthritis until several weeks or months after the initial bout with a gastrointestinal or genital/urinary infection. Your joints and their surrounding structures (ligaments, muscles, and tendons) may become swollen and tender. The joints of the lower extremities are more often affected, primarily the knees, ankles, and feet. The joints are affected in an asymmetrical pattern; in other words, only one knee may be involved, or one ankle. As in ankylosing spondylitis, you may have an enthesopathy, an inflammation of the places where your ligaments attach to your bones. This can cause pain around the ribs, in the sacroiliac joints, and in the lower back. You may also have pain in the heel of your foot and in the Achilles tendon, other places where ligaments attach to bone.

Your toes and fingers may become very swollen and are called sausage digits because of the way they look. Sometimes you'll have skin rashes on the palms or soles of the foot that may become thick and crusty, looking very much like psoriasis. Painless, shallow sores may develop on your penis or the vagina, and on the inside of your mouth and tongue.

Other associated symptoms include iritis and uveitis, two inflammatory conditions of the eye; cervicitis, an inflammation of the cervix; and prostatitis, an infected prostate gland.

Attacks of arthritis may last several months and then disappear completely, or they may recur on and off for years.

Cause

The cause of Reiter's syndrome is unknown, though there is apparently an interplay between the environment and someone who is genetically susceptible. I think that one piece of the history of Reiter's syndrome provides an interesting look at how serendipitous natural events can blend with scientific investigation to help unravel the secrets of disease.

In 1962 over a thousand crew members of a Navy cruiser, the U.S.S. *Little Rock*, went on a picnic to celebrate the ship's birthday. After their ship returned to sea, about half the crewmen came down with dysentery, which was eventually traced to two of the ship's cooks. Within sixteen days, nine of the affected men developed Reiter's syndrome. The ship's medical officer published a report of the episode in a medical journal.

In the next decade, it was subsequently discovered that a genetic marker, HLA-B27, was strongly associated with Reiter's syndrome. Scientists now wondered whether the nine men who contracted Reiter's syndrome aboard the Navy ship were positive for HLA-B27.

Tracking these men down over ten years after the fact was very difficult, but after much effort, five of the nine were located. Blood tests proved that four of them, indeed, were positive for HLA-B27. And even after all these years, some still suffered from recurrent eye disease and joint and back pains.

The link between an infectious disease, a genetic predisposition, and arthritis had been proved. Individuals with the HLA-B27 marker seem especially sensitive to infections that can cause arthritis. We now know that 80 to 90 percent of the patients suffering from Reiter's syndrome carry this marker—yet only 8 percent of the general population are positive for HLA-B27. Perhaps the offending bacteria contain proteins that resemble B27 or that somehow react to B27 itself in a way that sets off an impaired immune response in susceptible individuals.

Diagnosis

There are no specific tests for Reiter's syndrome. A diagnosis can usually be made on the basis of the medical history and the physical symptoms. If a patient complains of an eye inflammation or an intestinal or urinary tract infection before the onset of arthritis, I may suspect Reiter's syndrome. Routine laboratory tests help differentiate this from other forms of arthritis and can indicate whether an infection is present. X-rays may be taken to see if there are any changes in the bone around the sacroiliac joint. A test for the HLA-B27 marker can be performed in cases that are more difficult to diagnose.

Treatment

Nonsteroidal anti-inflammatory drugs are used to control the pain and inflammation of the arthritis. You should rest the affected joint when your condition is active; after that, I generally recommend physical therapy and range-of-motion exercises to build up your muscle strength and maintain the range of motion in your joints. Although Reiter's syndrome is likely caused by infections, antibiotics don't seem to be effective in treating it, although this is still being evaluated. Corticosteroid creams may be used to treat related skin problems.

Prognosis

For some, the disease runs a limited course of perhaps several months and then disappears. Others may have recurrent episodes over many years. Reiter's syndrome can usually be controlled with medication and rest and usually does not interfere with normal activities or result in joint damage or deformities.

Viral Arthritis

Joint pain is commonly associated with some viruses such as hepatitis and rubella. But we don't see many cases of virus-related arthritis from these diseases nowadays, because we have learned how to monitor our blood supply for hepatitis effectively and have developed a vaccine against rubella. I did, however, recently hear about a young medical student who was stuck with a needle while working in the hospital and several weeks later developed fever, joint pains, and a skin rash. A physical exam and blood work showed no obvious cause of the arthritis; but subsequently, this young woman became jaundiced and was diagnosed as having hepatitis.

This type of arthritis is usually self-limiting, since the body brings the viral infection under control, usually in a matter of weeks, and it may disappear on its own, before medical attention is sought. Usually the symptoms are milder, too. A person with a virus may have a fever, a rash, and flu-like symptoms, including joint and muscle aches. However, some develop acute symptoms of arthritis, usually in several joints. The arthritis is thought to occur from deposits of immune complexes in the joint tissues. Treatment usually involves NSAIDs.

Prosthetic Infections

As I mentioned earlier, infectious agents can enter the joint directly, as during an injury or surgery. In very rare instances, needle aspiration of a joint can introduce bacteria and cause an infection.

Infection may also be introduced into a joint as a result of artificial joint replacements. The prosthesis may behave as a foreign body. The resulting infection is often slower acting and less dramatic than other forms of infectious arthritis. It usually causes pain, but few other signs of infection.

One sixty-five-year-old patient at the clinic had very severe rheumatoid arthritis, and we recommended knee replacement surgery for her. After the surgery, she did extremely well and was able to get around without any pain. Two years after the surgery, she began to have increasingly severe pain in the knee. We took an X-ray of her knee, concerned that the prosthesis might be loosening, but found no evidence of that. We aspirated the joint with a needle and discovered the fluid was filled with pus, a sign that her joint was infected. Luckily, this woman responded to treatment with antibiotics, and we did not have to operate. Not infrequently, however, treatment of prosthetic infections is complicated because the body continues to react to the presence of a foreign object inside of it. Unfortunately, sometimes we must remove the artificial joint to eradicate the bacteria, although an artificial joint can successfully be reinserted later in some cases.

The vast majority of people with prosthetic joints do not develop problems with infection. To reduce the chances of infection, patients with joint prostheses should take prophylactic antibiotics whenever they go to the dentist or undergo medical procedures that would allow entry of bacteria into the bloodstream.

Fungi and Mycobacteria

Arthritis from infection with a fungus is very unusual, and the course of such a disease is very slow. It can develop as a result of many different fungal infections, the transmission of which differs. Some of these fungi are found in soil and plants, so gardeners and florists sometimes develop fungal infections. Fungal arthritis is usually a chronic disease. Because it develops so slowly, it is often difficult to diagnose. By the time the disease becomes apparent, a fair amount of joint damage may have already been done. There may be signs of fungal infection, for example, in the lung or skin, along with persistent inflammatory arthritis in one or more joints. Treatment involves the administration of antibiotics.

The mycobacteria that cause tuberculosis can in very rare instances cause a slow-growing arthritis that is very similar to fungal arthritis. In this instance, symptoms include evidence of TB in the lung along with a persistent type of arthritis in one or more joints.

AIDS

AIDS is associated with a variety of arthritic conditions, including severe joint pain, Reiter's-like arthritis, and muscle disease. It isn't clear whether these conditions are a direct result of the infection with the HIV virus itself or whether they result from other infectious microorganisms to which AIDS patients are so susceptible. HIV screening is usually done in patients with arthritis who are in a high-risk group. The arthritic complications are usually treated with NSAIDs.

The Ongoing Search for Microbes

We discussed a few of the less common types of arthritis that are related to previous infections. But what about major forms of inflammatory arthritis, such as rheumatoid arthritis and lupus? Can a bacterium, virus, or fungus be the cause?

The theory that an infection might cause rheumatoid arthritis is certainly not a new one. There was a time when rheumatoid arthritis was treated by draining infections elsewhere in the body—by removing abscessed teeth or gallbladders, for example, or by searching for an infected appendix. The theory was that an infection elsewhere in the body was "seeding" the joints. This turned out not to be true.

Still, the theory seems quite plausible. And scientists continue to search for infectious microbes. Their search is fueled by a few observations:

First, people with rheumatoid and other forms of inflammatory arthritis often have classic symptoms of infection, including fever, weakness, malaise, loss of appetite, and generalized aching and stiffness; they feel as if they have the flu and take to bed. When you do laboratory studies on these people, the results suggest the presence of an infection: white blood cell counts are high and sedimentation rates are elevated. The fluid in the joints seems to be filled with pus, but no microorganisms can be found in it.

Second, over the past few decades, scientists have discovered certain forms of arthritis that are linked to specific types of infectious agents. Lyme disease, for example, is caused by the spirochete bacteria; rheumatic fever is caused by an immune response to streptococci. These diseases are often successfully treated with antibiotics.

These precedents spur scientists in their continued research, but so far there is no proven link between rheumatoid arthritis and a foreign microorganism. The evidence remains purely circumstantial. Still, because this theory seems so reasonable, many physicians are attempting to treat certain types of arthritis with antibiotics.

At this time, I don't think there is convincing data on the role of antibiotics in the treatment of most forms of inflammatory arthritis, and it is not part of our routine care at Duke University. Inflammatory arthritis may be caused by any number of other factors; even if a microbe is responsible for the joint inflammation, it may already have invaded the body and disappeared by the time the symptoms of arthritis arise.

Rheumatology is a dynamic field that has made great strides in the last few decades. Research continues in many areas, including the search for infectious organisms. If we find that other microorganisms do indeed cause arthritis, then we can learn more about their transmission. We can then design more effective approaches to the treatment, cure, and prevention of many forms of arthritis.

INFECTION AND ARTHRITIS

Bacteria, viruses, and fungi can cause arthritis in a joint either directly (through a puncture wound or incision) or indirectly (from an infection elsewhere in the body that travels to the joints via the bloodstream). The cause, symptoms, and treatment vary, depending upon the microorganisms responsible for the infection and on the host's overall health.

LYME ARTHRITIS: A bacterial joint infection transmitted by a tick that feeds on mammals. Anyone bitten by the tick usually can get Lyme disease. The first symptoms may be fever and flu-like symptoms and a circular rash; heart inflammation, meningitis, and various neurological problems may follow. Arthritis doesn't occur until a later stage, and frequently affects the knees, though other joints can also be involved. The arthritis may be prevented or halted with prompt antibiotic treatment.

GONOCOCCAL ARTHRITIS: The most common form of infectious arthritis, caused by the gonococcus associated with gonorrhea. Bacteria spread from genitals to joints via the bloodstream. Young, sexually active people are prime candidates, especially women, who show fewer symptoms during initial stages of venereal disease. Joint pain is usually sudden, and arthritis appears to migrate from one joint to another on both upper and lower extremities. Cultures from genital, rectal, or oral discharges allow a firm diagnosis. Responds very well to antibiotics. Long-term joint damage is unlikely if treated promptly.

NONGONOCOCCAL INFECTIONS: Caused by bacteria other than gonococcus that spread through the bloodstream from another part of the body. Is quite rare and usually occurs in individuals with already weakened or damaged joints. Usually occurs very suddenly, with hot, painful swelling of one joint. Is a medical emergency, requiring prompt hospitalization and treatment with intravenous antibiotics and daily draining of the joint. May result in some loss of joint function, especially since most affected joints are already impaired.

RHEUMATIC FEVER: Caused by a streptococcal infection, primarily in children. Usually begins with a throat infection and fever. May progress to severe flu-like symptoms, migratory arthritis, and eventual heart damage. Prompt treatment of strep throat with antibiotics and better living conditions have nearly eradicated this disease from the developed world.

(continued)

REITER'S SYNDROME/REACTIVE ARTHRITIS: Often develops after a severe bowel or genital/urinary tract infection, though in some cases there is no evidence of previous infection. Occurs most frequently in young men and in those with an identifiable genetic marker, HLA-B27. Classic signs are arthritis, conjunctivitis, and urethritis or cystitis. Joints and surrounding ligaments may be swollen and tender, especially in lower extremities. Can affect attachment structures and sacroiliac joints. Treatment includes NSAIDs, exercise, and physical therapy. Usually does not result in joint damage.

VIRAL ARTHRITIS: A self-limited arthritis believed to result from deposits of immune complexes in joints. Disappears when the viral infection is cured.

FUNGAL ARTHRITIS: A rare and slowly progressive arthritis resulting from infection with fungi. Slow growth pattern is similar to that of tuberculosis arthritis. Difficult to diagnose which may lead to delayed treatment and joint damage.

AIDS: The HIV virus is associated with various arthritic conditions, including severe joint pain, Reiter's-like arthritis, and muscle disease. Arthritis complications are treated with NSAIDs.

12

Juvenile Rheumatoid Arthritis

Becky is an active four-year-old whose precocious chatter sometimes makes her sound years older than her age. Because Becky's parents both work, she spends her weekdays at a local child care center. The first person to notice some changes in Becky's behavior was Becky's teacher, Susan. Becky, a normally gregarious child, seemed more subdued than usual. On the playground she sometimes sat quietly on a bench instead of running around with the others. She occasionally seemed irritable, refusing to participate during storytime, normally one of her favorite periods. Susan also noticed that Becky seemed to favor her left leg, although she didn't complain of any pain and the leg looked normal.

Susan called the situation to the attention of Becky's parents. When they asked Becky if she hurt anywhere, Becky said no. Since Becky's mother had just gone back to work full time, they worried that their daughter might be having an emotional reaction to the child care center. They decided to try to give her more attention on the weekends and see if that might help the situation.

Over the next few weeks, Becky developed an obvious limp, and her parents noticed that her knee was swollen and hot. Becky, who usually woke up bright-eyed and eager to go to preschool in the morning, now woke up crying and saying that she hurt. Becky's parents took her to their pediatrician to see what was wrong.

When the doctor examined Becky's knee, he found evidence of swelling and ordered some laboratory tests. Results from these tests and from the physical examination and medical history pointed to juvenile rheumatoid arthritis.

Becky's parents were very upset. They couldn't believe that this was happening to their beautiful, healthy child. Didn't arthritis happen only to older people? They wondered if somehow they were at fault. Could Becky have gotten this illness at the child care center? Should Becky's mother have stayed home with her child?

The doctor had a lengthy consultation with Becky's parents. He told them that they shouldn't blame themselves for Becky's illness and that the disease is not contagious. Most children with arthritis do well, he said, although Becky might have some down periods. Although most children with arthritis do not have long-term joint damage or disabilities, the course of juvenile rheumatoid arthritis is different for each child, and there was no way to predict how long Becky's disease would last or how severe it would be. In the meantime, Becky's parents could help their daughter by seeing that she got the necessary medication, physical therapy, and exercise. This would help control her symptoms and allow Becky to remain as active as possible.

What Is Juvenile Rheumatoid Arthritis?

When parents are told their child has arthritis, they may at first be surprised or shocked at the diagnosis. Few people think of arthritis as a disease of young children. However, inflammatory types of arthritis can affect people of any age, from infants to centenarians.

When inflammatory arthritis affects people under the age of sixteen, we give it an entirely separate classification. That's because the course of arthritis in children is usually different from that in adults. Children experience symptoms differently, and in general they have a more favorable prognosis.

Childhood arthritis is not one disease but an umbrella term for at least three distinct types of arthritis that occur in young children. Each type has its unique set of symptoms and its pattern of onset. One form of childhood arthritis involves mainly swelling of the joints; another form affects mainly the spine; and a third type is marked by high fevers. Some cases of childhood arthritis may actually be early forms of adult disease.

Arthritis in childhood goes by several different names. Most doctors in the United States refer to childhood arthritis as juvenile rheumatoid arthritis, or JRA for short. This name is not entirely accurate. It implies that childhood arthritis is similar to the adult disease rheumatoid arthritis, or RA. Only one form of juvenile arthritis is similar to adult rheumatoid arthritis, but the disease in children is not usually as extensive or as deforming. Children with JRA usually don't have rheumatoid factor in their blood (an antibody found in the blood of many adult RA patients) or rheumatoid nodules (painless lumps that form under the skin).

Some physicians prefer to avoid the association between JRA and RA. They use the term juvenile chronic arthritis. However, this term is also inaccurate. Not all childhood arthritis is chronic. Fortunately, many cases subside after a number of years and have no lasting effects.

The name Still's disease is sometimes used to describe arthritis in childhood. The name comes from the English physician who described the disease in the nineteenth century. More frequently, Still's disease is the term used for one very specific type of childhood arthritis, which we will discuss later in this chapter.

For convenience, we will use the term JRA because this is the one most commonly used by doctors in this country.

Who Gets JRA?

JRA is not a rare disease: it affects approximately 50,000 to 200,000 children in the United States. It can develop at any age, but appears to peak between one and three years of age and during the early teenage years. Overall, girls are affected more than boys, but this can vary, depending upon which pattern of JRA we are talking about.

What Causes JRA?

We do not know what causes JRA. We do suspect genetic involvement and have found certain genetic markers occur more often among children who have some forms of this disease; however, it is very rare for more than one child in a family to have JRA. So while there may be a genetic predisposition toward the disease, there are clearly other factors that contribute to its development.

Symptoms

The symptoms of JRA vary greatly from child to child and even in one child from one day to the next. A child's symptoms may remain mild and never be overly troublesome. However, some children can be very stiff and sore. There can be periods of remission in which the disease disappears for weeks, months, or even years. Sometimes symptoms disappear completely and never return. Since it's so hard to predict exactly how severe or how long a child's arthritis will last, you may feel helpless and frustrated. However, many families learn how to work with their physicians to effectively control their children's symptoms, and their youngsters usually lead active and relatively normal lives.

It's hard to talk about the symptoms of JRA, since JRA is actually a number of different diseases grouped together for convenience. There are at least three major subsets of the disease, and each affects different joints and has its own distinct pattern of symptoms. However, these separate conditions do have some features in common.

In general, the major symptoms of JRA are inflamed joints that may be warm, swollen, and painful. The child may have morning stiffness that subsides with movement. He or she may also feel stiffness in the joints after sitting in one position for too long. This is known as the gel phenomenon.

Some children have systemic symptoms, including fever, malaise, anemia, loss of appetite, and a flu-like achiness.

Most of the time children do well and have no long-lasting disabilities. However, in some severe cases of JRA, if a child is in pain and does not move his or her joints, the muscles surrounding the joint may weaken, the normally elastic tendons may shorten, and the child may permanently lose full joint motion. This is called a contracture.

If the child's joint inflammation is very severe and persistent, there can, over time, be some damage to structures within the joint that can lead to deformities. Fortunately, this is not very common.

Sometimes severe inflammation can affect the growth centers within a child's bones. If the disease goes untreated or is especially severe, a child may not reach his or her full stature. Sometimes only isolated areas of the body may be affected, and a child may grow up with small hands, feet, or fingers. At times the inflammation can have the opposite effect, causing an overgrowth of bone. The legs, for example, may grow to be unequal in length. JRA may also cause a delay in sexual development. A child's growth may be altered during times of severe flare-up of the disease. However, the child's growth pattern should become normal again when the inflammation has subsided.

As I mentioned, these symptoms vary, depending on which subset of the disease you are talking about. There are at least three major subsets of the disease, which I will describe below. In addition, not every form of arthritis that occurs in childhood is JRA. Some children, for example, get arthritis as a result of Lyme disease or of an infection that has traveled to their joints. The three major subsets of JRA are polyarticular disease, pauciarticular disease, and Still's disease.

Polyarticular Disease

Polyarticular disease means a disease of many joints (*poly* = many; *articular* = joint). This type of JRA involves more than five joints and is most similar to adult rheumatoid arthritis. Girls are two times as likely as boys to have this disease.

The joints are usually affected symmetrically—in other words, if a joint on the right side of the body is involved, the corresponding joint on the left side will most likely also be affected. Often the small joints of the hands are affected, though other joints such as knees, ankles, hips, and feet can be affected too. The child may experience low-grade fever, weight loss, and anemia. In severe cases, he or she may have some growth problems.

Most children with polyarticular disease test negative for rheumatoid factor, an abnormal antibody that often appears in the blood of adults with rheumatoid arthritis. This group of children is said to have rheumatoid negative polyarticular disease. Their prognosis is generally good (see chapter 4 for a full discussion of rheumatoid factor).

A minority of children, however, do test positive for rheumatoid factor. This group may be more at risk for a more chronic, progressive form of the disease that can cause joint damage and is similar to adult rheumatoid arthritis. The medical term for this form of disease is rheumatoid positive polyarticular disease. Please keep in mind, though, that many children who test positive for rheumatoid factor can also expect to do well.

Pauciarticular Disease

Pauci means few, and this type of arthritis affects only four or fewer joints. The joints most commonly affected are the knees, elbows, wrists, and ankles. Joints are usually affected asymmetrically, so only a single joint on one side of the body is involved. This is the most common form of JRA, affecting over 50 percent of children who have the disease. This disease affects mostly girls.

Children with pauciarticular disease usually test positive for antinuclear antibodies (ANAs), antibodies to the cell nucleus (see chapter 3). Those who test positive for ANA are also more prone to an inflammatory eye condition called iridocyclitis, a potentially serious eye disease. With frequent eye checkups and good follow-up care, such eye trouble can be detected early and controlled. Children with pauciarticular disease generally do well.

While young girls are most prone to pauciarticular disease, it sometimes affects older boys, too. This group of boys has a somewhat different disease pattern from the girls. They generally do not have antinuclear antibodies and are less likely to develop eye disease. Their arthritis tends to affect the joints of the spine and hips. They also have the genetic marker HLA-B27, which is commonly found among young men with ankylosing spondylitis, an arthritis that primarily affects the spine. Perhaps this group of older boys has an early form of ankylosing spondylitis. Some doctors place this group in a separate category called B27 arthritis.

Still's Disease (Systemic Onset Arthritis)

This form of JRA begins with generalized systemic symptoms that can affect internal organs and parts of the body other than the joints. This is the least common type of JRA, affecting approximately 10 percent of children with the disease.

Still's disease commonly begins with fevers. You may find that your child has a high temperature, with chills and achiness, beginning in the late afternoon or evening. The fever may abate, only to return the next day. These fevers may last for weeks or months. They may be accompanied by a light-colored rash on the thighs and chest. In addition, your child may show other signs of inflammation before the joints become involved. He may experience enlargement of the spleen and lymph nodes, inflammation of the heart muscle (myocarditis) and surrounding tissues (pericarditis), a high white blood cell count, and anemia. He may feel fatigued and lose weight.

The prognosis for Still's disease is generally favorable, although children with systemic onset are more prone to problems with organs outside the joints, such as inflammation of the heart and liver. In 75 percent of cases, the disease subsides with no long-term effects.

How Is JRA Diagnosed?

There is no single test that can be used to diagnose JRA. The diagnosis is based upon a combination of clues gathered from the medical history, physical exam, and laboratory tests. It may take a number of weeks or even months for a pattern of symptoms to emerge that can help your doctor to classify the disease. In the meantime, your doctor will probably be able to determine how many of your child's joints are involved and whether the involvement is symmetrical or asymmetrical.

Your pediatrician may recommend you consult a pediatric rheumatologist if he or she suspects your child has JRA. Such specialists have a great deal of experience in diagnosing and treating arthritis in children.

The diagnosis of arthritis is somewhat more difficult to make for children than adults, because very young children may be unable to report symptoms, and children in general are less likely to complain about joint pain than adults. This was true of Laurie, a two-year-old I saw whose parents told me that she hadn't been acting herself for weeks. Laurie had been cranky, didn't eat well, and cried in the morning when her mother tried to dress her. She didn't seem to want to ride her tricycle or play with any of her friends, and she kept asking her parents to pick her up because she was too tired to walk. Laurie never complained of any pain. Her parents had no idea that Laurie's joints were stiff and achy until she started to run a fever and they brought her to a physician, whose examination showed swelling in her knees.

Your observations concerning your child's behavior can provide valuable clues in the diagnosis of his or her condition. Has he been especially irritable or fatigued? Has he run a fever, lost weight or shown a general loss of appetite? Have you noticed him moving his limbs in an unusual way? Does he seem to be walking with more difficulty than usual? Does he avoid using a particular joint or turn his head in an unusual way? Your doctor will perform a thorough physical exam to see whether your child shows evidence of inflammation in the joints; however, it's often hard to detect such swelling in little children because their knees and elbows are so naturally pudgy.

The laboratory tests conducted for JRA are essentially the same as those done for adults, including a complete blood count, the sedimentation rate, and a determination of rheumatoid factor and antinuclear antibodies (see chapter 3 for details). A thoughtful doctor will limit tests that are painful or traumatic for your child, and he or she will try to draw as little blood as possible as few times as possible.

Your child will not normally need an X-ray because children don't usually suffer the changes in the joints demonstrated by X-rays of adults. In addition, X-rays don't reveal whether the spine and sacroiliac joints in children with HLA-B27-related disease have been affected because children's joints look different from those of adults.

When a child has back pain and your doctor suspects B27 disease, he or she may sometimes perform tissue typing to identify this genetic marker. The presence of this marker would increase the likelihood of this diagnosis, but it is not definitive.

Because JRA is often linked with iridocyclitis, a potentially serious eye inflammation, I advise parents to take their child to an ophthalmologist (eye specialist) as part of the medical evaluation. He or she will perform a slit-lamp examination, a simple and painless test in which the opthalmologist shines a light into the child's eyes while looking through a magnification microscope.

The diagnostic workup for Still's disease may be long and involved, and quite frustrating for parents. Before the arthritis shows up, the child's doctor may suspect that an infection is causing the fevers. There is no one diagnostic test that can rule out infection, so the child frequently undergoes many laboratory tests as the doctor looks for possible infectious agents. That's what happened to three-year-old Amy, who was suffering from high fevers and a rash. Her pediatrician performed a complete examination of her ears, throat, and chest and couldn't find anything suspicious. He told the parents it was most likely a viral infection and would probably go away. But over the next few days the fever didn't abate, and Amy's parents brought her back. At this time the doctor ordered blood and urine tests and performed a throat culture, but the test results were negative. After several weeks of continued fevers, the doctor had Amy hospitalized for a more complete evaluation. A rheumatologist and hematologist were brought in for consultation. They found evidence of swelling in Amy's joints and concluded that she had a systemic onset arthritis.

Eventually signs of arthritis develop and the diagnosis becomes more clear-cut. Still's disease sometimes disappears after several weeks or months, but may then recur months or even years later for no apparent reason.

Drug Treatment

Aspirin is the drug most commonly used to treat JRA. Aspirin is a member of a group of drugs called nonsteroidal anti-inflammatory drugs (NSAIDs). This group of drugs is generally fast-acting and brings relief by reducing inflammation, pain, and fever.

You can give your child aspirin four times a day in liquid, chewable, or tablet form; however, chewable aspirin can cause gum inflammation and damage to the teeth and is not recommended by some physicians.

Children seem to do very well on aspirin, but the large dosages necessary can cause side effects in some children, including stomach upset. You may be able to prevent these stomach upsets by giving your child the aspirin with snacks or at mealtime, or in combination with an antacid. The aspirin may also cause a very mild liver inflammation that can be detected by routine blood screening. This inflammation usually doesn't cause any bothersome symptoms, and it reverses itself once the aspirin is discontinued. Since there are a limited number of NSAIDs approved for children, your doctor may sometimes continue administering aspirin despite laboratory evidence of liver inflammation.

Aspirin sometimes causes ringing in the ears (tinnitus), but this seems to be less of a problem for children than for adults. Other possible signs of excessive aspirin dosage include changes in mood, drowsiness, and changes in breathing pattern. The body metabolizes aspirin at different rates, depending upon how active the disease is, so the level of aspirin in a child's blood must be frequently monitored to avoid serious overdosage.

Children with certain viral infections—for example, chicken pox and influenza—who take aspirin may increase their risk for Reye's syndrome. This disease is marked by vomiting, mental confusion, and other neurological symptoms, as well as liver problems. I am not aware of reports of an increased incidence of Reye's syndrome among children with arthritis who are on long-term aspirin therapy. However, if your child develops the flu or chicken pox, you should consult your physician. He or she may recommend that the child temporarily stop taking aspirin. This brief discontinuation should not have any ill effects. Aspirin is a well-established therapy that is generally well tolerated.

If your child cannot tolerate aspirin, the doctor may want to try other nonsteroidal anti-inflammatory drugs. These are also effective and may have fewer side effects than aspirin. The choice of medications approved by the FDA for children with arthritis is much more limited than those approved for adult diseases, however. Tolectin (tolmetin sodium) and Naprosyn (naproxen) are both effective medications that have received FDA approval for use in JRA. Tolectin has a bitter taste and you may need to hide it in your child's food to get him to take it. Naprosyn is taken only two times a day, once in the morning and once at night. Your child can take the medication before or after school and avoid the embarrassment some children feel about taking medicine in front of their peers.

If NSAIDs don't bring the disease under control or if more severe disease is damaging your child's joints, your doctor may want to try the slower-acting, more potent remittive drugs (see chapter 14), particularly injectable gold. These may take weeks or even months to get results. Remittive drugs have potentially serious side effects, and the same warnings about drug safety given for adults pertain to children. These drugs must be used thoughtfully and their use must be clearly justified. Children taking remittive drugs must be monitored frequently to avoid serious side effects.

Corticosteroids such as prednisone are rarely used in JRA, except for serious, life-threatening complications of systemic disease or to treat inflammatory eye disease that is not responding to less extreme measures. Corticosteroids can slow the rate of bone growth, an especially serious side effect if JRA is already slowing your child's growth. They can also lower your child's resistance to infection. If used, these drugs should be administered in the smallest possible doses for the shortest possible time.

Eye Care

Because some forms of JRA are associated with eye disease, frequent regular eye examinations by an ophthalmologist are extremely important. Your doctor may recommend that your child have slit-lamp examinations as frequently as every six to twelve weeks. If the ophthalmologist detects iridocyclitis, he or she may prescribe corticosteroid eye drops. These drops result in fewer side effects than corticosteroids taken orally. The ophthalmologist may also prescribe drops that dilate the pupil and prevent the scarring that may occur in serious cases of iridocyclitis. These drugs are called mydriatics. Systemic corticosteroids are used only in the most serious cases. In most instances, with regular eye checkups and prompt treatment, your child won't have any long-term eye trouble.

Physical Activity

When a child's joints hurt, she may naturally try to avoid motions that bother her and limit her activity significantly. To prevent the muscles surrounding the joints from weakening and to keep the joints fully mobile, she has to be encouraged to perform range-of-motion exercises daily, which your doctor will prescribe specifically for the child. But children may not accept the routine of a conventional physical therapy program as readily as adults do. They're more likely to see physical therapy as a chore, like brushing teeth or making the bed; really young children won't even understand that concept. And as parents know all too well, children resist routines. Here's where an imaginative approach can really help with younger children. One father whose four-year-old daughter had a rather severe flare of JRA said he carried his daughter to the bathroom in the morning and set her in a tub of warm water to soak for twenty minutes or so. That helped to ease the pain in her muscles and to get her going. Afterward, they would do range-of-motion exercises together; he would tell jokes and stories to keep her interested. His approach—turning physical therapy into fun—worked very well.

Sometimes you can incorporate therapy into your child's regular activities. Riding a tricycle, for example, can be a good range-of-motion exercise, especially if the seat is raised to promote the full extension of the knee. Swimming is fun, exercises both the arms and the legs, and provides cardiovascular exercise without placing stress on the joints.

Some parents find that applications of heat—a shower or a bath, or warm compresses—help their child get moving in the morning and temporarily reduce the pain so that he or she can better perform his or her exercises.

Rest

Just as exercise is important to maintain the range of motion in a joint, rest is important during a flare to prevent more serious complications. It's easy to tell adults with rheumatoid arthritis to balance periods of activity with adequate rest. But telling your child that is a whole different matter. As one mother of a six-year-old patient of mine said, "Laura gets so engrossed in playing with the other kids that she doesn't know when to stop. If I make her come in for a rest, she cries and kicks and screams."

Children with JRA are just like any other children. They may balk when told to nap or to sit quietly in their rooms and entertain themselves. Enforced rest is not likely to work very well, and a rigid nap schedule that tears your child away from his or her playmates can make him or her feel different. You may have to encourage your child to rest at times, as you would any youngster who is overdoing it and needs some quiet time to wind down. Try introducing a special toy or activity just for quiet play in the bedroom. Share a good book, watch a video together, invent a new song—any game that at least gets your child to be quiet for a while. In general, try to let your younger child set his or her own pace of activity.

Similarly, encourage your older children to continue the sports and activities they enjoy. Obviously you don't want your child with arthritis being tackled on the football field, but except for certain activities that place undue stress on joints, such as basketball or gymnastics, your child can enjoy a wide range of sports.

Children, like adults, may deny their illness and try to show off in front of their peers. The son of one of my colleagues, for example, a boy with JRA, insists on playing basketball even though he is exhausted and limping. Like any teenager, he continues to test his parents, and the family has an ongoing battle over his apparent disregard for his worsening condition. In such a case, parents and child might want to sit down with the child's doctor and discuss the consequences of the child's actions.

If your child is older, you should discuss with him the importance of daily range-of-motion exercises and adequate rest; however, an older child, particularly a young teenager, should be allowed to assume some responsibilities for his own care and to set up his own rest schedule. Children usually rest and nap when they need to.

Splints

Your doctor may suggest your child wear a splint to alleviate pain, to hold the joint in a good position, or to prevent or reduce contractures. Splints are commonly made of plastic with a soft inner padding and are fashioned specifically to fit your child. They are usually worn at night, but may sometimes be necessary during the day as well. Splints are most commonly prescribed for knees and wrists, because these are the two most common sites of joint involvement. If your child has neck problems, he may have to wear a cervical collar, and a physical therapist may help him work to achieve better posture.

Surgery

Surgery is seldom necessary for JRA. Joint replacements for children are rare. Usually, childhood arthritis is not deforming, and such replacements are not necessary. In addition, joint replacement surgery may not be practical because young children's joints are not yet fully developed. Other surgeries that are occasionally performed are a synovectomy (to remove inflamed synovial tissue) and soft tissue release (to treat contractures).

School Activities

Many children with JRA do well and continue to go to school and participate in all their previous activities. There are times, however, when a child may have a flare and may hurt more than usual. Teachers and school administrators have to be made aware that your child has arthritis and may at times have some difficulties. For example, it may take longer to put on boots or to walk quickly from one end of the school building to another while changing classes.

The parents of a first grader with JRA told me a story about their daughter that shows what can happen when parents and teachers fail to communicate. Jennifer's parents got a letter from her first-grade teacher saying that Jennifer's behavior in class was disruptive. She would never stay in her seat, but got up, seemingly at will, and walked around the classroom. She was also uncooperative and refused to participate in class activities. Jennifer's parents had a long conference with the teacher. They explained to her that Jennifer had to move around at frequent intervals to prevent her joints from stiffening up. On days when she seemed cranky and irrational, Jennifer was hurting more than usual. She needed more patience and understanding from the adults around her. After the conference, the teacher was extremely cooperative, and Jennifer had a very positive first-grade experience. An understanding teacher can offer your child support if he or she feels sensitive about having to wear a brace, to walk more slowly than others, or otherwise to be different.

Parents of children with arthritis should be aware of the various federal laws that can help their children in school. According to these laws, all children are entitled to a free public education, regardless of their disabilities; and in order to receive federal funds, public schools must develop an individual educational plan (IEP) for every disabled child. This plan is developed with input from parents, the child's medical specialists, and the school specialists. It may include such adaptive learning aids as computers and typewriters, as well as elevators and transportation to schools. The Arthritis Foundation has literature describing these federal laws, and you may want to contact them for further details.

While a child with JRA may need some special considerations, school staff has to be careful not to treat him as an invalid. Most schoolchildren with arthritis can participate in many physical activities, so long as those activities don't involve a great deal of jumping or lifting and are pursued at a time when the disease is quiet. Open communication between you and the child's school nurse, principal, and teachers can make your child's time at school a positive experience.

The Family

Arthritis, like any medical illness, affects the entire family. This can be a difficult time for everyone. Illness brings out many different feelings. Many parents feel guilty or responsible for their child's condition. This feeling has no basis in reality: Parents do not cause their child's illness. Sometimes spouses blame each other, and the stress of having a sick child can strain a marriage.

Because you are so worried about your child, you may think you are helping him by protecting him from friends who may roughhouse with him, tease him, or ask questions. You may be afraid your child is going to get hurt. While your intentions may be good, this attitude can make your child excessively dependent on you and deprive him of the chance to assert his own identity through friendships with others. Your other children may resent a sibling with arthritis, because he appears to be getting so much attention and special treatment.

Children are individuals and react to illnesses in individual ways. Some may deny that they have a problem, others cope very well and take it in stride, and still others become angry and see the disease as an obstacle, refusing to take medications, rest, or do the necessary exercises. It's sometimes hard to tell why a child or teenager is acting out. Some testing of parents is a normal part of growing up, and the rebellion may have nothing at all to do with the arthritis.

In time, most families adapt. The medications, exercises, and other daily routines will become an accepted part of your child's life; and in most cases, the disease will be brought under control and the family can gradually resume a more normal living pattern. Even those with more serious disease appear to adapt with time. You might choose to accept the disease as a challenge and to focus on what your child *can* do, rather than on what he or she can't do.

The mother of one of my patients says she's dealt with her child's illness by becoming active in a parents' group, where families share information about what it's like to live with JRA. She has also learned to step away from the situation at times, to give herself a needed break. Taking a breather helps her to relate better to her child and to her husband.

Professional counseling can be a big help. A psychologist, psychiatrist, or social worker who is familiar with the issues of chronic disease in children may help you to understand the conflicts and to adapt to the situation.

Prognosis

The prognosis for JRA is generally favorable. Most children seem to outgrow this disease by the time they reach adulthood. Some who continue to have active joint disease retain good joint function. Fortunately, only a small minority have permanent limitations or active, long-standing disease.

JUVENILE RHEUMATOID ARTHRITIS (JRA)

A group of inflammatory arthritis diseases that affects children under the age of sixteen. JRA usually doesn't involve joint damage or disability, though it can. There are three major categories of JRA: (1) polyarticular disease, which affects more than five joints, usually on both sides of the body; (2) pauciarticular disease, which affects fewer than four joints, usually asymmetrically; and (3) Still's disease, a systemic onset arthritis that commonly begins with high fevers and may affect internal organs.

CAUSE: Unknown. Heredity may play a role.

SYMPTOMS: Specific symptoms vary depending on the disease category. General symptoms include warm, swollen, and painful joints; morning stiffness; sometimes fever, malaise, anemia, loss of appetite. In severe cases, growth may be affected and sexual development delayed.

WHO GETS IT? Can develop at any age, but peaks between one and three and again during the early teenage years. Most forms affect more girls than boys.

DIAGNOSIS: Diagnosis is based on combined evidence from medical history, physical exam, and blood tests.

TREATMENT: NSAIDs, most commonly aspirin; frequent eye exams; physical therapy; splinting to prevent contractures.

PROGNOSIS: Overall, favorable. Most outgrow the disease and have no lasting joint problems.

13

Tendonitis, Bursitis, and Other Soft Tissue Rheumatism

Ron, a thirty-six-year-old newspaper editor, decided to take up jogging because he'd gained some weight. He didn't have much time to run during the week. He had to be at the newspaper every morning by 7:00 A.M., and with high-pressure deadlines, he often ate lunch at his desk while he worked. So he tried to cram most of his exercising into the weekend. He bought a pair of running shoes and ran around the lake at a nearby park. Although quite winded, he pushed himself to do three miles a day on Saturday and Sunday. He followed this weekend routine for three weeks in a row.

Though Ron's leg muscles felt sore on Monday, the pain usually eased off during the week. By the fourth week, however, Ron felt a different kind of pain in his Achilles tendon. Thinking that the problem might stem from improper running shoes, he went out and bought a very expensive new pair. Although the tendon still bothered him, he went out and pushed himself hard, completing a six-mile run. His Achilles tendon felt okay while he was running, but really hurt him afterward. The back of his lower leg was so sore that he limped all week. He tried running shorter distances a few times more, but found it too painful.

After several weeks, when the pain still lingered, Ron sought the advice of his physician. The doctor carefully examined the affected area, asking Ron to move his foot up and down and sideways to make sure Ron still had a full range of motion in his ankle. He asked Ron about his sports activities and noticed that Ron's Achilles tendon was quite tender and swollen. The doctor diagnosed the problem as Achilles tendonitis, an inflammation of the tendon attached to the heel bone.

The doctor told Ron that if he stopped his running, the condition would probably heal itself in time. Ron could resume running when his tendon felt better; however, he should cut back on the mileage and increase it only very gradually as his body became more accustomed to exercise. Ron also needed to do some warm-up exercises to stretch his tendons before each run. In the meantime, Ron's doctor recommended a nonsteroidal anti-inflammatory drug for the pain and inflammation. Ron followed this advice, kept his mileage low, and was able to continue running without any difficulty.

What Is Soft Tissue Rheumatism?

Often, when I go to a social gathering and people hear that I am a rheumatologist, they'll say, "Oh, I have arthritis." If I ask, "What kind do you have?" the answer frequently is bursitis or tendonitis. While people commonly refer to any ache or pain in the body as arthritis, the term actually refers to a group of diseases involving inflammation of the joints. Bursitis and tendonitis, on the other hand, affect connective tissues that surround and support the joints. They are among a wide variety of conditions that affect the structures outside of the joints. As a group, these conditions are called soft tissue rheumatism. Some doctors also call them regional musculoskeletal disease or nonarticular rheumatism.

Soft tissue rheumatism differs from arthritis in several important ways. Many types of arthritis are systemic, causing generalized signs of inflammation such as fever and muscle aches. They may involve several joints and possibly other body organs. Soft tissue rheumatism, on the other hand, is a localized condition. It is usually confined to one area of the body.

While arthritis is frequently a chronic condition, lasting years or even a lifetime, soft tissue damage will often subside with treatment once you stop the activity that led up to it. Soft tissue problems sometimes take a while to clear up and may recur, especially if you repeat the motion that caused the problem; however, they usually leave no long-lasting disabilities or damage.

Soft tissue diseases such as bursitis and tendonitis are exceedingly common. Chances are you or someone you know has had one of these conditions at some point. They are sometimes associated with inflammatory and degenerative arthritis, but are most often caused by injuries on the job or from sports or leisure activities. With today's increased emphasis on fitness and sports, doctors are seeing many more patients with soft tissue rheumatism.

Soft Tissue Anatomy

In order to discuss soft tissue rheumatism, it's helpful to understand the tissues involved and where they're located relative to the joint. The following structures are often involved in soft tissue rheumatism:

1. The joint capsule: A protective capsule made of fibrous tissue. It completely surrounds the joint and encloses its contents.
2. Ligaments: The fibrous bands of tissue that connect bone to bone.
3. Entheses: The points where ligaments, tendons, and joint capsules attach to the bone.
4. Tendons: Fibrous bands of tissue that attach muscles to bone.
5. Tendon sheath: The tissue that surrounds and lubricates the tendon.
6. Bursa: A fibrous sac that acts as a small cushion between muscles and bones. It is lined with a membrane that releases fluid and smooths the movement of muscle across bone or muscle across muscle.
7. Fascia: Bands or sheets of connective tissue that surround muscles.

Individual soft tissue diseases are named after the structures affected. Bursitis, for example, is an inflammation of the bursae; tendonitis is an inflamed tendon; fasciitis refers to inflamed fascia; and so on.

What Causes Soft Tissue Rheumatism?

Soft tissue rheumatism can occur for a variety of reasons, the most common of which is injury or overuse of a joint. The structures that surround and support the joint may become irritated, inflamed, or torn from undue strain or stress placed upon them. Sometimes this occurs when people begin a new sport without getting themselves into shape gradually. One thirty-four-year-old patient, for example, developed tendonitis when she started a rigorous course in ballet after many years of being sedentary.

On the other hand, soft tissue problems can develop because of an anatomical weakness. In such cases, you needn't have had any previous

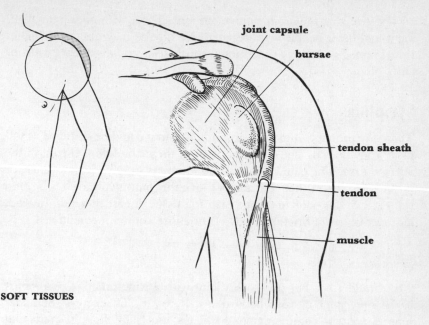

joint capsule

bursae

tendon sheath

tendon

muscle

SOFT TISSUES

trauma or injury. You may merely be mechanically predisposed to soft tissue problems because of the alignment of your joints.

These conditions can also develop as a result of improper body mechanics or posture, as in the case of the store clerk who lifted a heavy box of groceries with a sudden jerky motion and developed back pain.

Repeating the same motion over and over for long periods of time is thought to lead to soft tissue injury. A wide variety of sports and occupations have lent their names to various conditions; among them, ballet foot, golfer's elbow, housemaid's knee, jumper's knee, musician's hand, tennis elbow, weaver's bottom, welder's shoulder, soldier's heel, pipe setter's shoulder, and shopping bag syndrome.

While injury, overuse, and joint misalignment are the major causes of soft tissue rheumatism, they are not the only causes. Patients with rheumatoid arthritis can also have tendonitis and bursitis. Patients with Reiter's syndrome get Achilles tendonitis and plantar fasciitis. Gout can cause crystal deposits and swelling in the bursae.

Who Gets It?

Anyone can have soft tissue rheumatism. You may increase your predisposition to this condition if you are injured or involved in active sports or occupations that require repetitive motions. Those with poor joint alignment and older people with degenerative disease may also be at higher risk. Trained athletes in professional sports seem to have these problems fairly often.

Symptoms

There are probably hundreds of conditions that could be classified as soft tissue rheumatism. The chief symptom of these conditions is pain in the affected area. The pain can be so mild that it is simply an annoyance, or it can be so severe that you cannot move the joint involved. It is beyond the scope of this book to discuss each soft tissue disease in depth. Instead, let me give you a brief overview of the more common conditions.

Shoulders

The shoulder is a ball-and-socket joint with a wide range of rotation. It is the only joint in your body that can rotate 360 degrees. Shoulder injuries are very common among athletes, especially those in sports that require overhead motions, such as tennis or baseball. Possible problems with the shoulder joint include the following:

Rotator Cuff Tendonitis (Impingement Syndrome).
Three small muscles and their tendons hold the ball and socket of the shoulder joint firmly in place. These are the rotator cuff muscles and tendons. When you hold your arm straight up, the rotator cuff tendons can rub against the bone beneath and become irritated. Overuse can result in an inflammation of the tendons called rotator cuff tendonitis, tendonitis of the shoulder, or impingement syndrome. Sometimes the bursae are also inflamed. This is a very common cause of shoulder pain. Swimmer's shoulder is one example of a tendonitis of the shoulder.

A person with tendonitis of the shoulder may have soreness in his shoulder and may find it difficult to dress himself or put on his coat. Often he may find it difficult to sleep because he can't find a comfortable position.

Rotator Cuff Tear.
This occurs when a rotator cuff tendon ruptures or tears. The shoulder pain varies, depending upon whether the tear is small or large. This

condition can be chronic and occurs more commonly in older people. It generally follows excessive use of the shoulder.

Frozen Shoulder (Adhesive Capsulitis).

The ball-and-socket area of your shoulder joint is held together by a sleeve-like structure. When you raise your arm, this sleeve gets tighter; when you lower your arm, the sleeve loosens up. The pushing, pulling, and reaching movements of daily living keep the sleeve stretched and operating normally. A frozen shoulder typically follows an inflammation or injury that keeps you from moving your arm for a prolonged period of time. During a lengthy period of inactivity, the sleeve can form tiny adhesions that freeze the shoulder so that motion becomes difficult. If you have a frozen shoulder, you may experience a great deal of pain whenever you try to move your arm in any direction.

Shoulder Bursitis (Calcific Tendonitis).

This condition results when too much pressure is placed on the shoulder bursae and they become irritated and inflamed and expand with excess fluid. This happens to patients who play sports, such as baseball, that require a throwing motion. But I've also seen patients get shoulder bursitis from painting their ceilings or pruning their hedges. Sometimes calcium deposits form in the rotator cuff tendons and irritate the bursa sac, causing it to produce too much fluid. A patient with shoulder bursitis usually feels most comfortable holding his arm close to his body, with the forearm across the stomach. It may be very painful for him to try to move his arm away from his body.

Elbows

Tennis Elbow (Lateral Epicondylitis).

Obviously, this condition often affects tennis players, particularly those who use a top-heavy racket that is strung too tightly and who play with an improper backhand stroke, leading with the elbow. The impact of the ball travels from racket to forearm muscles to the elbow, causing the muscles and tissues of the elbow to swell from excess strain. Playing tennis on a concrete surface can add to the problem, because bouncing off of a hard surface increases the ball's velocity and impact. And when you use only your wrist to hit the ball instead of your entire arm, as you do with an improper swing, your elbow receives the brunt of the force. You don't have to be a tennis player to get tennis elbow, however. Many occupations result in overuse of the arms. Gripping tools improperly can tighten the muscles of your hand and forearm. Carpenters, gardeners, mechanics, plumbers, and dentists can get tennis elbow, too.

Most people with tennis elbow feel pain and tenderness over or near the affected area. Some say it hurts to shake hands or to lift a shopping bag or briefcase.

Golfer's Elbow (Medial Epicondylitis).
This is similar to tennis elbow, but is less common and usually less disabling.

Wrists and Hands

Carpal Tunnel Syndrome.
This condition is caused by pressure on the median nerve that supplies half the hand. The compression of the nerve results in pain, weakness, burning, tingling, or aching in the wrist and hand that may spread to the forearm and shoulder. Carpal tunnel syndrome is seen most commonly in women, especially during pregnancy and menopause. Symptoms may result from an injury or be part of rheumatoid arthritis. Some believe the condition can be caused by repetitive motions of the wrist such as those employed by supermarket scanners, seamstresses, or poultry workers. Shaking or rubbing the hand frequently makes it feel better, but some people with carpal tunnel syndrome have symptoms that don't seem to abate. If untreated, it can be quite debilitating.

de Quervain's Tenosynovitis.
This condition results from repetitive thumb use and injury and involves pain on the thumb side of the hand above the wrist. It is much more common in women than in men. The pain is usually dull and aching and develops slowly. The pain may radiate several inches up the forearm and down into the thumb. If you try to touch your thumb to your fifth finger, it may be quite painful. One forty-year-old I know developed de Quervain's wrist after the birth of her first child. She had to use a splint to reduce the movement of that hand, and was treated with a nonsteroidal anti-inflammatory. The problem eventually resolves itself.

Dupuytren's Contracture.

A thickening or fibrosis of the sheaths of connective tissue that may make it difficult to straighten the ring and little finger in one or both hands. Alcoholics and diabetics appear to have a predisposition for this problem. It is hereditary and occurs mostly in men.

Trigger Finger.

Tendons in the fingers may become inflamed, and bumps may develop on the tendons, preventing your fingers from flexing normally. You may even hear a snapping sound when you straighten your fingers. Trigger finger may result from repetitive tasks, such as doing needlepoint or peeling potatoes.

Lower Extremities

Prepatellar Bursitis.

The patella is the kneecap, and this condition is caused by an irritation to the bursa situated in front of the kneecap. The condition is usually caused by overuse and results in pain and swelling of the kneecap. Prepatellar bursitis is also known as housemaid's knee because it frequently occurs in women who spend a great deal of time on their knees scrubbing floors. It can also develop in people who have to stand on their feet a great deal or who have occupations, such as carpet laying, that require them to be on their knees a lot. The pain is usually not too severe unless you apply direct pressure to the area.

Patellofemoral Pain Syndrome.

This condition is also known as chondromalacia, which means a softening or wearing away of the cartilage behind the kneecap. It is thought to result from a misalignment of the knee joint. It can occur when a jogger or weight lifter puts too much pressure on the knee. However, you don't necessarily have to overuse your joints to develop this condition. One thirty-five-year-old patient of mine, a jogger, had abnormal knee alignment and started to develop pain even though he was running relatively short distances that normally wouldn't hurt most people. Pain is usually felt behind the kneecap, and any motion that requires bending, such as sliding in and out of a car or climbing stairs, may be difficult, and makes the pain worse.

Lower Leg

Shin Splints.

This condition involves a pain in the front of your lower leg and is common among athletes who do a lot of running. Shin splints result from several causes, among them a rip in a muscle in the back of your leg (this is the muscle that allows you to point your forefoot up); an inflammation of the membrane surrounding your shin; or small stress fractures of the shinbone. Movement usually makes the pain worse. You can treat shin splints with simple rest.

Feet

Achilles Tendonitis.

The tendon connecting the heel bone to the calf muscles is called the Achilles tendon. It is the largest tendon in your body. Achilles tendonitis is common in runners who overtax their bodies, but can also occur as a result of overexertion in other sports, such as basketball, squash, and baseball. Running on concrete and wearing shoes with poor support in the heels can contribute to the problem. The condition usually causes pain, swelling, and tenderness in the back of the heel. The tendon may feel stiff in the morning.

Achilles tendonitis can also occur in people with spondyloarthropathies, a type of arthritis that involves the attachment structures connecting ligaments and tendons to bone (see chapter 8). One of my patients, a twenty-eight-year-old jogger, developed pain in his Achilles tendon despite the fact that he ran only a modest amount, increased his mileage gradually, and did a proper warm-up before exercising. He tried new running shoes and then finally stopped jogging, but the pain persisted. Several months later, he developed a pain in his knee. This time he went to a rheumatologist, who took X-rays and noticed evidence of Reiter's syndrome. This patient's Achilles tendonitis had nothing at all to do with his running.

Plantar Fasciitis.

This condition is common in runners and involves a partial or complete tear where the ligament in the arch attaches to the heel bone. Bony growths or heel spurs may also develop. In fact, for no apparent reason some people develop only the heel spurs. This condition causes pain in the bottom of the heel. It may hurt to rise on your toes or walk on your heels. Plantar fasciitis can also occur from prolonged walking or from wearing shoes without adequate support for the arches (an orthotic insert can sometimes correct the problem). Like Achilles tendonitis, this condition can also accompany a spondyloarthropathy. A rheumatologist can help you establish the proper diagnosis.

Hip

Trochanteric Bursitis.
This condition occurs mostly in middle-aged and older people, and more often in women than men. It results from inflammation of the trochanteric bursa, near the hip joint. You'll feel the pain in both the hip and the thigh, and it may feel worse when you walk, rise from a chair, or lie on the affected side. Sometimes people who develop this condition have a disparity in leg length or osteoarthritis of the hip or spine.

Diagnosis

Since soft tissue conditions are so common, where should you go for a diagnosis? Your general internist or family practitioner will probably be able to diagnose and treat many of these problems. If you have a sports-related injury, you may want to go to an orthopedic surgeon who specializes in sports medicine. You might also want to consult a rheumatologist, because while these problems may be isolated local conditions, they can also be part of a systemic inflammatory disease. Margaret, a seventy-year-old woman, for example, came to our clinic after being treated for a swelling in the tendon of her hand. The swelling had developed very gradually, and her local physician thought it might be due to the fact that Margaret had been doing too much sewing. Her doctor placed her on a number of nonsteroidal anti-inflammatory drugs, but none seemed to bring relief. He referred her to Duke when Margaret's hand became reddened and her pain grew worse. It turned out that Margaret had an infection, which we were able to treat.

Your doctor will make the diagnosis based on a physical examination and medical history. Laboratory tests may be useful only to rule out other diseases. Soft tissue conditions can usually be diagnosed straightforwardly; extensive X-rays and lab work aren't generally called for.

Treatment

Treatment may vary somewhat, depending upon the condition. However, your doctor will probably recommend a combination of the following:

Rest.

Reduce your activity until the pain subsides. You may need to use a sling or splint to immobilize the area so that it may begin to heal.

Medication.

You'll probably use a nonsteroidal anti-inflammatory drug to help relieve pain. Though some doctors prescribe aspirin, many prefer other faster-acting NSAIDs such as Indocin, Motrin, and Naprosyn. To avoid gastric side effects, try taking your NSAIDs with your meals or together with an antacid.

Sometimes, if your condition doesn't respond to rest, splints, and NSAIDs, your doctor may suggest injecting corticosteroid drugs directly into the affected tissue. Corticosteroids act quickly, but can have potentially serious side effects when taken in high doses for prolonged periods of time. Corticosteroid injections, however, have less serious side effects than corticosteroids taken by mouth. Sometimes your doctor will also inject a local anesthetic such as Xylocaine into the area.

Heat or Cold.

You can try using ice packs during the initial stages of an acute condition to bring down the inflammation and swelling. Later on (usually after forty-eight hours), try heat treatments to ease the discomfort and encourage the flow of blood to the area.

Physical Therapy.

Exercise can be very important in the treatment of some forms of soft tissue disease, especially for more chronic and persistent problems, such as frozen shoulder. A joint that is held in one position for too long can rapidly lose its muscle tone and range of motion. To prevent this from happening, begin gradually exercising as soon as the initial pain subsides. Your doctor can suggest some gentle range-of-motion exercises for you to do at home. Do them faithfully so you don't lose any functioning in your joints. Sometimes your doctor may refer you to a physical therapist, who will assist you with exercises several times a week. In addition, the physical therapist may prescribe various immobilizing splints, orthotics for foot problems, and elbow wraps for tennis elbow.

Surgery.

Most of the conditions I've discussed are self-limiting and do not require surgery. However, for such conditions as carpal tunnel syndrome and shoulder impingements, you may need surgery. Surgery for carpal tunnel syndrome is relatively simple, involving a small incision around the wrist to release the nerves. Shoulder impingement surgery is a major operation that requires weeks of recuperation. Some shoulder impingement surgery is now done via arthroscopy.

Liniments.

Soft tissue problems are very common, and there are many over-the-counter medicines available to treat them. The most common medicines are liniments or creams, marketed for temporary relief of arthritis and rheumatism. These preparations usually contain a mild irritant, commonly methyl salicylate, which stimulates the skin's nerve endings to decrease your sensation of pain. Creams and liniments are not usually prescribed by physicians.

Prevention

Prevention is the best treatment of all. If you have been injured while playing a sport, I suggest you cut back on the intensity of your activity or try a new sport that does not stress your muscles and tissues as much. Then once you have healed and are feeling good again, you can go back and try the initial sport once more. Don't go back to exercising until you're pain-free; then proceed with caution.

Injuries often happen when you exceed your own physical limits. In fact, there's one case I am intimately involved with that illustrates this point—my own. I had been running 20 to 25 miles a week when I decided to increase my mileage in order to train for a marathon. I had two months to prepare myself, and over the next few weeks I worked up to 40 to 50 miles a week. At this point I noticed extreme pain in my Achilles tendon; in fact I couldn't even walk for several days. I had to take NSAIDs and stop running for a month. Needless to say, I didn't get to participate in the marathon. Though I consider myself in good shape, I learned that I am not a 50-mile-a-week runner.

It's never wise to exercise when you have persistent pain following exercise or when you have recurrent injuries. I know that others feel differently, but I think it's really not smart for the ordinary recreational athlete who's not involved in a competitive sport to exercise with pain. There is a difference, however, between the acceptable level of pain that results from vigorous exercise and the pain that results from being injured. I am especially concerned about young people pushing themselves beyond their physical limits. We don't know that much about the relationship between injuries and the development of degenerative diseases. There may be long-term consequences of overexercising that we're not yet aware of, so I'd advise you to play it safe and be cautious.

My prescription for sensible exercise and sports is this: Pay attention to your body and to the pains you're experiencing. And if you are embarking on a new exercise program, don't try to jump into it too quickly. Instead, learn to pace yourself and build up your strength gradually. Also, take time out before an activity to do warm-up exercises. By stretching your muscles beforehand, you can avoid most damage to tissues.

You should also practice good body mechanics. How you bend, lift, grip, and so forth can play a large role in whether you'll damage yourself. A physical therapist can teach you how to do certain jobs or sports with less strain.

Sometimes faulty equipment can add to injuries. If you have tennis elbow, try switching to a lighter-weight racket. Also, be sure you have the right size grip and are using the proper stroke, and use elbow wraps when you play. Wear good-quality shoes appropriate for your sport, and replace them often. Sometimes foot and heel problems can be corrected with orthotic devices prescribed by your physician.

Try not to do tasks that require prolonged repetitive motions. Vary your positions and take frequent breaks. If you have a chronic, recurring problem that is exacerbated by your job, ask your physician or physical therapist for advice on ways to modify your work so as to produce less physical strain. Perhaps you can rearrange your work surfaces or alter the way you perform a task. A person with wrist problems who works at a supermarket scanner all day, for example, can learn to pass products over the scanner using his entire arm rather than just his wrist. You may need to notify your employee health services about your work-related problem and get assistance from your employer for this preventive effort.

Prognosis

Many of these local conditions heal by themselves with adequate rest and therapy, usually analgesics and anti-inflammatory drugs, though some can recur and may take time to respond to physical therapy and retraining of body mechanics. With the proper therapy and exercise, most people are able to return to their former activities. Reinjuries can be prevented if you heed your body's signals and stop an activity that gives you pain.

SOFT TISSUE RHEUMATISM

Soft tissue rheumatism refers to a number of conditions that involve localized inflammation or injury of the tendons, bursae, muscles, and other soft tissues surrounding the joints.

CAUSE: Usually caused by injury or overuse from improper body mechanics and prolonged repetitive motions. May also accompany inflammatory joint diseases such as rheumatoid arthritis.

SYMPTOMS: Over a hundred conditions are classified as soft tissue rheumatism. Most involve pain in the affected area. Pain may range from mild and annoying to severe and disabling.

WHO GETS IT? Anyone who is injured or involved in active sports and in occupations that require repetitive motions.

DIAGNOSIS: A physical exam and medical history aid in diagnosis. Laboratory tests may be used to rule out other diseases.

TREATMENT: Generally a combination of rest, NSAIDs, applications of heat or cold, physical therapy, and exercise to strengthen muscles and retain motion of joints. Avoid reinjury through proper body mechanics; use of appropriate sports equipment; slow, gradual conditioning when embarking on a new sport; warm-up stretches before exercising. Avoid excessive increases in level of activity.

PROGNOSIS: Many conditions are self-limiting and will respond to adequate rest and therapy.

PART THREE

Treating Arthritis

Introduction

The Duke University Basic Arthritis Program

Duke University Medical Center is a nationally recognized center for patient care, research and teaching. Immunology and rheumatology have always played an important role in the university, and our arthritis clinic, established in the 1930s, was one of the first to deliver services in the Southeast. In 1989, to further highlight the importance of arthritis, Duke established the Duke University Arthritis Center to conduct specialized programs for arthritis treatment and research. This center embodies Duke's commitment to excellence in the care of arthritis patients and our leadership role in arthritis research and the education of medical students, physician trainees, and other health care professionals.

Part of our excellent reputation for treating arthritis comes from the fact that we are extremely systematic and thorough in our approach to patient care. We treat each person as an individual and tailor a specific program to meet his or her needs. We try to get to know our patients well and to help them understand their condition. This partnership between doctor and patient increases the likelihood for a positive outcome.

Although each patient receives individualized care, there are certain basic components that are part of every patient's diagnosis and treatment plan. We call this unified approach the Duke Basic Program, although similar programs may be followed in other institutions. Here are the elements of the basic plan that are used in most major arthritis centers across the country.

Thorough Patient Assessments

The first visit to the clinic is a very important time for both the patient and the physician. We take a great deal of time with our patients so that we can get to know them better and learn what impact their disease is having on their lives. We ask them about their work, their family and social relationships, and the recreational activities they enjoy. Physical, social, and emotional aspects of arthritis are all important, and must be considered together if we are to develop a treatment strategy that can be realistically followed. For example, it makes no sense to counsel the mother of an infant and a toddler to take several rest periods during the day unless you also help her figure out how to get help from neighbors and family so that she can get this rest.

We combine this personalized approach to arthritis with a detailed and thorough clinical assessment. We gather as much objective information as we can in order to make an intelligent treatment decision. We perform a thorough physical exam, and then, depending upon what we think the condition might be, we may order laboratory tests, X-rays, and biopsies. Sometimes we call in additional specialists for further consultation. When all of the data are assembled, we can design an appropriate treatment plan and set objective goals for treatment.

Multidisciplinary Team Approach

Another important component of the Duke Basic Program is our team approach to arthritis. Our health care team includes the rheumatologist; the nurse, who helps oversee the treatment therapies, such as gold injections; the physical therapist, who gives patients with arthritis exercises appropriate for their condition; and the occupational therapist, who teaches patients how to perform the tasks of daily living more easily. In addition, other specialists on the hospital staff are called in for consultation as necessary. If we have a patient with osteoarthritis who looks as if he might need hip surgery somewhere down the road, we'll send him to see our orthopedic surgeon. That way doctor and patient can get to know each other from the beginning. The orthopedist can follow the patient's progress with us, so that if we must decide whether surgery is appropriate or not, we can make the decision together. We may also refer patients to neurologists, neurosurgeons, psychologists, psychiatrists, and various other specialists.

One of the major advantages of working in a medical center is that we can talk to other specialists and get other opinions. Within the group, we present difficult cases to each other to review the results of important biopsies and X-rays. This team approach assures us that patients with specialized problems will get the most precise diagnosis and the most appropriate and up-to-date treatment possible.

The Duke Basic Treatment Plan

After the physical examination, laboratory tests, and appropriate consultations, we'll sit down with the patient and develop a treatment plan. The Duke Basic Program treatment plan has the following components:

- Use of nonsteroidal anti-inflammatory drugs to treat inflammation.
- Daily rest periods to conserve energy and prevent joint damage.
- Physical therapy and joint protection to maintain full range of motion in the joints and to prevent joint damage.
- Pain relief through medication, physical therapy, and psychological approaches.
- An emphasis on good health habits, including diet, exercise, and mental health.

In many cases, this basic approach to treatment is all you'll need to keep many forms of arthritis under control. However, some patients with more active disease may need to try some of the more potent medications. Occasionally they may also require surgery.

Patient Follow-up

Patient follow-up is an important part of the Duke Basic Program. We like to see patients at regular intervals to review laboratory studies and establish goals for therapy that can be verified by objective means. Regular monitoring for the side effects of drugs is important to make sure we are treating the condition effectively while minimizing the side effects. We try to keep the lines of communication open between health care providers and patients. When our clinic patients have questions or problems, they're encouraged to call the physicians here. We also like to keep the patient's referring doctor abreast of developments, and we work closely with him or her in the patient's treatment.

Research and Training

Duke University Arthritis Center is a prominent teaching and research center. Our researchers played a major role in developing allopurinol, a drug used to treat gout. And we are currently seeking better treatments for rheumatoid arthritis, lupus, scleroderma, and vasculitis.

Research and direct patient care go hand in hand. We get a better understanding of the disease process by following our patients carefully. Patients in turn benefit from our growing knowledge of better treatment techniques. Since we are also a major teaching center, medical residents, interns, and fellows gain valuable experience in the Duke approach both by observing our patterns of patient care and by treating arthritis patients.

The information in this section of the book is drawn from the main elements of our treatment plan at Duke. It should serve as a guide to help you discuss your own treatment options with your doctor.

14

Drugs

Since arthritis is not one, but over a hundred different diseases, there are naturally many different ways to treat it. In deciding which therapy is right for you, your doctor has to consider the form of arthritis you have, the severity of your condition, and the likelihood that it could get worse. Many people do well with the Duke Basic Program, in which case the only drug they'll need to take is a nonsteroidal anti-inflammatory. However, in some cases your doctor may recommend more potent medications that have a greater likelihood for serious side effects.

When you sit down with your doctor to discuss which treatment is best for you, you should review with him or her the relative benefits and risks of each drug. Which one is best for your particular form of arthritis? In what dosages? How often should you take it? What are the possible side effects? What are the alternatives to this treatment?

Your role in any drug treatment plan is crucial: You must take the prescribed drug as recommended by your physician and report any possible side effects promptly. When you adjust drug dosages on your own, you may render your treatment ineffective, even dangerous. By working together, you and your physician will likely find the therapy and the dosage that works best for you.

If your condition is under control, you may need no drugs at all; then again if you have a more severe case of arthritis, you may require a combination of drugs from different groups. This chapter provides a general overview of the five drug groups: aspirin and nonsteroidal anti-inflammatories (NSAIDs); analgesics; remittive (slow-acting) drugs; corticosteroids; and immunosuppressives (see tables 1 and 2).

Table 1. DRUGS USED TO TREAT ARTHRITIS

Aspirin

Drug	For What Condition?	How It Works	How Given	Side Effects	Reminders
Aspirin/acetylsalicylic acid. Many brand names.	For pain and inflammation of most types of arthritis (not used in gout).	Suppresses the production of the inflammatory substances that cause pain, swelling, warmth, and redness in many forms of arthritis.	Plain, buffered, enteric tablets. Much higher doses are called for when it is used for inflammation (12 to 20 tablets a day) than when it is used for pain relief alone.	Side effects common to aspirin and other NSAIDs include gastrointestinal irritation and upset, bleeding, fluid retention, liver inflammation. At toxic levels aspirin can cause salicylism (ringing in ears, hearing loss, and mental confusion).	Take with meals to reduce stomach irritation. Don't increase or decrease dosages on your own.

DRUGS USED TO TREAT ARTHRITIS *(continued)*

Non-aspirin NSAIDs

Drug	For What Condition?	How It Works	How Given	Side Effects	Reminders
See the list of NSAIDs on page 243.	For pain and inflammation of most types of arthritis.	Same manner as aspirin.	Available in tablet and capsule forms. Far fewer tablets required than with aspirin.	Most commonly gastrointestinal irritation, stomach pain, bleeding, fluid retention, change in kidney function.	Do not take if allergic to aspirin or other NSAIDs. Take cautiously if you have poor kidney function and if you are taking other drugs that affect the kidney (e.g., diuretics). Take with meals to reduce gastrointestinal irritation.

DRUGS USED TO TREAT ARTHRITIS (continued)

Corticosteroids

Drug	For What Condition?	How It Works	How Given	Side Effects	Reminders
Synthetic steroids that include prednisone, hydrocortisone, dexamethasone, methylprednisolone. Many brand names.	RA, SLE, polymyositis, polymyalgia rheumatica, giant cell arteritis.	Blocks release of inflammatory substances, suppresses white blood cell function. Quickly reduces swelling and inflammation.	By mouth, injection into the joint, locally on skin, intravenously. Dosage and form depend on type and severity of condition.	Increased appetite and weight gain; deposits of fat in chest, face, upper back, and stomach; water and salt retention; high blood pressure; osteoporosis; thinning of the skin; cataracts; acne; muscle weakness; increased susceptibility to infection; stomach ulcers; depression. Side effects for short-term therapy are less common.	Wear a Medic Alert bracelet. Adhere to your schedule; if you are unable to take the medication for some reason, notify physician.

DRUGS USED TO TREAT ARTHRITIS *(continued)*

Immunosuppressive Drugs

Drug	For What Condition?	How It Works	How Given	Side Effects	Reminders
Azathioprine. Brand name: Imuran.	Severe, progressive RA not responsive to NSAIDs or other remittive drugs; lupus with severe, progressive renal disease.	Blocks cell growth and suppresses white cells.	Tablet form, given as a single dose or twice daily.	Gastrointestinal problems, nausea, heartburn, increased incidence of infections, easy bleeding and bruising.	Take with food. Have regular blood tests. Report unusual symptoms and signs of infection immediately.
Cyclophosphamide. Brand name: Cytoxan.	RA (rarely used), SLE (occasionally), vasculitis. Used mostly in severe progressive cases, especially with organ damage.	Binds with cell DNA and interferes with cell growth and division.	Tablet (usually 1 to 2 tablets daily); intravenously (usually once a month).	Low blood counts, bleeding, infections, hair loss, bladder inflammation, and bleeding.	Drink plenty of fluids when taking orally. Have blood counts checked regularly. Report signs of infection immediately.
Cyclosporine	RA—though rarely.	Appears to suppress immune response and selectively inhibit white cells.	Swallowed in liquid form.	Prolonged use can cause kidney damage.	Is still experimental. Blood levels must be carefully monitored. Report signs of infection immediately.

DRUGS USED TO TREAT ARTHRITIS *(continued)*

Remitive Drugs

(Also called second line, slow-acting, and disease-modifying)

Drug	For What Condition?	How It Works	How Given	Side Effects	Reminders
Gold. Brand names: Solganal, Myochrysine (injectable); Ridaura (capsules).	Rheumatoid arthritis patients with serious, progressive disease who have not responded to NSAID therapy.	Works on immune system. May slow tissue destruction.	Injections, at first weekly, then more spread out. Also available orally (1 to 2 capsules a day).	Skin rash, mouth sores, kidney damage, problems with blood cell production. Oral dose may cause diarrhea.	Always have appropriate lab tests before each gold injection.
Penicillamine. Brand names: Depen, Cuprimine.	Serious, progressive RA unresponsive to NSAIDs, frequently after a trial of gold.	Probably affects immune cell function.	Orally. Doses start low and increase slowly from 250 milligrams a day during the first 3 months up to 750 milligrams a day after 6 months (full dose).	Similar to those of gold. Skin rash, mouth sores, loss of taste, stomach upset. Also, possible kidney damage and lowered blood count.	Take on empty stomach at least 1 hour before meals. May take several months to work. Have appropriate laboratory tests.

DRUGS USED TO TREAT ARTHRITIS *(continued)*

Remittive Drugs

(Also called second line, slow-acting, and disease-modifying)

Drug	For What Condition?	How It Works	How Given	Side Effects	Reminders
Hydroxychloroquine. Brand name: Plaquenil.	Serious, progressive RA unresponsive to NSAIDs; SLE, especially that causing skin and joint problems.	Probably affects immune cell function.	Orally. Tablet form, 1 to 2 tablets daily.	Rarely, visual impairment and eventual blindness, but this can be prevented by regular eye exams.	Need eye exam.
Methotrexate. Brand name: Rheumatrex.	Serious, progressive RA unresponsive to NSAIDs.	An antimetabolite that inhibits cell growth.	Tablets, usually taken once a week at 12-hour intervals, but sometimes given in one dose.	Nausea, vomiting, loss of appetite, mouth ulcers, scarring of liver (fibrosis), jaundice, diarrhea, infections.	Liver function tests must be performed regularly. Avoid alcohol.
Sulfasalazine. Brand name: Azulfidine.	For RA, but its use is restricted to clinical trials.	Unknown. Is a combination salicylate and antibiotic.	Tablet and liquid form.	Nausea, vomiting, diarrhea, loss of appetite.	Avoid if allergic to sulfa drugs or aspirin. Take after meals.

Table 2. DRUGS COMMONLY USED TO TREAT ARTHRITIS

	Nonsteroidal Anti-inflammatory Drugs (NSAIDs)	Corticosteroids	Remittive Drugs*	Immunosuppressives (Imuran, Cytoxan)
Rheumatoid arthritis	X	X (systemic and local)	X	X
Osteoarthritis	X	X (local)	O	O
Lupus	X	X (systemic)	X (Plaquenil)	X
Ankylosing spondylitis	X	O	O	O
Reiter's disease	X	O	O	O
Polymyalgia rheumatica	X	X (systemic)	O	O
Giant cell arteritis	X	X (systemic)	O	O
Scleroderma	X	X (systemic)	X (penicillamine)	O
Fibromyalgia	X	O	O	O
Soft tissue rheumatism	X	X (local)	O	O

X indicates drug may be useful for that condition.
O indicates drug is not usually used.

*Remitive drugs include gold, penicillamine, methotrexate, and Plaquenil.

Aspirin and the Other NSAIDs

Aspirin is truly a wonder drug in the treatment of arthritis: It relieves pain, prevents or lessens inflammation, and lowers fever. Many other drugs have been developed to mimic the actions of aspirin. As a group, these drugs are called nonsteroidal anti-inflammatory drugs, or NSAIDs. (The word *nonsteroidal* distinguishes these drugs from corticosteroids, which are more potent anti-inflammatories; *anti-inflammatory* refers to their role in reducing inflammation.)

Aspirin and NSAIDs are useful for virtually all arthritic disorders. Aspirin, however, remains the standard against which all other drugs in this class are measured because of its long record of safety and efficacy.

How Do Aspirin and NSAIDs Work?

All NSAIDs, including aspirin, reduce pain and inflammation because they inhibit cyclooxygenase, an enzyme that helps your body produce prostaglandins. Prostaglandins are chemicals that appear to play a key role in inflammation. They dilate your blood vessels and allow an increased blood flow to sites of injury or infection; they also interact with other substances released during inflammation, causing pain and fever. These actions contribute to the cardinal signs of inflammation—redness, warmth, pain, swelling, and loss of function. In addition, prostaglandins indirectly promote weakening of the bone and loss of cartilage, and may add to the tissue destruction in some forms of arthritis. By reducing prostaglandin production, aspirin and NSAIDs reduce the pain, swelling, and tenderness that usually accompany arthritis.

While all NSAIDs operate in basically the same way, their actions are not identical. One of these drugs may be more effective for you than another, and your doctor may want to try several before settling on the one that's best for you.

Aspirin

The active ingredient in aspirin is acetylsalicylic acid, a close relative to salicylic acid, which was first derived from the bark of a willow tree and was used to treat arthritic pain in eighteenth-century England.

Since aspirin is readily available without a prescription and costs so little, some patients wonder how effective it can really be. Aspirin is a very powerful and effective agent. It has two basic properties—it relieves pain (analgesic) and it alleviates inflammation (anti-inflammatory).

How Is Aspirin Given?

The size of a regular aspirin tablet is 325 milligrams, or 5 grains. The number of tablets you need depends upon whether you are taking aspirin to relieve your pain or to treat the inflammation. If you're taking aspirin for pain, you may need to take only two 5-grain tablets every four hours until you obtain relief. These doses are considered safe without a prescription. However, higher doses of aspirin are required to relieve inflammation and should be taken only under the supervision of your physician; they may cause serious side effects and require adjustment. In order for aspirin to work against inflammation, blood levels must be kept constant at 20 to 25 milligrams of aspirin per 100 milliliters of blood—20 to 25 milligram percent. That translates into approximately twelve to twenty tablets a day. The exact number varies, depending upon your size.

Prescribing the right amount of aspirin can be a little tricky, since no set dose of aspirin uniformly produces a therapeutic blood level. Most doctors take an educated guess and then adjust the dosage as necessary according to how you respond to it. I usually use the following scheme: I start a patient on twelve aspirin a day, divided into four doses at three tablets each every four hours. Each day thereafter, I ask the patient to add an additional tablet to one of the doses. As the aspirin in their bloodstream reaches the anti-inflammatory level, many patients report a ringing or buzzing in their ears. This is called tinnitus. At that point, I recommend they drop back by one tablet a day until the ringing stops and then have their blood levels checked. This usually happens within a day or two. Usually, they are close to the 20 to 25 milligram percent level, and this simple adjustment of one to two tablets is all that is needed. (Patients should never attempt this type of therapy on their own, since the process requires monitoring of the blood to be safe.)

Your doctor will check your aspirin levels with a simple blood test called a salicylate level. When the levels of salicylate in your blood get too high, your body may not be able to break down and excrete the aspirin adequately; any additional aspirin may cause your salicylate blood level to rise rapidly. For example, a dose of twelve pills a day may result in a blood level of 10 milligram percent. At thirteen pills, blood levels may rise to 20 milligram percent. At fourteen pills, it may be 30 milligram percent.

If you were to continue taking aspirin beyond that point, the blood salicylate level might soon be toxic.

If you are on long-term aspirin therapy, you must have your blood levels checked regularly. When I am starting my patients on a course of aspirin therapy, I may have their blood levels checked every few days. Later, when the aspirin program has stabilized, I may check their blood levels at less frequent intervals, possibly every few months or even just once a year. If a patient develops tinnitus, I have him or her reduce the dose of aspirin by one or two tablets a day.

If you are taking high doses of aspirin to treat inflammation, you have to be very careful not to take any more aspirin inadvertently. This is trickier than it seems. Many over-the-counter preparations, including cold medicines, headache remedies, and some stomach-relief preparations, contain aspirin. Read all medicine labels carefully. (See table 3 for common drugs containing aspirin.) When reading labels, look for the words *acetylsalicylic acid,* which means aspirin, or for *salicylate, salsalate,* or *salsamide*—close relatives of aspirin. *Do not exceed your prescribed dose of aspirin!*

Sometimes people will decide on their own to cut back on aspirin because of unpleasant side effects. For example, one of my patients experienced ringing in her ears and decided independently to cut back from sixteen to twelve tablets daily. The tinnitus disappeared, but her joints became swollen and tender. I recommended the addition of one and then two additional tablets a day, and at fourteen tablets her blood level was fine and the ringing disappeared. Please inform your physician before you make any changes in your aspirin dosage. Sometimes a small change is all that is needed to reduce unpleasant side effects without affecting the drug's anti-inflammatory action.

Side Effects

Though aspirin is generally safe when taken as prescribed, it and the other NSAIDs have several possible side effects. Aspirin inhibits the production of pain-causing prostaglandins. Prostaglandins, however, play other roles in the body: They protect the stomach lining, promote clotting of the blood, regulate salt and fluid balance, and maintain blood flow to the kidneys when kidney function is reduced. By decreasing the levels of prostaglandins in the blood, NSAIDs can impair these normal body functions. In fact, stomach irritation, bleeding, fluid retention, and decreased kidney function are the major side effects of NSAIDs.

Table 3. COMMON DRUGS CONTAINING ACETYLSALICYLIC ACID (ASPIRIN)

Alka-Seltzer
Aspirin (generic and brand names, including Anacin, Bayer, Excedrin, etc.)
Aspergum
Axotal
Azdone Tablets
B.A.C. Tablets
Darvon with A.S.A.
Empirin
Equagesic Tablets
4-Way Cold Tablets
Fiogesic Tablets
Fiorinal
Gelpirin
Lortab ASA Tablets
Norgesic Tablets
Orphengesic
Oxycodone w/Aspirin Tablets
Percodan
Roxiprin
Soma Compound
Talwin Compound
Vanquish
Zorprin

SOURCE: *Physicians' Desk Reference*

Gastrointestinal problems are quite common in patients on long-term high doses of aspirin and NSAIDs. Approximately 5 to 10 percent of patients have some physical evidence of stomach irritation when the stomach lining is examined with a fiberoptic scope (endoscopy). Though this may sound alarming, a mild gastric irritation shouldn't be confused with the serious ulceration that causes bleeding and hospitalization. Only one in every few thousand patients will experience this kind of ulceration; you're far more likely to have only the occasional heartburn if you feel any side effects due to aspirin at all.

Since aspirin and other non-aspirin NSAIDs can affect kidney functioning, you should avoid them if you already have kidney trouble. You should also avoid them if you use diuretics (water pills) or have congestive heart failure, kidney disease, or cirrhosis of the liver. Older people who have decreased kidney function due to age-related changes need to exercise caution when using NSAIDs. In general, NSAIDs have only mild effects on kidney function, and these usually reverse when you discontinue the drug. Occasionally, however, there may be serious renal problems.

Certain side effects seem more unique to aspirin and other salicylate compounds. These effects are known as salicylism and include tinnitus. Some people may even lose their hearing while on high doses of aspirin. Older patients who already have hearing problems may essentially become deaf on aspirin. However, when these patients stop taking the aspirin, their hearing will be restored to what it was before. In very rare cases, high doses of aspirin can cause salicylate toxicity, whose symptoms include mental confusion, excitability, abnormal breathing, chemical imbalances, seizures, coma, and—even more rarely—death. However, regular monitoring of your blood levels can help prevent this serious consequence.

Aspirin Preparations

Aspirin comes in three basic forms: plain, buffered, or enteric-coated. Buffered aspirin contains an antacid to reduce the acid content of your stomach and prevent irritation. The enteric-coated preparation has a special covering to prevent aspirin from dissolving until it has left your stomach. I prefer enteric-coated aspirin because it's less irritating, but other doctors may have their own preferences.

Always take your aspirin and other NSAIDs with meals because food will help reduce stomach irritation. Some doctors recommend that you sandwich your aspirin within a meal: eat something, take your aspirin, and then eat some more.

Sometimes your doctor will prescribe other drugs that you can take with aspirin and other NSAIDs to protect the stomach lining. These include the anti-ulcer medicines cimetidine (Tagamet) and ranitidine (Zantac), which block stomach acid production; and carafate (Sucralate), which coats the stomach lining. Recently, a new synthetic prostaglandin, misoprostol (Cytotec), has been approved and is being used to help patients avoid gastrointestinal ulceration and bleeding. This may prove a good alternative for people with serious previous gastrointestinal problems, allowing them to take NSAIDs more safely.

Many patients ask me whether it would be helpful to take "arthritis strength" or "maximum strength" aspirin. These over-the-counter preparations contain more aspirin per tablet than regular aspirin (there are usually 500 milligrams per tablet in extra-strength aspirin versus 325 milligrams in a regular tablet). So taking an extra-strength pill is almost the same as taking two regular aspirin tablets (although the extra-strength pill is probably more expensive). The maximum recommended dosage on the bottle (usually eight tablets a day) is still below the level needed to control inflammation adequately. I feel that if a person with arthritis has sufficient pain to warrant taking such products, he should see a physician who can evaluate his condition and prescribe appropriate treatment.

Patients also ask me whether brand-name aspirin is better than the generic brands. All such preparations have the same aspirin content and are equally effective. They may, however, differ somewhat in the number of impurities present and in the composition and consistency of tablets. Therefore you may be able to tolerate some brands better than others. Generic aspirin is generally cheaper than brand-name aspirin (less than a penny a tablet), while buffered or enteric-coated aspirin can cost three to five cents each.

Other Nonsteroidal Anti-inflammatory Drugs

While aspirin is still one of the most effective anti-inflammatory drugs we have at our disposal today, it does have its drawbacks. You have to take many tablets to get a therapeutic effect, and you have to remember to take them frequently (every four to six hours) to keep your blood levels high. That's because aspirin is quickly metabolized by your body and stays active in your bloodstream only a short length of time. In scientific terms, we say it has a short half-life (the time it takes the drug to go down to half of its beginning level). Aspirin also has some annoying and potentially dangerous side effects.

In view of these drawbacks, scientists have searched for drugs that are similar to aspirin, but that cause fewer problems. These are the nonsteroidal anti-inflammatory drugs. So far, about a dozen such drugs have been approved for use in the United States (see table 4 on page 243).

Most NSAIDs are available only through prescription; however, one non-aspirin NSAID, ibuprofen (the ingredient in Motrin), has been released for over-the-counter use. The amount of ibuprofen in over-the-counter preparations is lower than the amount you would get in a prescription. Ibuprofen has an excellent record of safety and efficacy. As with aspirin, long-term use of NSAIDs for treatment of arthritis requires the guidance of a knowledgeable physician.

As previously mentioned, non-aspirin NSAIDs also act by inhibiting prostaglandin production; and like aspirin, they relieve pain, inflammation, and fever. They also have similar side effects, including gastrointestinal upset, bleeding, fluid imbalances, and disturbances in kidney function. People with serious allergies to aspirin are usually sensitive to NSAIDs as well.

A major benefit of NSAIDs over aspirin is that NSAIDs have a higher potency and a longer half-life, and you need far fewer doses to achieve a therapeutic effect. In other words, 100 milligrams of a particular NSAID

Table 4. NON-ASPIRIN NSAIDs

	Brand Name(s)
Diclofenac sodium	Voltaren
Diflunisal	Dolobid
Fenoprofen	Nalfon
Flurbiprofen	Ansaid
Ibuprofen	Motrin, Advil, Nuprin
Indomethacin	Indocin
Ketoprofen	Orudis
Meclofenamate	Meclomen
Mefenamic acid	Ponstel
Naproxen	Anaprox, Naprosyn
Phenylbutazone*	Azolid, Butagen, Butazolidin, Butazone
Piroxicam	Feldene
Sulindac	Clinoril
Tolmetin	Tolectin

*No longer commonly used for initial therapy because of serious side effects with blood toxicity.

may produce the same anti-inflammatory action or pain relief of 1,000 milligrams of aspirin. So you may need only take one or two tablets of an NSAID a day versus twelve to sixteen tablets of aspirin. This makes it much easier for you to remember to take your medicine. In addition, some NSAIDs are less toxic and may cause fewer gastrointestinal disturbances than aspirin, and salicylism is not a problem with non-aspirin NSAIDs.

Every medication, however, has its own set of problems, and it sometimes takes many years until a drug's side effects are fully known. Over the last decade, three NSAIDs—Zomax, Suprol, and Oraflex—have been withdrawn from the market because of the high rate of accompanying side effects. New NSAIDs come on the market often and patients want to try them; however, I would not switch a patient from his current medication to a newer NSAID until its safety is well established, especially if the patient was responding well to current treatments.

Non-aspirin NSAIDs are usually more expensive than aspirin, though enteric-coated aspirin, usually prescribed for long-term treatment, approaches NSAIDs in price. Some would argue that if aspirin causes more stomach ulcers than other NSAIDs, you have to include the expense of hospitalization as a hidden cost. All things considered, I don't feel the differences in cost between drugs should be the usual deciding factor in planning long-term therapy.

You and your doctor should base the decision to switch from aspirin to a different NSAID on the following:

- Any intolerance you may have to aspirin because of its side effects (usually gastrointestinal trouble, tinnitus, and decreased hearing).
- Difficulty in complying with the high and frequent dosages required for an aspirin regimen.
- Failure to respond adequately to aspirin therapy (sometimes an NSAID may be combined with aspirin, although their actions are similar).

The decision to switch to an NSAID may also depend upon which condition you have. Many doctors believe that aspirin is the most effective treatment for rheumatoid arthritis and that indomethacin is best for treating ankylosing spondylitis and gout. It is not clear whether there is a scientific basis for these common preferences.

Not everyone responds the same way to a particular NSAID. You may find that while a certain drug brings you relief, someone else may derive little benefit from that same drug. This means that your doctor may have to try a number of NSAIDs before he or she finds one that is effective for you.

Things to Remember

If you're on aspirin to treat inflammation, remember to have your blood levels monitored regularly. Read over-the-counter medication labels carefully and avoid taking preparations containing aspirin. As with all prescribed medications, take NSAIDs regularly, according to schedule.

Analgesics

Acetaminophen

Relief of pain is an important part of our treatment program at Duke, and the major painkiller used, other than aspirin and NSAIDs, is acetaminophen. This analgesic is known by the brand name Tylenol, and appears in many over-the-counter drugs, including Datril and Tempra.

How Does It Work?

Acetaminophen does not inhibit prostaglandin production and is therefore not effective for treating inflammation. It acts instead on the brain, blocking pain perception and lowering fever.

How Is It Given?

Acetaminophen is taken orally in tablet or pill form four times a day.

Side Effects

Acetaminophen does not have the same side effects as aspirin and does not cause stomach irritation. I think it's an excellent choice for pain relief, especially for those with degenerative joint disease. Like aspirin, acetaminophen is available in regular and extra-strength forms. The most serious side effect is liver damage at high doses. Warning signs are abnormalities in liver function and jaundice.

Things to Remember

Acetaminophen is not an anti-inflammatory and will not relieve inflammation.

Narcotics

Sometimes arthritis patients with severe pain need the stronger relief from pain afforded by narcotics. Though effective, narcotics can be addictive, and are used only when other drugs such as NSAIDs have proven unsuccessful in alleviating pain. They are used only for temporary pain relief and are not substitutes for long-term therapies.

How Do They Work?

Narcotics work by blocking pain messages to the brain. You may eventually need more and more of a narcotic drug to get the same painkilling benefits, so you must be monitored closely while you are taking a narcotic.

How Are They Given?

Narcotic preparations can be given by prescription alone or in combination with aspirin or acetominophen as well as caffeine (for example, Darvon, Darvon Compound, Tylox, and Tylenol with Codeine). Dosages vary, but I always try to give the lowest dose for the shortest period of time.

Side Effects

Side effects of narcotics include drowsiness, mood changes, and constipation. Excessive doses can cause breathing difficulties, and narcotics should be avoided by those with a history of respiratory problems. The fact that you can become addicted to narcotics is also a matter of concern, especially in the treatment of chronic diseases; however, when you take them orally, as arthritis patients generally do, your doctor can control the amounts you take, and problems with addiction are unlikely.

Who Should Take Narcotics?

Narcotics may be necessary for temporary pain control pre- or postoperatively, or for occasional problems with severe pain. For example, I recently prescribed a narcotic for Joseph, a sixty-five-year-old patient with advanced RA who had to wait several weeks before a joint replacement operation for his left hip joint could be done. Joseph was in such excruciating pain that he was not able to sleep. A prescription of Tylox effectively eased his pain and allowed him to get his rest. After the surgery was done, the joint pain abated and Joseph no longer needed the medication.

Unfortunately, some people have problems with drugs and may use complaints of pain as a way of getting a narcotics prescription. A thirty-two-year-old man, Jim, came to my office requesting an injection of Demerol to treat his lower back pain. Jim had previously visited several doctors, none of whom was able to find an organic cause for his back pain.

Jim had a previous history of alcoholism and was taking a sedative three times a day without relief. When I examined Jim, I too was unable to find a physical basis for his complaints. I wondered if his drug use had become excessive and whether he might not benefit from psychological counseling. Jim and I had a long talk, during which I expressed my concerns; he followed my advice and scheduled a consultation with our psychology service.

Things to Remember

In view of the fact that you can become addicted to them, narcotics should be prescribed only when there are no other alternatives and should be taken only as directed by your doctor.

Muscle Relaxants

Who Should Take Them?

Muscle relaxants are usually not a major component of arthritis therapy. Some physicians prescribe them for low back pain and various musculoskeletal disorders, especially those associated with muscle spasm.

How Do They Work?

These drugs block the body's pain messages to the brain and may act as sedatives.

How Are They Given?

Muscle relaxants are given orally, in pill form. Some commonly used muscle relaxants are Parafon Forte, Flexeril, and Robaxin.

Side Effects

Side effects may include drowsiness, confusion, difficulty in concentrating, and visual problems.

Things to Remember

These are not anti-inflammatory drugs and aren't intended for long-term therapy, though some people with arthritis find that they provide temporary relief.

Remittive (Slow-acting) Drugs

Drugs in this group are used primarily to treat rheumatoid arthritis and only rarely for other conditions. These drugs are your doctor's second line of defense, used only when other, less potent drugs fail. They go by a variety of names, including *remittive, slow-acting, disease-modifying, anti-rheumatic drugs (DMARDs)* or *second line*. None of these terms is totally accurate, but each tells you something about the way these medicines work. Some physicians call these drugs remittive because they may slow the disease process down (though they only occasionally result in a complete remission). They are called slow-acting because it may take six to eight months for the drug to produce a response (though I've seen patients have good responses to some of these drugs in just a few weeks). They are referred to as second line because they are very potent and are therefore tried only after aspirin and other NSAIDs have been proven ineffective. I prefer the term remittive, since it describes the dramatic improvement some patients experience after treatments.

How Do They Work?

Though not generally anti-inflammatory, remittive drugs do decrease some of the signs of inflammation and may prevent or slow the process of joint erosion. Unlike NSAIDs, they don't reduce the body's production of prostaglandins and don't directly relieve pain or reduce fever. They appear to modify the body's immune system in some way that helps to slow the disease process. However, we don't understand exactly how they work.

Who Should Take Remittive Drugs?

Remittive drugs are usually reserved for patients with severe active rheumatoid arthritis. In rare cases, remittive drugs may be used for other diseases when all other measures fail; for example, ankylosing spondylitis and psoriatic arthritis with peripheral joint involvement. Joint and skin problems of lupus are sometimes treated with the remittive drug Plaquenil.

People with RA who are most likely to be prescribed remittive drugs are those who have failed to respond to NSAIDs; whose X-rays show they have joint erosion; and who have signs of poor prognoses, including high levels of rheumatoid factor or rheumatoid nodules. Since remittive drugs may reduce the immune mechanisms responsible for inflammation, they are also sometimes used to decrease a patient's need for corticosteroids, which should always be taken for the shortest possible time in the smallest possible dose because of their side effects.

If your arthritis is troublesome, but not causing progressive joint damage, the risk of side effects from remittive drugs may outweigh their potential benefits. Similarly, I don't think pain by itself is a sufficient reason for taking these drugs unless it is accompanied by signs of active inflammation.

Rheumatoid arthritis has its ups and downs, so I like to observe my patients for several months before starting this course of therapy. If a patient is not improving, I'll try a different NSAID first. I always continue NSAID therapy when I start a patient on remittive drugs; this is a combination therapy, attacking arthritis on several fronts.

Since remittive agents often take several months to work, trying them requires patience, commitment, and time. The rewards can be substantial, however, and often justify the wait. I have prescribed remittive agents for patients with active inflammatory rheumatoid arthritis who are in such pain that they must use a wheelchair. After only a few months on remittives, I've seen them undergo what is essentially a complete remission, such that they are able to get up and around with little pain and only minor morning stiffness.

A number of remittive drugs are used in rheumatology. The one you and your doctor choose will depend upon the severity of your disease and on any other medical problems you may have. Your choice will also depend on your willingness to take injections, your ability to get to the doctor's office for regular laboratory follow-up, and cost. Once you start treatments, your blood count, liver, or kidney function must be monitored carefully, depending on the drug you take.

Common Misconceptions

Before reviewing the available remittive drugs, I think it's important to discuss some common misconceptions regarding remittive therapy. First is the question of efficacy. Until recently, it was thought that remittive agents such as gold were not very effective. Studies have since demonstrated that remittive agents can be very powerful and effective. In fact some patients do get complete remissions when treated with them.

Second is the issue of safety. Many patients tell me stories about friends or acquaintances who have had bad reactions to these drugs. Sometimes my patients' fears are so extreme that they deny themselves the benefits of this therapy. One patient at the Duke University clinic, Bill, an insurance salesman with severe rheumatoid arthritis and joint damage, resisted gold therapy because he hated injections and because someone he knew had taken gold and had developed a severe rash from it. Bill's joints were highly inflamed, and he was in a great deal of pain. He had to take a great deal of time off from work, and it was hard for him to get around at home without his wife's help. Much of his time at home was spent in bed. None of the other drug treatments had brought Bill any relief, and after several months he finally agreed to the gold therapy. Bill was relieved to find that he didn't have any of the untoward side effects experienced by his friend, and after several months on gold, he was in much less pain and was able to go back to work and to return to many of his previous activities.

While serious side effects can result from use of a remittive drug, they are uncommon and are usually reversible once the drug is discontinued. Frequent laboratory monitoring will largely keep them from happening. You must always weigh the possibility of side effects against the risks of the disease itself. If left untreated, rheumatoid arthritis can result in deformity and prolonged pain. Its seriousness often justifies the use of remittive agents.

A third misconception concerns the length of time you will have to be on these medications. In the past, physicians used to prescribe brief courses of remittive therapy. When the drug was stopped, it was not unusual for a patient to experience a relapse of arthritis. We now understand that remittives must be used long-term to control symptoms. Once your symptoms have abated, you may have to stay on remittive agents indefinitely, though your doctor may try to decrease the dosage. So if you've used gold in the past and were discouraged when your symptoms returned, don't automatically discount another course of gold.

Finally, because some of the remittive drugs have been used to treat cancer, some people worry that they have cancer or that cancer has caused their arthritis. You might also have these fears, especially if you've looked these agents up in an encyclopedia of drugs or a medical textbook, where their role in cancer treatment is emphasized. Remittive drugs help slow the progress of arthritis by slowing down the rapid growth of synovial cells. Though slowing down the growth of cells is a useful action in controlling cancer, you are using remittive drugs to treat arthritis, not cancer. Hundreds of medicines can be prescribed to treat more than one condition.

Gold

Gold salts have been used for the treatment of arthritis for over fifty years. The discovery that they could be used as a treatment for arthritis was accidental. Jacques Forrestier, a French physician acting on the theory prevalent in his time that metals could treat infections, injected gold salts into tuberculosis patients who also happened to have arthritis. After a number of months, the patients' arthritis started to improve. Gold has been used for the treatment of arthritis ever since.

Who Should Take Gold?

In the past, gold was the first choice of many physicians as a remittive drug for patients with rheumatoid arthritis not responsive to NSAIDs alone; however, some physicians now prefer to prescribe methotrexate or Plaquenil first. Though response rates to gold differ, I find it works extremely well for about ten percent of my patients, and very well for another 30 to 40 percent. About 50 percent of all patients will discontinue the drug either because they experience side effects or because it doesn't work for them. Results are usually best when gold is taken early in the course of the disease, though it can be used at any time.

How Does It Work?

It's not known how gold works, though it appears to interfere with some functions of the white cells responsible for joint damage and inflammation. Though the drug may slow tissue destruction, it can't correct existing joint deformities.

How Is It Given?

The gold you'll be given isn't in pure, elemental form; it's part of a compound. Two gold-salt preparations are injectable and are usually administered into your buttock muscle. Myochrysine is soluble in water, and Solganal is oil-based. When you start gold salts, you'll receive a small test dose first. If you experience no ill effects, you'll receive gold injections on a regular weekly basis in increasing amounts: 10 milligrams, 25 milligrams, 50 milligrams, then 50 milligrams each week for a total of 1,000 milligrams. Thereafter, you'll receive 50-milligram gold treatments once every two weeks, then every three weeks, and then less often. Today gold is administered on a continuous maintenance basis. Each time you come in for your gold injection, your blood and urine will be tested.

Some patients find injections unpleasant and inconvenient. As of 1986, gold has also been available in oral form under the trade name Ridaura. The usual dose is one or two capsules a day. Initial patient monitoring for oral drugs is usually less frequent than for injectable gold. I may test a patient's blood and urine levels once a month.

Side Effects

The most common side effects of injectable gold are an itchy rash on the lower extremities and mouth ulcers that can be painful and annoying, but which usually disappear when you stop taking the medicine. Laboratory tests during each office visit help your doctor identify potential side effects at an early stage, before any damage is done. Protein in the urine and lowered blood counts signal possible kidney damage and problems with blood cell production, and require prompt evaluation and cessation of therapy. Occasionally you may have a more severe skin rash or lung inflammation.

Gold taken orally has fewer serious side effects, although many people who take the capsules have transitory diarrhea or loose bowel movements.

Things to Remember

- Gold can be used along with other drugs (NSAIDs).
- Always have your laboratory tests *before* you have your next gold shot.
- If gold works for you, but you develop a rash and have to discontinue treatment, you may be able to continue therapy again once the rash subsides.

• Myochrysine injections may cause a curious type of hypotension (low blood pressure). If you have heart disease or a history of stroke, you may prefer a different type of medication.

Penicillamine

Penicillamine (Cuprimine, Depen) became available to treat RA during the seventies. Penicillamine is distantly related to penicillin but has entirely different effects. It is called a chelator because it can bind heavy metals in the body. Penicillamine has actually been used to treat gold overdoses as well as conditions caused by copper buildup in the body. Patients allergic to penicillin can take penicillamine.

Who Should Use Penicillamine?

In my practice, patients with rheumatoid arthritis who have not responded to NSAIDs alone may try penicillamine, frequently after a trial of another remittive agent. It is effective in about 30 percent of patients.

How Does It Work?

The exact mode of action is not known, but penicillamine is thought to alter the function of certain white blood cells responsible for joint damage in rheumatoid arthritis. Penicillamine may become more active when it combines with the copper naturally present in your body.

How Is It Given?

Penicillamine is given orally. You begin with low doses and increase them very slowly: 250 milligrams a day during the first three months; 500 milligrams a day during the next three months; 750 milligrams a day (full dose) after six months. Thereafter, you must stay on this course of treatment indefinitely.

Side Effects

Many of the side effects of penicillamine are similar to those observed for gold. The most common are skin rashes, mouth sores, loss of taste, odd tastes, and gastrointestinal upset.

More serious side effects include kidney damage, signaled by protein in the urine and lowering of the blood count. Penicillamine has been associated with rare autoimmune problems that can cause damage to the skin or muscle weakness.

Things to Remember

- Take penicillamine on an empty stomach or at least one hour before or after meals.
- Penicillamine can be used together with NSAIDs, but the NSAID should be taken during meals.
- Be patient: The penicillamine may take several months to work.
- You may lose your sense of taste while taking penicillamine, but this usually improves after you've taken the drug for a while and is not a reason to stop the medicine.
- Since protein in the urine is an early symptom of kidney damage, some physicians instruct their patients to test their urine occasionally using a special strip of paper called a dipstick, which turns colors and indicates the presence of blood or protein in the urine.

Hydroxychloroquine (Plaquenil)

Plaquenil has been available for many years and was originally developed to treat malaria. It is simple to use and has few side effects. It does not require monitoring with blood tests.

Plaquenil is used for patients with rheumatoid arthritis who don't respond to NSAIDs. It's effective in about 30 percent of patients. Since it's simple to use, some physicians are more willing to give it a try early in the course of RA. It's valuable for patients who would benefit from a remittive agent but who have trouble getting to the doctor or the laboratory with great frequency. Plaquenil is also useful for patients with systemic lupus erythematosus, especially those with skin and joint problems.

How Does It Work?

We don't know exactly how it works, but Plaquenil appears to interfere with immune-cell function.

How Is It Given?

Plaquenil is given orally. The usual dose is one to two tablets a day.

Side Effects

Plaquenil is a relatively safe drug with few side effects. The one rare serious side effect is deposit of the drug in the retina, which can lead to visual impairment and blindness. This condition can be diagnosed by a fundoscopic eye examination before it can cause any damage. An ophthalmologist simply projects a beam of light through your pupil and then looks at the back of your eye through a microscope. This exam should be performed by an ophthalmologist every six months.

Things to Remember

NSAIDs can be taken along with Plaquenil and are frequently given together.

Methotrexate (Rheumatrex)

Methotrexate has been available over forty years and is widely used in the treatment of psoriasis, a skin disorder that can also affect the joints. It is also used in the treatment of cancer. More recently, methotrexate has been approved for the treatment of rheumatoid arthritis and is being marketed under the brand name Rheumatrex. It is rapidly becoming the drug of choice of many physicians for RA when NSAIDs fail to provide relief. Methotrexate works more rapidly than other remittive agents and can bring improvement in a matter of weeks, rather than months.

How Does It Work?

Methotrexate is an antimetabolite, which means that it interferes with the way cells utilize essential nutrients, in this case folic acid, one of the B complex vitamins. As a result, methotrexate may inhibit the activity of the immune system, thereby reducing inflammation. It may also slow the rapid growth of cells in the synovial membrane that lines the joint.

How Is It Given?

Methotrexate may be taken in tablet form. The entire weekly dose (7½ to 15 milligrams per week) is usually given once a week, frequently over a twenty-four-hour period (three doses at twelve-hour intervals; for example, at 8:00 A.M., 8:00 P.M., and 8:00 A.M. the next day). Some doctors prefer to give it in one dose. You may wish to start taking the drug on a Saturday morning so the possible side effects (mainly gastrointestinal disturbance) will not interfere with your work week. Though methotrexate can also be injected or administered intravenously, it is not usually given this way for rheumatoid arthritis.

Side Effects

Less serious side effects include nausea, vomiting, loss of appetite, and mouth ulcers. These problems often disappear or decrease with usage.

The most serious complication of long-term methotrexate therapy is a scarring of the liver called fibrosis. While you're taking this drug, your liver functions will be monitored by a few simple blood tests, usually every two to four weeks. In addition, a liver biopsy will be performed every one to two years after initiation of therapy.

Some physicians recommend a liver biopsy before starting methotrexate, but we don't do this at Duke unless a patient has a history of liver disease or heavy alcohol use. During a biopsy, a small piece of tissue is removed from the liver with a needle introduced through the abdominal wall. The procedure is not especially painful and is done under local anesthesia. It is often done in the hospital, because occasionally it may cause bleeding. However, it can also be performed on an outpatient basis if you can be monitored throughout the day. After the biopsy, you must lie still in bed on your right side for several hours. Such immobility can be unpleasant and even painful for some patients with rheumatoid arthritis. The local anesthesia may also cause some local burning.

More serious side effects may require a decrease in dosage. Approximately 10 percent of patients have to discontinue the drug altogether.

Other side effects of methotrexate include jaundice, diarrhea, mouth sores, and infections. It has also been associated with serious lung reactions, especially in smokers.

Things to Remember

- Liver function tests are best performed several days after your last methotrexate dose. This delay in testing prevents your doctor from confusing transient abnormalities in liver function that may be caused by the drug with real damage to the liver.
- Methotrexate and alcohol do not mix. Reduce or eliminate your

alcohol intake. With your physician's permission you can have an occasional drink.
• Methotrexate can be taken along with NSAIDs.

Sulfasalazine

Sulfasalazine is a combination salicylate and antibiotic that has been around since the forties and was originally used mainly to treat patients with inflammatory bowel diseases, such as ulcerative colitis. At one time it was used to treat rheumatoid arthritis, but its use was limited because of concern about side effects. It has been tried in a number of clinical trials as an alternative to gold, and there has been renewed interest in its use as a remittive agent that does not have the toxicity problems associated with gold and penicillamine. However, sulfasalazine has not yet been officially approved for arthritis treatment and its role in treatment remains uncertain at this time.

How Does It Work?

We do not know exactly how sulfasalazine works, although it has two potential actions—to block inflammation as well as to inhibit the growth of bacteria.

How Is It Given?

Sulfasalazine comes in tablet and liquid form.

Side Effects

Patients with allergies to other sulfa drugs or to aspirin and other salicylates should avoid this drug. Nausea, vomiting, diarrhea, and loss of appetite are common side effects. More serious side effects include urine problems, blood diseases, and severe allergic reactions.

Corticosteroids

In 1948, the Mayo Clinic in Rochester, Minnesota, treated a group of arthritis patients with daily injections of a corticosteroid. The results were startling. Within days, patients who had been stooped over and incapacitated by arthritis were standing, walking, and even dancing. These events, captured on film, were presented at scientific meetings, where they were greeted with great enthusiasm. The doctors who developed this drug received the Nobel prize. It seemed a cure for arthritis had been discovered.

Over the years, as the use of corticosteroids expanded, certain side effects of the drug emerged. The initial rejoicing about corticosteroid therapy gave way to the realization that these drugs had considerable toxicity when given at high doses for prolonged periods. The medical pendulum then swung in the opposite direction. Patients were warned of the hazards of these drugs, and their use became restricted. Some patients became so frightened of corticosteroids that they declined treatment.

In view of the history of this drug, you may feel confused if your doctor recommends corticosteroids for the treatment of your arthritis. Are these drugs miracle workers, or do they just cause more problems than they solve? The answer lies somewhere in between. Corticosteroids are potent drugs that can be of value when administered under proper guidelines. It is important to understand when they are needed, how they work, and how they can be taken most safely.

What Are Corticosteroids?

Corticosteroids are very potent and effective drugs that can quickly reduce swelling and inflammation. They are closely related to cortisol, a hormone naturally produced in the outer layer (cortex) of your adrenal glands, one of which sits on top of each of your kidneys.

Cortisol plays an important regulatory role in your body, including control of salt and water balance and regulation of carbohydrate, fat, and protein metabolism. It is released in increased amounts during times of stress or injury and can produce a feeling of well-being, sometimes even exhilaration.

When your body is stressed, the tiny pituitary gland at the base of your brain releases a chemical, ACTH (adrenocorticotropic hormone), which in turn stimulates your adrenals to produce cortisol. This extra cortisol allows your body to cope effectively with any stress, including infection, trauma, surgery, and even emotional disturbance. When the stress is over, your adrenal hormone production returns to normal.

The adrenal glands usually produce about 20 milligrams of cortisol daily, but can increase their production to five times that level when necessary. Most cortisol is produced in the morning. This so-called diurnal variation probably reflects the increased energy needs of the body early in the day.

How Do They Work?

Corticosteroids were first developed because scientists noticed that the symptoms of women who had rheumatoid arthritis often improved during pregnancy. Scientists began to search for the hormones produced during pregnancy that might be responsible for that improvement. Cortisol emerged as a likely possibility.

Corticosteroids exert a powerful action on the immune system. They block the production of substances that can trigger allergic and inflammatory actions, including prostaglandins. But they also dampen the function of white blood cells that destroy foreign microorganisms and help keep your immune system working smoothly. Indeed, one of the serious side effects of corticosteroids is an increased susceptibility to infection, frequently with unusual microorganisms that the immune system normally handles with ease. These infections are similar to those encountered by patients on immunosuppressive drugs.

Who Should Take Corticosteroids?

Corticosteroids are valuable in the treatment of rheumatoid arthritis, systemic lupus erythematosus, polymyositis, polymyalgia rheumatica, and giant cell arteritis. They are not used systemically for osteoarthritis, though they are sometimes injected directly into a painful joint.

How Are They Given?

These drugs are among the most versatile of medications. They can be given by mouth, injected into the vein or muscle, applied locally to the skin, or injected directly into sites of painful inflammation. Some corticosteroid preparations can be purchased over the counter for treatment of minor rashes.

Corticosteroids are valuable when used with other drugs because of their powerful anti-inflammatory and immunosuppressive actions. They are prescribed for both short- and long-term relief of symptoms, but are not usually given as an initial therapy for rheumatoid arthritis.

The most common corticosteroid prescribed for arthritis is prednisone, a synthetic agent that usually comes in tablet form. Prednisone is four to five times as potent as cortisol, so that approximately 5 milligrams of prednisone provide the equivalent of the body's daily output of cortisol. Many other synthetic corticosteroids, including hydrocortisone, dexamethasone, and methylprednisolone, are also available. All have anti-inflammatory properties, but differ in their potency and half-life.

At Duke, we often prescribe a brief course of corticosteroids for patients with severe, active inflammatory arthritis that is not responsive to adequate doses of NSAIDs or to the Duke Basic Program. Patients with severely swollen joints and severe systemic symptoms who have tried several NSAIDs with no success often respond within days to corticosteroids. Martin, a fifty-seven-year-old patient with rheumatoid arthritis, had been bedridden and running fevers when he was given corticosteroids. Within days his pain was completely gone and he even felt "a little giddy" about the dramatic improvement. His doses were subsequently lowered, and he was able to return to work for the first time in weeks.

Short-term Corticosteroid Therapy

When used on a short-term basis, prednisone or an equivalent corticosteroid is usually started at a moderate dose and then reduced over the course of one to two weeks. This is called a steroid taper. Its purpose is to achieve a prompt improvement in symptoms. Indeed, many patients experience striking benefit in a day or two.

In our clinic, a steroid taper is usually begun with 20 to 30 milligrams of prednisone a day, with dose reductions every two to three days (20 milligrams for three days; 15 milligrams for three days; 10 milligrams for three days; 5 milligrams for three days). Prepared dose packs allow patients to follow a steroid taper easily; some physicians inject long-acting steroid preparations that essentially accomplish the same thing.

Many patients continue to show improvement even after they discontinue steroids. It's possible that their flare would have resolved by itself and that the steroids simply reduced the severity and hastened their recovery. However, steroids may have the effect of "shaking up" the immune system, preventing a turn for the worse. In fact we may never know for sure how corticosteroids do their work.

Some patients find that, after a course of steroids, their severe pain and stiffness may return and can be as bad or even worse than before. This is not necessarily a rebound reaction. Such patients were probably not experiencing a flare of disease when they first started taking corticosteroids; rather, their disease may have been progressing to a new, more serious stage. Even though steroids have powerful effects, they may be unable to interrupt this progression.

Steroid tapers can be prescribed at any point in the therapy of rheumatoid arthritis. However, the doses of corticosteroids given at the peak of treatment far exceed the amount of cortisol the body normally produces, so tapers should not be given too frequently, since they can have serious side effects.

Unfortunately, some patients may request boosts of corticosteroids because these are so effective, and this can lead to their use as a mainstay of therapy. This can happen quite inadvertently. If a patient's medical care is fragmented, he can also receive far too much of the drug. For example, a patient may be seeing several physicians, each of whom will independently prescribe corticosteroids. He may be in great discomfort and will plead with his doctor to have the dosage increased, or he may boost the dose on his own. Even though it can be difficult, you must adhere to your doctor's prescribed dosage schedule to avoid becoming dependent on this medication.

Your doctor may prefer to inject synthetic ACTH instead of using corticosteroid tapers. The injected ACTH stimulates the adrenal glands to produce high levels of cortisol. Some physicians view this as a more natural or physiological way of achieving the same end.

Long-term Therapy

Sometimes patients with severe and persistent rheumatoid arthritis need prolonged treatment with corticosteroids. The doses used in long-term treatment are usually much lower than those used in tapers. Between 5 and 7½ milligrams of prednisone a day is sufficient for this purpose—the equivalent of the body's daily production of cortisol.

Often you may start your treatment with low doses of steroids along with a remittive agent. The corticosteroids can relieve your symptoms until you receive the benefits of the remittive agent. A forty-eight-year-old patient at Duke with severe and unrelenting rheumatoid arthritis in a number of joints was placed on an initial dose of prednisone to "cool" his arthritis down. When he returned to the clinic for a second visit, he was started on a course of gold therapy. He continued to take low doses of prednisone because we anticipated that it might take several months for the gold to be effective, and we wanted to help him bridge the gap. He understood that use of the corticosteroids would be tapered off, and hopefully eliminated altogether, as soon as possible. After several months he was doing very well and I gradually lowered his dose of steroids.

Once you are stabilized on a remittive agent, your doctor will gradually lower the dose of corticosteroids so that you are taking as little of the drug as possible. Eventually your doctor should be able to eliminate the corticosteroid entirely.

Patients who do not respond to remittive agents and the Duke Basic Program may be placed on an indefinite course of low-dose corticosteroid therapy. The long-term use of low-dose corticosteroids along with a remittive agent may have some advantages. It can lessen your pain and stiffness, thus permitting you to work and carry on with your normal activities, and it can improve the overall quality of your life. It may even prevent disease complications. Though steroids are intended to alleviate the symptoms while the remittive drug takes effect, the combination of therapies may be more effective than either alone and could hasten improvement of your condition.

Long-term low-dose steroids do involve a trade-off: they can produce great benefits, but they can also have serious side effects. However, when corticosteroids are used at the lowest possible doses, the risks of side effects can be minimized.

When you take corticosteroids on a long-term basis, you'll be taking a tablet of 5 to 7½ milligrams each day in the morning, to duplicate your body's natural rhythm in cortisol production. The usual tablet size is 5 milligrams.

Unfortunately, some patients will readjust their doses of corticosteroids on their own, without consulting a physician. They may discover that they feel better when they split the dosage, for example, or may decide on their own to take extra doses of the drug when their symptoms grow worse. These changes can have serious consequences. Splitting the dosage can increase the risk of side effects, as can an inadvertent escalation in the amount of the drug you are taking. Every decision you make about corticosteroids should be made in consultation with your physician.

High-dose Steroids

Only the most severe forms of inflammatory disease, often requiring immediate action, merit high-dose steroids. These include severe cases of systemic lupus erythematosus, polymyositis, and giant cell arteritis. Only in rare cases of rheumatoid arthritis so severe that it can cause serious tissue damage is such treatment required. In these circumstances, high-dose steroids are tapered as soon as possible.

High-dose steroids are daily doses of prednisone at 1 milligram per kilogram of body weight, or about 60 milligrams per day. (This is the usual starting dose and you taper down gradually.) This represents approximately ten times the normal level of cortisol in your body. Initial dosages are usually divided over the course of a day and then, as the condition improves, are consolidated into a single daily dose. Sometimes a preparation can be injected into your vein for even faster action. High-dose steroid therapy, especially in divided doses, is the most effective to date of any drugs as regards anti-inflammatory and immunosuppressive actions.

You may be asked to take high-dose steroids for weeks or even months at a time to control the symptoms of serious inflammatory disease. At such doses, side effects can be substantial, so your doctor may sometimes prescribe additional immunosuppressive agents, such as Imuran and Cytoxan, to get the inflammation under better control and to spare you the effects of high-dose steroids. Another strategy is to take high doses of steroids every other day, although this may be difficult if your condition is very painful on the days when you're off the drug.

Side Effects

Since corticosteroids have such a powerful effect on the body, it's not surprising that their side effects may be serious. Many of the side effects mimic Cushing's disease, a malfunctioning of the adrenal glands that results in an overproduction of cortisol. In fact, a combination of some of the side effects of corticosteroids is known as Cushing's syndrome. The list of potential side effects is rather lengthy, and includes:

- Increased appetite and weight gain.
- Deposits of fat in the chest, face (moon face), upper back, and stomach.
- Water and salt retention, leading to swelling and edema.
- High blood pressure.
- Diabetes.
- Osteoporosis.
- Cataracts.
- Acne.
- Muscle weakness.

- Thinning of the skin.
- Increased susceptibility to infection.
- Stomach ulcers.
- Psychological problems, ranging from depression to psychosis.
- Adrenal suppression and adrenal crisis (see below).

You can minimize side effects by working very closely with your doctor and avoiding self-regulation of your dosage, either adjusting or dividing doses without medical guidance. If you're being treated by more than one doctor, you need to keep each informed about your medications so that you don't inadvertently receive additional doses of corticosteroids.

Adrenal Crisis

Corticosteroids are in a sense addictive substances. High doses can cause your own adrenal glands to stop production of cortisol and can lead to a dependency on the drug. Then, when you come under stress, you may not produce enough cortisol to meet your body's demands. This is called adrenal insufficiency or crisis, a serious, life-threatening condition characterized by weakness, disturbance of salt and water balance, low blood pressure, and eventually shock.

Adrenal insufficiency can occur any time your body is heavily stressed, as during an infection, after surgery, or after a heart attack. It can happen during an illness, when you might be unable to take your daily corticosteroid pills because of stomach upset, nausea, or vomiting. It can also develop when you become unconscious and the physician caring for you is unaware of your drug regimen.

Fortunately, physicians can effectively treat adrenal suppressions as long as they are aware of the problem. They'll increase your corticosteroids to "stress levels" temporarily, balance your body's fluids, and treat your underlying condition.

A patient on corticosteroids should wear a Medic Alert bracelet or necklace indicating that he or she is taking corticosteroids so they can be administered in the event of an accident or serious illness.

Side effects of steroids are more severe when corticosteroids are given in frequent high doses; that's why doses are kept as low as possible and given once a day.

Coming Off Steroids

When steroid dosages are reduced or eliminated, they have to be decreased gradually so as to permit your own glands to resume production of cortisol. If doses are lowered too rapidly, adrenal insufficiency problems will occur.

When your disease is under control, your doctor will gradually reduce your dosage of steroids, watching to see if your disease symptoms recur. There's no single laboratory test that can show whether rheumatoid arthritis is active; so if you have RA, your doctor will base his or her decisions on the appropriate dosage largely on your symptoms, the physical exam, and the sed rate and other blood work. However, if you have other forms of arthritis, your doctor can use more objective tests to see how active the condition is. In the case of lupus, your doctor can gauge disease activity by measuring complement and anti-DNA levels; he can check CPK levels to assess activity levels in polymyositis (see chapters 3 and 10).

When corticosteroids are given in low doses for long periods of time, the tapering process can continue for months or even years. Sometimes your dosages will be lowered by only 1 milligram at a time. Any larger amount may lead to a flare. It's amazing that the body can sense the difference between 4 and 5 milligrams, but it does. When you take corticosteroids for only short periods of time, the tapering process is more rapid, and decreases in dosages can be much larger.

Another possible problem when coming off steroids is steroid withdrawal syndrome, your body's exaggerated response to removal of the drug from your system. This drug's rebound effect can cause fever, muscle pain, and joint pain. Your physician may find it hard to distinguish between withdrawal symptoms and a return of disease. A doctor may put the patient back on a dose of steroids to control the symptoms and then try the taper again more gradually.

Steroid Injections

Corticosteroids can be injected directly into the joints. This is called intra-articular therapy. It is a great advance in treatment, because it permits doctors to use very high doses of corticosteroids directly at the site of inflammation, but spares the rest of the body from high concentrations of the drug.

Intra-articular steroids are used when your joint inflammation has failed to respond to the Basic Program or to remittive agents and possibly to systemic corticosteroids. Usually only a single joint will be injected at a time, although several joints can be treated at once if you have serious, active disease. Joints of all sizes can be injected. Steroid injections are also useful for treating the inflamed bursae and tendons of rheumatoid arthritis and for the localized pain of bursitis and tendonitis.

Joints severely damaged by long-standing disease are usually not treated by injection unless they are inflamed, because injections are frequently ineffective in such instances. In addition, you would not inject a joint that is infected because there is a danger that the infection will spread or worsen; when possible, your doctor should examine your joint fluid for signs of infection before administering steroid injections.

The intra-articular injections can be done on an in- or outpatient basis. Your skin will be cleansed with iodine antiseptic, followed by a topical local anesthetic that freezes the skin where the needle is inserted. If there is enough fluid inside the joint, it may be withdrawn first for examination. Removal of fluid from the joint provides more room there for the corticosteroids (the extra fluid from the injection can sometimes cause joint pain). The injectable corticosteroid preparations are crystalline. They dissolve slowly and are long-acting.

Prolonged relief from pain often follows an intra-articular injection. There may also be a decrease in swelling and inflammation of the synovial lining. Some physicians call this a chemical synovectomy. These responses may reduce your need for a remittive agent or enable you to delay surgery.

As with any procedure, joint injections have potential side effects. These include the small possibility of introducing an infection into the joint or inducing a reaction to the drug crystals, producing a kind of synovitis. Frequent injections into the same joint can cause cartilage damage. In view of these side effects, intra-articular injections are used sparingly and physicians avoid repeated injections into the same joint. As a general principle, I don't like to inject each joint more than once every six months, with a total of only a few injections throughout the course of therapy.

Many patients find the first joint injection produces the greatest benefits, providing months or even years of relief. Successive injections seem less effective, and subsequent relief may last only days or weeks. I don't like to give intra-articular injections when the benefits are so short-lived and at that point will consider the alternative of surgery.

Things to Remember

Avoid frequent injections into joints and take it easy for a few days after the injection. Call your doctor if your joint feels worse after the injection.

Immunosuppressive Drugs

Immunosuppressive drugs are potent drugs that can suppress the immune system and are therefore useful in treating rheumatoid arthritis and other immune system diseases. However, because they can have potentially serious side effects, especially when used in conjunction with corticosteroids, they are used sparingly in the treatment of arthritis; they are reserved for cases in which patients fail to respond to corticosteroid therapy or in which there is very serious potential for tissue injury. Immunosuppressives are routinely prescribed for lupus patients with severe kidney disease and may also be used in the treatment of rheumatoid arthritis and polymyositis.

Some immunosuppressive drugs are also called cytotoxic, because they kill rapidly dividing cells. They seem to act by suppressing the body's immune response, thereby blocking the actions of potentially damaging cells. In the process, they may also reduce the body's ability to fight injury and infection. The major immunosuppressive drugs used for arthritis are Imuran, Cytoxan, and cyclosporine. Some physicians place methotrexate within this group as well.

Azathioprine (Imuran)

Imuran is called an antimetabolite because it interferes with the utilization of essential nutrients by cells. It works by blocking your body's production of purines and by inhibiting the growth of rapidly dividing cells. Imuran is also called an immunosuppressive drug because it suppresses white blood cells and lowers the body's response to infection and foreign microorganisms.

Who Should Use Imuran?

Imuran's major use has been to prevent rejection of grafts in kidney and heart transplantation. It has also been used over the past fifteen years to treat severe unremitting rheumatoid arthritis. It is also used in other instances where immune suppression is desired—for example, in treatment of lupus and other serious immune disorders. It is used far less frequently for rheumatoid arthritis than the other drugs I have discussed, probably because of concern about its side effects.

How Is It Given?

Imuran is given in tablet form, usually once a day in doses of 1 to 2 milligrams per kilogram. In some cases, as for chronic rheumatoid arthritis, it may be prescribed indefinitely; in other cases, it may be tapered or discontinued.

Side Effects

Approximately 10 percent of patients have serious side effects that may force them to discontinue use of the drug. These side effects include:

- Gastrointestinal disturbances such as nausea, vomiting, and heartburn.
- Increased incidence of infections (caused by the decreased number of white blood cells).
- Easy bruising and bleeding (caused by the decreased number of platelets).

When Imuran was used along with corticosteroids to prevent organ rejection in patients undergoing kidney transplants, the drug was associated with an increased risk of cancer. No such increase in the incidence of cancer has been observed so far in patients being treated with Imuran for rheumatoid arthritis. Still, this observation makes doctors increasingly vigilant during follow-up monitoring.

Things to Remember

- Take this drug with meals to reduce gastrointestinal discomfort.
- Have regular blood counts performed, approximately every two to four weeks.
- Report any unusual symptoms, including infections, fever, headaches, and breathing problems.
- Aspirin and NSAIDs can be taken together with Imuran.

Cyclophosphamide (Cytoxan)

This is a very powerful drug with major side effects. Cytoxan is reserved for only the most serious immune-related disorders. In cases of rheumatoid arthritis, this is usually only when there is widespread and life-threatening blood vessel inflammation that causes major organ damage. Fortunately, cyclophosphamide is rarely needed to treat RA, although it is commonly used to treat severe systemic lupus erythematosus that has not responded to corticosteroids and a group of conditions related to arthritis called vasculitis.

How Does It Work?

Cytoxan is called an alkylating agent because it directly binds (alkylates) DNA in the cell, causing permanent genetic damage. This chemical reaction interferes with cell growth and division. This drug is also called cytotoxic because it kills cells (*cyt* = cell, *toxic* = poison). Specifically, Cytoxan appears to kill lymphocytes.

How Is It Given?

Cytoxan is generally given in tablet form, usually one to two tablets per day (1 to 2 milligrams per kilogram). It can also be given intravenously in higher doses of 3 to 5 milligrams, given approximately once a month. The latter form of administration is known as pulse Cytoxan and is being increasingly used for severe cases of lupus. Pulse Cytoxan may help patients avoid exposure to continuous doses of the drug and decrease chances of bladder problems or malignancies.

Side Effects

Cytoxan destroys or inhibits rapidly growing cells. It can't distinguish between the "bad" cells that you want to destroy and the "good" cells that keep you healthy. As a result, it may damage rapidly dividing cells in the bone marrow (where your red blood cells are formed), gastrointestinal tract, and hair. This can result in bone marrow suppression with low blood cell counts, bleeding, and infections. Cytoxan can also cause severe inflammation and bleeding from the bladder (hemorrhagic cystitis), the first signs of which are painful urination and blood in the urine. There may be extensive hair loss—though the hair usually grows back once therapy is stopped. Over time, alkylating agents may cause an increased incidence of certain cancers related to chromosome damage, as well as decreased fertility. Your doctor will monitor you extremely carefully while you're on Cytoxan to minimize or prevent these side effects.

Things to Remember

- When Cytoxan is taken orally, it is important to drink enough fluids (1 to 2 quarts a day) to keep the concentration of the drug in the urine low. This will help prevent bladder damage.
- Report any symptoms to your doctor—for example, bruising, bleeding, weakness, and fatigue.
- Blood counts must be performed regularly, usually every few weeks.

Cyclosporine

Cyclosporine, formerly called cyclosporine A, is a new drug currently used to prevent organ transplant rejection. Since it appears to suppress the body's immune response, it is also being used experimentally for rheumatoid arthritis patients and for patients with other immune-related disorders. It is not usually used for rheumatoid arthritis patients unless they haven't responded to remittive drugs.

How Does It Work?

Other immunosuppressive drugs indiscriminately inhibit or destroy fast-growing cells. However, cyclosporine acts selectively on white blood cells. It works especially well on helper T cells and some B cells, the cells that play a large role in the inflammatory action that can damage the joint and its surrounding tissues. Because it does not affect the bone marrow, it does not cause serious low blood counts like other immunosuppressives.

How Is It Given?

Cyclosporine comes in an oil. It is mixed with fluids and swallowed. The length of treatment varies according to your condition. In view of its side effects, however, doctors prefer to prescribe cyclosporine for the shortest time possible.

Side Effects

Patients on cyclosporine must be closely watched for side effects. The possibility of kidney damage is a major limitation on its use for long-term therapy. Other side effects include muscle tremors, gum problems, excessive hair growth, and hypertension.

Things to Remember

- Cyclosporine is still an experimental drug. Its long-term effects are unknown.
- Treatment is very expensive and may cost thousands of dollars a year.
- Your blood levels must be carefully monitored to prevent kidney damage. The frequency of monitoring depends on whether you have underlying renal or heart disease and on how you are responding to treatment.

Drugs to Treat Crystal-induced Arthritis

In general, NSAIDs are the drugs of choice for pseudogout and may also be used to treat gout. Colchicine, probenecid (Benemid), and allopurinol (Zyloprim) play a prominent role in the treatment of gout. Please turn to chapter 9 for a full discussion of these drug treatments.

New or Experimental Drugs

Table 1 summarizes the many drugs I've discussed in this chapter.

Scientists continue to investigate the causes of arthritis and experiment with new and better drugs that may one day help prevent or slow the progress of these diseases. Different types of arthritis require distinctly different strategies, and progress is ongoing in a number of different areas.

There has been an enormous increase in the knowledge of immunology within the last ten years. Scientists are looking for ways to alter rheumatoid arthritis either by interrupting the abnormal cell processes promoting this disease or by blocking the many stages of the inflammatory response itself. For RA and lupus, efforts are being made to develop immunosuppressive drugs that would target the cells directly responsible for arthritis without damaging other cells. In osteoarthritis, there is much interest in studying the effects of various therapies on cartilage and in developing agents that can promote cartilage growth and inhibit its breakdown. We are also investigating the possible role of infectious agents in and use of antibiotics to treat such diseases as Reiter's syndrome.

We have made great strides in the prevention of arthritis related to rheumatic fever, so that such cases are virtually unheard of today. We have also learned how to manage gout very well. The NSAIDs we've developed are really quite effective, and their side effects are generally well tolerated. As research continues in this field, new and better strategies for combating arthritis will undoubtedly soon emerge.

15

Rest and Exercise

Rick, a fifty-five-year-old professional photographer, has active rheumatoid arthritis. His symptoms have been kept under good control with the nonsteroidal anti-inflammatory drugs I prescribed for him. Lately, however, he'd been having problems with his shoulders. They've been hurting him a great deal and interfering with his ability to work in his studio. Because of the pain, he'd been avoiding movements involving his shoulders. When I examined Rick, I noticed that he was having difficulty moving his shoulder joints through their full range of motion. I became concerned and sent him to see the physical therapist on staff, who prescribed a few exercises for Rick to do daily. These involved "walking" his fingers up a wall while facing the wall and again with his side to the wall. These exercises helped Rick gradually raise his shoulders above his head. When I examined him a month later, I noticed that he had a much greater range of motion. Two months later, his shoulder movements were essentially back to normal, and he said he felt very satisfied with the results of his exercise program.

Arthritis patients in the Duke Basic Program are given two seemingly contradictory pieces of advice: namely, to rest and to exercise. How can you rest your joints and exercise them at the same time? The key here is to understand the principles of proper rest and exercise and to strike a balance between the two.

At Duke, the physical therapist is the person on the health care team who teaches patients about the physical aspects of disease and the importance of physical training and exercise in promoting recovery. The physical therapist may work not only with arthritis patients but also with those recovering from injuries, heart attacks, strokes, and other medical conditions.

Often, the physical therapist will spend a good hour or two with you, evaluating your particular condition and special exercise needs. Working in conjunction with your physician, the therapist can set up a daily exercise program to keep your joints as healthy and mobile as possible. The physical therapist can also advise you on how much exercise to do and when to cut back and rest. When necessary, he or she can also prescribe splints, canes, and special shoes and may administer pain relief measures such as heat, cold, and ultrasound treatments (see chapter 17).

Benefits of Rest

While activity is important in maintaining the health of your joints, so is getting the appropriate amount of rest. If you have a systemic inflammatory disease, such as rheumatoid arthritis or lupus, you may notice that you tire more easily and that you have to learn to pace yourself. Some days may be better than others; and when you're feeling weak and fatigued, it pays to heed your body's signals and conserve your energy.

I encourage my patients to incorporate several rest periods into their daily routines; to take a brief nap daily, if possible, and to try to get adequate sleep. Sometimes these suggestions are difficult to follow, especially if you have a demanding job or are the parent of young children. However, I've had executives tell me that they have managed to push some of their work aside and slip a brief nap or rest period into their day. One corporate CEO says he gets a thirty-minute nap on a sofa in an empty conference room at lunchtime every day.

How do you know if you're not getting enough rest? If you feel fatigued, and if an activity causes you pain for more than two hours after you stop, then you need to slow down. Ideally, you should rest *before* you tire. You might also try planning your day so that you tackle the more difficult tasks when you have the most energy.

Energy conservation may also mean being less of a perfectionist. One fastidious homemaker felt she had to vacuum and mop the floors every day so the house would come up to her high standards. At the end of each day she felt stiff and sore, and her arthritis continued to grow worse. When she reviewed her daily activities with the physical therapist at our clinic, it became apparent that she was driving herself too hard. She was advised to reorder her priorities and to talk to her husband and children about her need for several uninterrupted rest periods during the day.

Adequate rest is also important during a flare-up of your arthritis, when your joints are highly inflamed. Continued stress to your joints under these circumstances can be painful and may even accelerate joint damage.

On the other hand, too much inactivity can itself be a problem. If you've ever spent a few days in bed with illness, you know how stiff and weak your joints can feel after a period of inactivity. When a joint is immobilized for too long, its functioning may become impaired—sometimes permanently. This is true for everyone, not just those with arthritis. People who break an arm or a leg, for example, find that after several weeks with the limb in a cast their muscles have grown smaller and weaker.

In the past, we used to treat arthritis with bed rest and instructed patients to lead restricted lives. Unfortunately, many patients experienced an unnecessary loss in functional capacity, sometimes with long-term results. Physicians learned through observation that even rest can be overdone and needs to be balanced with exercise.

Benefits of Exercise

While vigorous exercise is not possible for everyone with arthritis, a physical therapist can work with you to design a program appropriate for your needs and abilities.

Exercise has special advantages as far as your joints are concerned. By moving your joints daily, you help keep them fully mobile. You also strengthen the surrounding muscles, which means added joint support. Weight-bearing exercises help keep your bones strong and so reduce your chances of osteoporosis, a disease characterized by thinning bones, sometimes associated with arthritis. Joint movement also transports nutrients and waste products to and from your cartilage, maintaining the health of this resilient material that protects the ends of your bones.

The benefits of exercise extend far beyond your joints. Aerobic exercise is a superb cardiovascular conditioner, keeping your lungs and heart functioning well. It is a natural relaxant and mood elevator and can make you feel happier and more in control of your life. Exercise promotes more refreshing sleep and aids digestion and elimination. It can also help you keep your weight in check, which means you put less stress on your joints. One patient who joined a water exercise class says it is a way to see friends and talk to people and is one of the most enjoyable parts of her day.

Exercise clearly has many advantages. It's good for your overall health; and if you have arthritis, it can help keep your joints healthy and prevent loss of mobility. As with rest, however, exercise can be overdone. Sometimes when people feel good they push themselves too hard. One forty-four-year-old patient told me he felt so good one day that he went out and played touch football with his young sons for almost an hour. The next morning he paid the price. He felt terrible. His joints hurt worse than they had for months.

So while some exercise is good, you have to respect your own limitations. In addition, you may need to cut back on your activity when your joints are inflamed and painful. In such instances, exercise can make joints feel worse.

Before You Begin: Evaluation by a Physical Therapist

No one with arthritis should embark on an exercise program without first consulting his physician. I highly recommend that you receive a full medical evaluation first. Many arthritis patients are older and may have heart problems that have not been apparent because of a sedentary lifestyle. Depending upon your condition and history, your physician may want to consider doing a stress test. During a stress test, you'll walk on a treadmill or pedal a stationary bicycle while your pulse and blood pressure are monitored by an electrocardiogram machine. The test takes about fifteen minutes and is usually done in the doctor's office or in a hospital laboratory. (This type of test may be more difficult for some arthritis patients because of physical limitations.)

Your doctor may refer you to a physical therapist who can design an exercise program suited to your particular needs. Physical therapists practice in the hospital and in outpatient settings. You don't necessarily need a physician referral to be treated by a physical therapist; however, I think you should have a complete evaluation by a rheumatologist before you consult a physical therapist. This assures a sound diagnosis and treatment plan and the proper coordination of your future care.

The physical therapist will begin with a complete assessment of your joints, determining the range of motion in each one and the strength of your muscles. These will be recorded to serve as a baseline against which to gauge future improvement. The therapist will observe your gait to see if you have a limp or imbalance. He or she will examine your feet, since problems with the feet can cause considerable pain and may prevent you from participating in an appropriate exercise program. Based on this exam, the therapist may recommend a cane, special shoes, or splints to aid your mobility.

If you have a mild form of arthritis, you may need to see the physical therapist only once or twice for education and occasionally thereafter for exercise review. However, some patients, especially those who are hospitalized with more severe joint problems, may need to see the physical therapist several times weekly and may need physical assistance with exercises. If you've had joint surgery, the physical therapist will play a major role in your rehabilitation, helping you to walk again. The goal of therapy is to enable you to do your exercises independently, at home or at work.

The specific goals of your exercise program depend upon your condition. The emphasis with rheumatoid arthritis, for example, may be on range-of-motion exercises. If you have osteoarthritis, the emphasis will be on exercises to strengthen the muscles around your affected joints as well as range of motion. The goal in ankylosing spondylitis is to promote good posture and back flexibility.

Types of Exercise

There are three basic types of exercise:

Range-of-motion Exercises.

Range-of-motion or stretching exercises aim to move each of your joints as far as possible in all directions. These are gentle stretching exercises that need to be done on a daily basis. They help keep joints fully mobile and prevent stiffness and deformities. Such exercises are especially beneficial for rheumatoid arthritis patients, who tend not to want to move their inflamed joints. During the course of your normal daily activities, you may not move your joints through their full range of motion, so such activities are no substitute for these exercises.

Strengthening Exercises.

These exercises strengthen the muscles that support and move the joints. They can help you move more easily and with less pain. There are two types of strengthening exercises—isometric and isotonic. During isometric exercises, you exercise a specific muscle by squeezing it tightly without moving the joint itself. These are especially valuable when joint motion is impaired. One of my patients who was being considered for knee surgery was able to use isometric exercises to strengthen his knee muscles, which had been seriously weakened by years of disuse. He began to do quad sets (contracting the quadriceps, the large muscle in front of the thigh) and these muscles got much stronger. If he hadn't strengthened them before the operation, his recovery after surgery would have been slower and more difficult.

Endurance Exercises.

Endurance or aerobic exercises are physical activities that bring your heart rate up to your optimal target level for at least twenty to thirty minutes (your target heart rate is computed on the basis of your age and physical condition). You should perform such exercises at least three times a week in order for them to be effective. Exercises that raise your heart rate are especially valuable because they boost your cardiovascular fitness. They may also bring some other surprising benefits. Many arthritis patients who do them report increased physical strength, a better mental attitude, and even an improvement in their arthritis symptoms. Not all arthritis patients, however, are able to perform endurance exercises. If you are overweight and have a mild form of dengenerative arthritis, this is a good form of exercise for you. On the other hand, if you have had rheumatoid arthritis for twenty years and your shoulders, knees, and hips have functional limitations, you will not be able to participate in this type of activity.

Endurance exercises for arthritis patients have to be chosen carefully to avoid joint injury. The vigorous jumping and pounding that goes on in many aerobic exercise classes is inappropriate for most patients. Swimming, walking, and bicycle riding are safest and most effective, and can be done without undue stress on the joints. Stationary bicycles are good alternatives. They have seat adjustments and tension controls, and allow you to exercise safely and regularly indoors, without fear of falling or regard to the weather.

Some people find exercise to be more enjoyable when they do it with a friend or in a class. Others say that walking or exercising while listening to music or a radio talk show is pleasant. You might even park a stationary bicycle in front of the TV and pedal during your favorite program.

Exercise needs to be done year-round if you are to reap its full benefits. There are many gyms and community centers where you can exercise indoors during the winter months. Some communities sponsor water exercise classes especially for arthritis patients. These are done in a warm pool that is comfortable for people with arthritis who don't like the cold. The water provides buoyancy and can take the stress off your joints as you perform gentle stretching movements. Your local chapter of the Arthritis Foundation can provide you with information about classes near you.

Exercise Guidelines

Many arthritis patients find exercise to be an enjoyable part of their treatment. It does require some commitment and perseverance, but as many exercise enthusiasts will tell you, the results are well worth the effort.

The following guidelines can help you get the most benefit out of your exercise program.

1. *Be consistent.* Exercise is one commitment you can't keep putting off until tomorrow. It takes time to see results, and in order for your program to be effective, you must exercise every day. Exercise done sporadically can't provide you with full benefits. If you have to miss a few days, you may have to begin at a lower level of intensity and build back up again.

2. *Build up gradually.* Don't rush into your exercise program too quickly: Too much exercise can worsen symptoms, at least initially, and that could discourage you from continuing. The best exercise program is one that starts at low intensity and gradually is built up as your symptoms allow.

3. *Exercise when your symptoms are least troublesome.* It's best to exercise when your pain and stiffness are at a minimum. Some say the morning is the best time, especially after they've had a warm shower to help limber them up. Others like to wait until their morning stiffness is past and their morning medication has taken effect. Afternoons are not usually the best time to plan an exercise session, because you may feel fatigued. Some people like to exercise throughout the day as opposed to having one rigidly scheduled time.

4. *Don't overdo it.* Most programs recommend that you perform strengthening and range-of-motion exercises in sets of three to ten repetitions, with each set repeated one to four times. This is a broad recommendation. There is no magic number that works for everyone. The number of repetitions you should do depends upon how well you feel. If your disease is active, you may have to decrease the amount of exercise you do. Too much activity during a flare can aggravate your symptoms.

5. *Pay attention to your body's signals.* A certain amount of discomfort during exercise is acceptable and may even be inevitable, especially for

patients with long-standing active disease. If you experience pain that lasts two hours or more after you exercise, however, you overdid it. Perform fewer repetitions until your symptoms abate.

6. *If your joint feels hot, don't use it.* Exercise can make a swollen and tender joint feel even worse. Modify your activity until your arthritis is under better control. The rubric "no pain, no gain" certainly does not apply to this situation.

7. *Set realistic goals.* For example, perform an aerobic activity for a set time instead of aiming to cover a certain distance. If you've been sedentary, don't start out with immediate plans to walk a mile each day. Instead, plan to start with a daily ten-minute walk and then gradually increase the time by a few minutes each week.

8. *Exercise in a smooth, steady rhythm and relax between repetitions.* Coordinate your exercise and your breathing. Don't bounce or use jerky motions, as these can put stress on your joints.

9. *Alternate rest with activity.* This way you'll reap the benefits of both.

Foot Problems and Exercise

Arthritis can sometimes cause painful foot problems that may prevent you from walking or doing other forms of exercise. Rheumatoid arthritis, for example, may distort the shape of the foot so that the shock of each step is borne by the ends of the bones in the foot rather than dispersed and cushioned by the sole.

Your physical therapist may have several suggestions on foot care. For example, he or she may recommend that a metatarsal bar be glued to the bottom of your shoe. This thin strip of shock-absorbent material relieves pain by cushioning the impact of each step and deflecting it away from painful spots.

Women should avoid pointy-toed shoes and high heels that squeeze their toes unnaturally and shift the balance of their weight. Sensible shoes that fit properly can decrease pain, improve mobility, and make exercising easier. Well-cushioned running shoes may be all that you need. Or you may need a prescription for a pair of extra-depth, extra-width shoes. Those with severely deformed feet may need to obtain molded, custom-made shoes that conform to the exact shape of your foot.

Measures to increase the comfort of your feet can dramatically improve the quality of your life.

Exercises

The following stretching and strengthening exercises are used in the Duke Basic Program. They maintain the range of motion in each joint and keep the surrounding muscles strong. After you have your doctor's okay, I recommend that you perform them in sets of three to ten repetitions, repeating each set one to four times. Remember to do the exercises slowly and rhythmically, to rest in between, and to breathe deeply and regularly while exercising. Hold each stretch for a count of five to ten. You may need to reduce the number of repetitions if you are having a flare.

SHOULDER EXERCISES

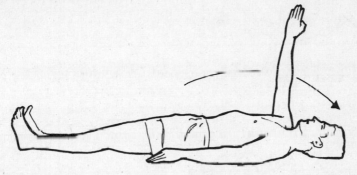

1. *Lie on your back, arms at your sides and with your palms facing your body. Keep your elbows straight. Lift your right arm toward the ceiling until it's perpendicular to the floor. Repeat with the left arm. You can do this exercise in bed.*

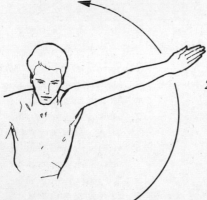

2. *Lie on your back, arms at your sides and palms facing up. Slide your left arm along the floor in an arc until you've raised it above your head. Repeat with the right arm. You can do this exercise in bed.*

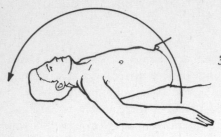

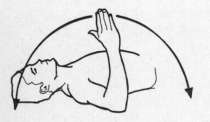

3. Lie on your back, with your arms perpendicular to your sides at shoulder level, palms facing up. Rotate your right forearm down toward the bed, then up toward your head. Keep your elbow on the floor or bed. Repeat with your left forearm.

ELBOW EXERCISES

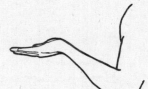

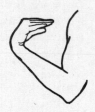

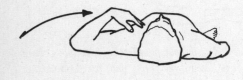

1. Start with your arms at your sides and your elbows straight. Bend your left elbow and bring your left hand as close to your shoulder as possible. Straighten the elbow completely. Repeat with the right arm.

2. Stand with your right elbow bent and fingers in a loose fist with your thumb pointing up toward the ceiling. Turn your fist so that your thumb faces your side. Then turn your fist so that your thumb points away from your side. Repeat with the left hand.

ANKLE EXERCISES

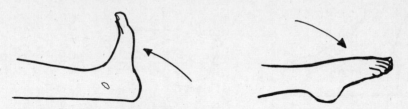

1. *Lie on your back with your legs straight. Bend your left ankle, pulling your toes up toward you. Then point your toes away from you. Repeat with the right foot.*

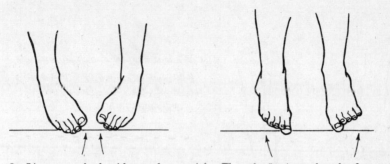

2. *Lie on your back with your legs straight. Turn the feet in so the soles face each other. Turn the feet out so the soles face away from each other.*

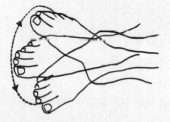

3. *Lie on your back with your legs straight. Make inward and outward circles with your left foot. Do 5 circles in each direction, then repeat with the right foot.*

ARCH EXERCISES

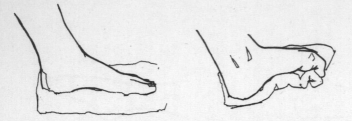

1. *Sit with your feet resting on a towel. Curl your toes and gather the towel under the arch of your foot. Rest frequently to avoid cramping. Repeat with the other foot.*

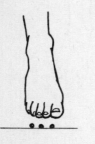 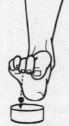

2. *While sitting, try to pick up a marble with your toes and drop it into a dish near your other foot. Pick up several marbles with each foot.*

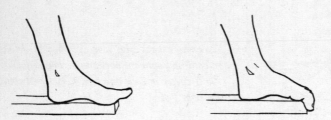

3. *Stand with your toes over the edge of a board. Bend your toes down over the edge. Straighten them and relax.*

HIP EXERCISES

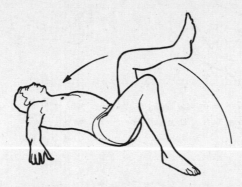

1. *Lie on your back with your knees bent. Lift your left leg, bending at the hip. Bring your left knee toward your chest as far as possible. Lower the leg. Relax. Repeat with your other leg. (This exercise also helps to strengthen back muscles.)*

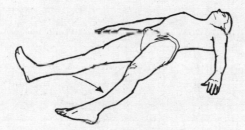

2. *Lie on your back with your legs straight. Slide your right leg along the floor to the right, then slide it back toward the other leg. Keep the knee straight and toes pointing up toward the ceiling. Relax, then repeat with the other leg.*

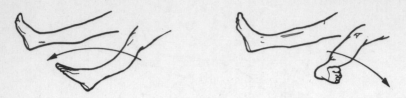

3. *Lie on your back with your legs straight. Roll your right leg in (knees facing), then out (knees turned out). Relax and repeat with the other leg.*

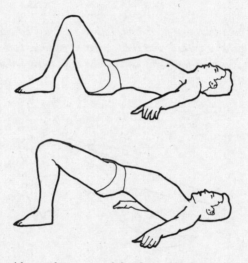

4. *Lie on your back with your knees up and feet flat on the floor or bed. Tighten your buttock muscles and lift your bottom up 2 to 3 inches. Do not push with your arms or shoulders.*

KNEE EXERCISES

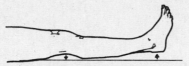

1. *Lie on your back with your legs straight. Tighten the muscle just above your knee by straightening your knee completely. Hold for the count of 5 and relax. When this exercise is done properly, your heel should come up off the bed. Repeat with your left knee.*

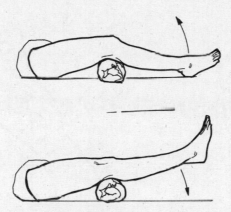

2. *Lie on your back with your legs straight. Bend your right knee slightly by placing a roll under it. Straighten the knee as far as you can; then hold for a count of 5. Slowly lower the leg to the starting position. Repeat with the opposite leg.*

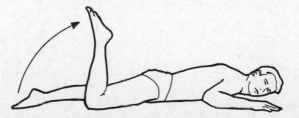

3. *Roll onto your stomach. Bend your right knee so that the heel of your foot moves toward your right buttock. Lower your leg to the starting position. Repeat with the other knee.*

HAND AND WRIST EXERCISES

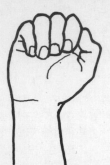

1. Make a fist. Straighten your fingers. Repeat with the other hand.

2. Touch your fingertips to the line on the bottom of each finger. Keep the big knuckle straight. Hold for a count of 5. Repeat with the other hand.

3. Touch your thumb to the tip of each finger. Repeat with the other hand.

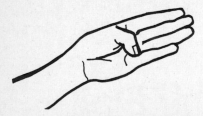

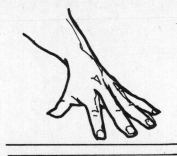

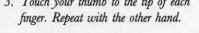

4. Place your hand flat with the palm up. Touch your thumb to the bottom of the little finger. Repeat with the other hand.

5. Place your hand and forearm flat on a table, palm down. Spread the fingers apart, then pull them together. Repeat with the other hand.

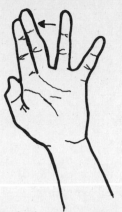

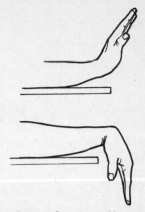

6. Start in the same position as in the previous exercise. Bring each finger individually over toward the thumb. Repeat with the other hand.

7. Place your forearm flat on a table with the wrist and hand over the edge. Flex your wrist up and down as far as possible. Repeat with the other hand.

BACK EXERCISES

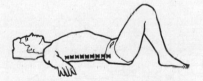

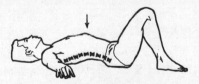

1. Lie on your back with your knees bent. Now tighten your stomach and press your back against the floor. Hold this position for a count of 10 and relax, then repeat. You can also practice this exercise in a standing position while standing 5 to 10 inches away from a wall. Press your lower back firmly against the wall until there is no space between your back and the wall. Stand away from the wall and repeat.

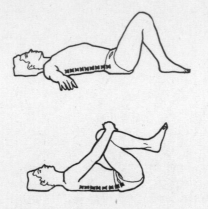

2. *Start with the pelvic tilt. Slide your feet along the floor to your buttocks. Slowly bring your knees toward your chest and pull your knees even closer with your hands. With your knees slightly separated, hold for a count of 10 and repeat.*

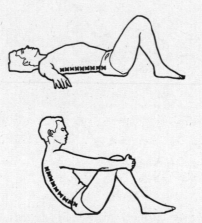

3. *Start with the pelvic tilt. Reach for your knees and partially sit up. Hold for a count of 10. Relax and repeat. When this becomes easy for you, change the way you do it by starting in the second position and slowly lowering your upper body down to the mat. Keep your back rounded. Don't flop down!*

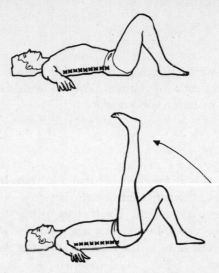

4. *Start in the pelvic tilt position. Straighten your right leg above your body. Get your knee as straight as possible. Hold for a count of 10 and then return to the starting position. Repeat the exercise with the left leg. (You may feel a slight pulling sensation behind your knees when your leg is straight up.)*

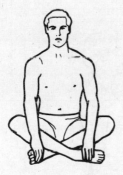

5. *Sit with your legs crossed in front of you. Hold your feet with your hands. Stretch forward slowly, moving your nose toward your ankles. Do not bob.*

Posture

Good posture while walking, sitting, and even lying down can also minimize pain and strengthen your muscles. The following are some guidelines to help you to maintain good posture.

Sitting

- Try to keep one or both knees higher than your hips by placing your
  feet on a footstool, box, or other object.
- Keep your upper back straight. Use a chair with a straight back for
  firm support. Don't round your back into a cushiony easy chair.
- Avoid bending your arms at the elbows by resting them on a work
  surface or armrest.
- Keep your shoulders relaxed.

Standing and Walking

- Hold yourself erect but relaxed, with your spine lengthened, shoulders
  back, and hips tucked under. Visualize a string coming up from the
  top of your head holding you straight and tall.

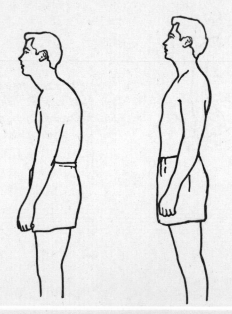

- When standing for a long time, raise one foot slightly on a footstool to take the stress off your lower back. You'll find this especially helpful when you're in the kitchen preparing a meal.
- Wear comfortable shoes with flat heels. Avoid high heels and platform shoes.
- Wear thick rubber soles to cushion your feet on hard surfaces.

Lifting

- Always bend your knees (squat) and keep objects close to your body when lifting.
- Don't lift heavy objects above your waist.
- Avoid sudden, jerky movements when lifting.

CORRECT   **INCORRECT**

correct

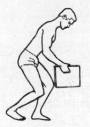

correct

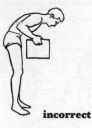

incorrect

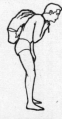

correct

incorrect

incorrect

incorrect

Sleeping

- Sleep on a firm mattress.
- Sleep on your side, not on your stomach or back.

CORRECT

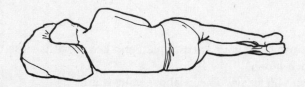

INCORRECT

Driving

- Sit close enough to the wheel so your legs are not fully stretched out.

CORRECT   **INCORRECT**

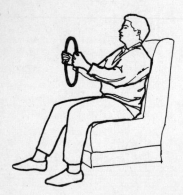 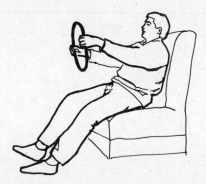

Canes, Walkers, and Wheelchairs

The goal of physical therapy is not only to help you exercise but also to help you get around. Canes and walkers can be invaluable aids. They take the stress off weight-bearing joints during a flare and can help relieve pain, increase your mobility, and postpone the need for surgery.

Your physical therapist should help you select a cane of the appropriate height. Generally speaking, when you extend your arm, the head of your cane should be even with your wrist.

You should use the cane on the side opposite your affected joint. So, for example, if your left hip, knee, or ankle is affected, you should hold the cane in your right hand.

Walkers are often most helpful for older individuals with arthritic knees or hips who would otherwise not be able to get around. Again, your physical therapist will help you select a walker adjusted to the correct height. You can hang a fabric pocket from the crossbar to help you carry small objects from one part of the house to another.

Wheelchairs and motorized scooters are sometimes useful for people with advanced disease who feel considerable pain when they move, but you don't want to become too dependent on them if you can help it. If you rely on these aids too heavily, you'll miss out on the beneficial effects of walking and weight-bearing exercise. Motorized scooters can be very useful, but can be difficult to maneuver in some situations—for example, while getting into or out of a car; two people are often required to handle the scooter.

Summary

I can't stress enough the importance of exercise to your health and the optimal function of your joints. Your physical therapist can play a key role in helping you devise an exercise plan appropriate for your particular condition. While exercise is beneficial, don't forget to get enough rest and to slow down if you feel fatigued. Remember also to start exercising slowly and to build up gradually. As you begin, keep in mind all the benefits that a daily program conscientiously followed will bring. After a while, exercise should become an integral and enjoyable part of each day.

16

Diet

Michael, a fifty-four-year-old systems analyst, has had rheumatoid arthritis for a number of years. I've followed his condition closely and treated him with NSAIDs and gold injections. Although he seems to be responding well to treatments, he frequently looks for other therapies and brings me newspaper articles about new treatments and diets. The last article on diet that he showed me recommended eating nightshade vegetables (the nightshade family includes such familiar plants as the potato and the tomato). Michael wanted to know what I thought of this diet. I told him that this isn't a standard therapy; the value of such a diet hasn't been proven and therefore I couldn't recommend it. Michael seemed very disappointed that I couldn't be more supportive, but he was nevertheless thinking about trying the diet.

Patrick, a sixty-two-year-old lawyer, has osteoarthritis in his left knee. The pain in his knee developed several years ago and has slowly gotten worse. To minimize his discomfort, he stopped walking during his golf games and has been avoiding other physical activities. Slowly he began to put on weight, going from 180 pounds to 230. The problems with his knee got even worse, and he came to my office for an evaluation. During our consultation, I told Paul I wanted to refer him to a dietitian and have him go on a weight-loss program. He had a strong family history of heart disease, and the added weight not only placed excess stress on his knee joint but increased his risk for heart disease as well. Paul agreed to try to lose some weight. He met with the dietitian, and within a year he got down to 190 pounds. His knee pain became less severe, so he was able to increase his activities. He has kept to his diet and continues to walk regularly every day.

Diet and Health

Patients frequently ask if there is any connection between diet and arthritis. The answer to this question is not a simple yes or no. It depends on the type of arthritis you have and the kind of diet you are talking about. There is evidence that diet can influence many forms of arthritis. But many of the diets advocated in the media or via word of mouth are actually remedies that have not been clinically tested; the support for these diets comes solely from testimonials by those who have tried them.

Some people interpret medical caution about unproven diet remedies as a dismissal of the importance of diet. In fact, the opposite is true. Certainly, physicians know that a healthful diet can be valuable not only in the treatment of arthritis but also in the prevention of many other diseases as well, including heart disease and cancer.

Nearly anyone who watches television or reads newspapers and magazines today knows that diets low in fiber and full of fat can contribute to obesity, high blood pressure, and heart attacks. This growing emphasis on healthy eating is very gratifying to health professionals. We have seen a drop in the number of deaths from cardiovascular disease that appears to be related to relatively simple changes in lifestyle and diet. Concerns about the contributions diet makes to cardiovascular disease and cancer and the move toward more natural foods have led to less reliance on preservatives, additives, and saturated fats, and I think that's great.

Dietary changes may also contribute to improvements in some forms of arthritis. A diet low in alcohol and purine-rich foods can lower blood uric acid levels and reduce the likelihood of a gout attack. If you have osteoarthritis and maintain your ideal weight, you may reduce joint stress and help prevent additional degenerative changes. In addition, a well-nourished person with arthritis may be able to tolerate medication and therapy better; and if he or she has to undergo surgery, he or she is likely to recover more quickly.

But arthritis patients sometimes have a different agenda in mind when they talk about diet. Rather than asking whether a good diet can improve arthritis, they may want to know if a specific diet they've read or heard about can cure their disease. One fifty-six-year-old I know who was thirty pounds overweight had been under treatment for high blood pressure at Duke for nearly ten years when he developed rheumatoid arthritis. For years doctors had suggested he lose weight and stay on a low-salt diet. Despite consultations with our dietitian and discussions with his doctor, he continued to add lots of salt to his foods and to eat fatty fast foods. Instead of losing weight, he had gained several more pounds. When he was told he had arthritis, he asked, "Well, Doc, do you have a diet I can follow?"

Many of my patients are highly motivated people who conscientiously follow their treatment plans. They read widely, and often discuss with me the alternative diets they find mentioned in various sources. When there are no scientific studies supporting the diet, I explain my reservations. Such diets are often really nothing more than unproven remedies or fads. In addition, the media often blur different forms of arthritic diseases, as if arthritis were a single entity rather than a number of different conditions. Most doctors prefer to give you advice based upon your particular disease, their clinical experience with diet, and evidence from scientific literature and animal studies.

In reviewing the evidence for a relationship between arthritis and diet, you must ask yourself several questions. First, what type of arthritis do you have? If you had a gout attack right after you'd gone out and had a big, rich meal and a lot to drink, I'd say there is a likely connection between your diet and arthritis. If you have rheumatoid arthritis or another type of inflammatory arthritis, however, the connection is far less clear.

Second, what expectations do you have regarding diet? If you have osteoarthritis and are overweight and want to know whether a sensible weight-loss diet can help your condition, the answer is that it most likely will. Certainly a patient with rheumatoid arthritis who may not be eating well would benefit from a nutritious and well-balanced diet. I can't respond as positively to the patient who comes to my office with a clipping from a magazine or testimony from a friend about a miracle diet. I'm interested in treating arthritis and in helping to make you better, not in having you distracted from a good program of therapy.

Will diet cure your arthritis? That depends on what you mean by *cure* and on what your condition is. You can significantly improve certain conditions, such as gout, by good diet; and by keeping to your ideal weight, you may decrease symptoms of degenerative disease. When you eat properly and are well nourished, you are more likely to be able to cope with a chronic disease.

The Arthritis/Diet Connection

Investigators are currently studying many possible links between diet and arthritis. Before looking at some of these areas of research, let's review some of the commonly believed ideas about diet and arthritis for which there is some reasonable evidence.

First, rheumatologists believe that body weight does influence arthritis. Our clinical experience tells us that those who are overweight or obese (defined as 20 percent over normal body weight as listed in standard height-weight tables) seem to have more problems with arthritis. Patients who become overweight may increase the load on their joints. This increased stress can make hip and knee joints more painful and may lead to a more sedentary lifestyle and further weight gain.

Obesity is much more of a problem for people with osteoarthritis than for those with rheumatoid arthritis (although I've treated many thin patients with severe OA). Rheumatoid arthritis patients may in fact have problems with lack of appetite and weight loss, probably due to the effects of the inflammatory substances released in their blood; an exception might be RA patients on corticosteroid therapy, since one of the side effects of corticosteroids is appetite stimulation and fluid retention. Though rheumatoid arthritis patients taking steroids are cautioned about the tendency to overeat while on steroids, the ensuing weight gain is often unavoidable.

We also have evidence that purines and alcohol can set off a gout attack. Purines are natural substances found in certain foods, including organ meats, sardines, and anchovies. Excess purine intake can raise uric acid levels in the blood and can lead to gout attacks in some individuals. Alcohol appears to contribute to gout by altering the purine metabolism. If you have gout, you may be advised not to eat purine-rich foods or to drink excess amounts of alcohol.

Many books and articles offer diets that claim to cure arthritis. Most of these claims are directed toward rheumatoid and other inflammatory forms of arthritis, but people with OA may also give them a try. Some of the more popular food "cures" include eating honey and vinegar, poke-berries, blackstrap molasses, and cranberry juice. Such claims are usually backed by testimonials from arthritis patients who say they have eaten these foods and have noticed an improvement in their condition.

Several reports in the medical literature suggest that a change in diet may actually help some arthritis patients, although the basis for this effect is uncertain. It is sometimes impossible to tell whether improvements are due to a particular food or to natural fluctuations in the course of the disease. Sometimes patients respond to inactive pills or ineffective diets because of a psychological phenomenon known as the placebo effect. That is, a patient's condition improves because he or she has faith in the treatment. The only way to know for sure if a diet works is to test it scientifically. That means administering the diet to a group of arthritis patients and comparing the response of this group to that of a matched group of patients who are not on the diet. Only a limited number of such studies have been performed, and the results thus far have been inconclusive.

Some people think that certain foods may act like allergens, triggering arthritis in sensitive individuals. This is a possibility, but it's rather difficult to prove. The situation could be similar to food allergies. Some people are allergic to shellfish, some to chocolate, some to milk products, and so on. Any number of foods could possibly trigger arthritis as well, but the variety of possible foods would make their identification difficult.

You could try testing patients on an individual basis, to see if a certain allergen is acting as the trigger. The usual approach is to place patients on an elimination diet, in which their main sustenance comes from a mixture of nutrients without the suspect food substances, and see if their arthritis improves. Then ordinary foods are added back to the diet one at a time, to determine whether one of them makes the arthritis worse. The food causing the disease is then identified. This is exceedingly hard to do. Arthritis symptoms can take a long time to develop. As an example, an inflammatory gastrointestinal disease called gluten-sensitive enteropathy is caused by gluten, a wheat protein. If gluten is eliminated from the diet, improvement occurs only after weeks or months. You can see how difficult an accurate diagnosis can be and what time and patience it can take.

Though no specific food or group of foods have yet been implicated as causes of arthritis, physicians like to keep an open mind. There is no doubt that what you eat can modify the function of your immune system. Foods are clearly linked to a variety of immune-mediated reactions, including asthma, rashes, and hives. We've seen examples of immune responses to foods in laboratory animals. And in humans, the most extreme example occurs in malnutrition, which produces a state of immune deficiency and susceptibility to infection that can be clearly documented in the laboratory. It would not be surprising, then, if arthritis in some patients resulted from a similar immune system response.

If one of my patients asks whether a particular food in his diet causes arthritis, I may suggest that he pay attention to his body's signals. If a patient notices that he feels worse after eating a certain food, he might try eliminating it from his diet, as long as in doing so he does not cause any significant nutritional problem. At a later time, he can try the food again, to see if the hunch was right. I do not recommend that patients try any drastic dietary manipulations on their own without consulting a physician.

Other dietary changes may also improve arthritis. When laboratory animals with experimentally induced arthritis are fed diets low in saturated fats and rich in fish oils, their arthritis may improve. Fish oils contain a large amount of a highly unsaturated fatty acid called eicosapentanoic acid (EPA) that may play a major role in modifying the inflammatory process. There is some evidence that this therapy may have similar effects on humans, but the evidence is not fully in yet. However, it would certainly be to your benefit to follow a diet low in saturated fat. We already know that such a diet can lower blood cholesterol and decrease the risk of heart attacks. Diets high in saturated fat are also associated with an increased incidence of cancer. So reducing fat intake makes good medical sense, regardless of its effects on arthritis.

I find it intriguing that foods that increase the risk of cancer and heart disease also seem to aggravate arthritis. I hope that more definite evidence will emerge over the next few years so that the current general recommendations on a diet lower in fat can be made stronger and more specific for arthritis.

Seven Dietary Guidelines

As a doctor, I don't treat just arthritis—I treat the whole patient. Good nutrition as well as exercise are part of maintaining good general health, and may make it less likely that you will have high blood pressure or cardiovascular disease. A good starting point for any recommendations on diet is the Government Dietary Guidelines for Americans, originally published by the U.S. Department of Agriculture and the U.S. Department of Health and Human Services.

1. *Eat a variety of foods.* To stay healthy, you need over forty essential nutrients. You can make sure that you are getting these nutrients when you choose a variety of foods from each of the four major food groups: whole grains (bread and cereals); fruits and vegetables; meat (poultry, fish, and lean meat); milk (low- or nonfat milk, cheese, and yogurt). If you rely too heavily on foods from any one group, you may not be getting all the nutrients you need.

2. *Maintain your ideal weight.* Less weight means less strain on your heart, circulatory system, and weight-bearing joints.
3. *Avoid too much fat, saturated fat, and cholesterol.* The American diet relies too heavily on these, and there is strong evidence that fat can contribute to obesity and to an increase in heart disease and certain types of cancer.
4. *Eat food with adequate starch and fiber.* Starches include bread, rice, beans, pasta, and potatoes; these give your body energy. Fiber is the undigested portion of the plants we eat. Both starches and fibers add bulk and aid in the process of elimination.
5. *Avoid too much sugar.* Sugary snacks provide empty calories that add little in terms of nutrition and contribute to excess weight gain.
6. *Avoid too much sodium.* Excess salt consumption may contribute to high blood pressure and water retention. Learn to enjoy the natural taste of foods.
7. *Avoid alcohol.* Alcohol can rob the body of essential vitamins and minerals. It is also high in calories and may interact with medications you are taking for arthritis.

Strategies for Weight Loss

Sensible eating patterns are not always easy to establish and maintain. It's hard to break poor lifelong eating habits. You may also find that your condition can sometimes make it difficult to prepare meals or eat properly.

One patient at Duke, a seventy-two-year-old man, never bothered to learn to cook and now lives alone; he has taken to relying on prepared foods and fast-food restaurants for his meals. Lacking much to do, he often goes to the cupboard or the refrigerator to reach for salty or sugary snacks without even being aware of it. If you are bored and spend a lot of time at home, you may not pay attention to what you eat, and you may eat poorly and end up gaining too much weight. If this is a problem for you, talk about it with your physician. He or she may suggest ways for you to increase your activity and may refer you to a dietitian, who will help you set up a more sensible eating plan. Diet has to become a medical focus for you, just like taking your medication.

On days when you're tired and your joints hurt, the last thing you may want is to be in the kitchen preparing meals. Some patients rely heavily on prepared frozen or canned foods or on meals from fast-food restaurants. These foods may be tasty and inexpensive, but they are usually high in salt and fat. Sometimes an occupational therapist can help you to devise ways of performing kitchen tasks that are more comfortable. Using a high stool at the kitchen counter instead of standing, for example, can take the stress off your hips and knees. If you must eat processed foods, read the labels carefully. Look for foods that are low in sugar, fats, and salt. Cooking a frozen dinner that is low in sodium and fat takes the same amount of effort as cooking one that is highly salted and smothered in gravy or butter sauce.

Physicians, medical centers, and dietitians have all become involved in weight reduction programs for hypertension, cardiovascular diseases, and diabetes. Duke University Medical Center was in fact among the first medical centers to develop a diet to treat hypertension. The success of this approach has led to the development of several programs for diet research, weight reduction, and lifestyle modification in the city of Durham, North Carolina. Durham is probably the diet center of the United States, if not the world. There are many strategies for weight loss, and this book will not attempt to duplicate the information found in so many other good books available on the subject today. Instead, I'll review some behavior modification techniques that can help you to watch your weight and teach you how to figure out your calorie requirement.

Behavior Modification and Weight Control

Behavior modification techniques can help you change your eating behavior patterns so that you feel in control. The following suggestions are made by Diane A. Gelman, a nutritionist on the staff of the Duke University Preventive Approach to Cardiology (DUPAC), a program combining diet and exercise (see table 5). Similar techniques have been used in other hospital programs.

The major principles of dietary behavior modification are:

- Decrease your food intake by reducing the cues that lead you to eating.
- Limit the amount of available food by buying in smaller quantities and measuring out your portion sizes.
- Eat only at mealtimes.
- Plan nutritious snacks.
- Set reasonable goals for yourself.
- Accept failures.
- Increase your level of physical activity.

Table 5. DIET: SUGGESTIONS FOR BEHAVIOR MODIFICATION

Self-Monitoring. (1) Keep a record of your daily food and calorie intake. Record when and where you eat, and what you eat. (2) Chart your weight. (3) Set small goals for weight reduction (five or ten pounds). Reward yourself when these are met.

Food Shopping. Never shop when you're hungry; it encourages impulse buying.

Food Preparation. Prepare reasonable quantities of food so you won't have too many leftovers.

Storing Food. (1) To reduce food cues, store food in opaque containers or out of sight. Store low-calorie food in the same way so you'll get out of the nibbling habit. (2) Keep all food in the kitchen, so that it takes effort to get at it.

Quantity Control. (1) Use small, measured portions. (2) Don't go back for seconds. (3) Don't serve "family style." Keep food in the kitchen or on the stove and eat in another room. (4) Eat slowly; savor what you eat. Pause 30 seconds between bites, putting down your fork in between. (5) Do not finish the food on your plate. Leave at least one mouthful. (6) Stop eating as soon as you feel full. (7) Don't do other things while you are eating, such as reading or watching TV. (8) Eat only when sitting in your accustomed place at the dinner table.

Snacking. (1) Limit snacks to small quantities of low-calorie foods. (2) Limit snacking time: never eat after 10:00 P.M., or only two to five minutes each hour. Progressively reduce the time allotted.

Goal Setting: Set realistic short-term and long-term weight-loss goals. Also, set goals for specific behavioral changes, such as:

1. This week I will not eat any fried food or gravies.
2. This week I will take a walk when I get angry or bored.
3. This week I will not eat while standing.
4. This week, when eating out, I will ask that my salad dressing be served on the side so that I can control the amount I use.
5. This week I will only eat ——— servings of sweets.
6. This week I will not eat while I do other things.
7. This week I will not shop when hungry.

DIET: SUGGESTIONS FOR BEHAVIOR MODIFICATION *(continued)*

8. This week I will take at least 25 minutes to eat each meal.
9. This week I will practice control over my food intake by putting my fork down between bites of food.
10. This week I will not skip any meals.
11. This week I will eat an average of _____ calories per day.
12. This week I will leave a bite of food on my plate at two meals.
13. This week, when returning for seconds, I will serve myself low-calorie vegetables instead of higher calorie foods.
14. This week I will limit my intake of alcoholic beverages to _____.

Reward yourself for achieving your goal with praise and/or a concrete reward such as a new book, a hot bath, etc.
Try to overlook temporary setbacks and concentrate on the positive aspects. If you succumb to one piece of candy on an occasion, don't consider this license to forgo your eating plan. Forgive yourself and persevere. (Dieters are too hard on themselves!)

Physical Activity. Arthritis patients may have to modify their exercise, but will benefit from exercising within prescribed limits. If you are not in an exercise program, you may want to get together with a physical therapist and, in conjunction with your physician, design an exercise plan (see chapter 15).

Substitutions. Substitute other enjoyable pursuits for eating.

Adapted from *Behavior Modification* by Diane A. Gelman, R.D., M.Ed., in *Diet for Living: A Healthy Low-Calorie, Low-Sodium, High-Complex-Carbohydrate Diet Plan.*

Your Food Diary

Since many overweight people often eat without thinking about it, you might find it helpful to write down everything you eat during the course of a day. The following Food Diary may help you to become aware of how much you actually eat. (You may want to make several additional photocopies.) Record everything you eat and note when and where you ate it.

FOOD DIARY

Day	What	Where	Planned/Unplanned	Calories
Monday				
Tuesday				
Wednesday				
Thursday				
Friday				
Saturday				
Sunday				

How Many Calories Are Enough?

When planning a diet, you must know your daily calorie requirement. Calorie needs are highly individualized and depend on your sex, age, weight, height, and physical activity (see table 6). There are several ways of estimating your specific daily requirement for weight maintenance. The system used at DUPAC is as follows:

your weight × activity factor = number of calories to maintain
current weight

Table 6. ACTIVITY FACTORS TO DETERMINE CALORIC REQUIREMENTS

Physical Activity	Factor
Extremely inactive	10
Inactive	11
Sedentary, with occasional activity	12
Fairly active several times per week	13
Fairly active every day	14

Example: A fairly active (several times a week) person weighing 150 pounds would require 150 × 13 = 1,950 calories to maintain his or her present body weight.

In order to lose one pound of body weight, you must eat 3,500 calories less than required. Stated in another way, a deficit of 500 calories a day results in a weight loss of 1 pound a week. A deficit of 1,000 calories a day results in a weight loss of 2 pounds a week. Without additional exercise, most people would lose an average of 1 to 2 pounds a week on the 750-calorie DUPAC diet. Take heart! Exercise burns up additional calories, and the more you weigh, the more calories you burn.

Summary

We still have a lot to learn about the precise role different foods play in arthritis. In certain instances diet clearly does matter. On the other hand, many dietary claims do not have enough evidence to recommend them, and doctors are justifiably concerned about diverting people away from good therapies. A well-balanced, nutritious diet can improve your overall health and feeling of well-being. You'll have more energy and more resilience. By keeping to your ideal weight, you can also spare your joints unnecessary stress. The association between arthritis and diet continues to be an intriguing area of scientific investigation.

17

Better Daily Living with Arthritis

A chronic disease can influence many facets of your life, including your home, work, and leisure activities. The number of adjustments you and your family may have to make in your daily lives depend a great deal on the kind of arthritis you have and on its severity. You may also find that you have good days, when you feel perfectly fine and energetic, and bad days, when you hurt more and have to minimize use of your joints and rest more.

One of the health professionals who can help you learn how to organize your daily living habits most effectively is the occupational therapist (O.T.). At Duke University, the occupational therapist is an integral part of our health care team. This specialist is a licensed professional who works along with your doctor and physical therapist to evaluate the impact of arthritis on your daily activities at home and on the job. Occupational therapists can help you devise plans to overcome your physical limitations; they can teach you how to perform various tasks in ways that place less strain on your joints, prevent further damage, and in general make your life more pleasant. They can also help design and prescribe splints and assistive devices.

Most occupational therapists practice within a hospital or as part of a medical practice. Sometimes the occupational therapist works with a physiatrist, a professional certified in rehabilitative medicine. Physiatrists in some hospitals coordinate the work of occupational therapists and physical therapists.

This chapter takes a very broad look at techniques you can use to make living with arthritis easier. Some of these techniques are reserved for more advanced forms of disease; others, such as stress management techniques, can be used by almost anyone. Not all of the therapies described in the following pages fall under the province of the occupational therapist. In different contexts physical therapists, trained arthritis nurses, mental health counselors, or other medical professionals may be involved.

Since occupational therapy is often an important facet of arthritis care, I'd like to begin with an explanation of the role of the specialist in this area.

Being Evaluated for Occupational Therapy

In order to understand your particular needs, an occupational therapist will ask you detailed questions about your life, including how old you are, whether you work outside the home, and whether you are married, have children, or have social supports. You may be asked to recount everything you usually do over a twenty-four-hour period—from when you get up in the morning to when you normally go to bed.

You'll be asked many questions about your home and work situation. Do you live alone or with a spouse or children? How do you divide the chores in your family? Who does most of the cooking and cleaning? If you work, what are the physical demands of your job? Do you have to use your affected joints? What sort of work schedule do you have? One of our patients had a sedentary job that required a lot of sitting. He complained of nagging pains in his joints whenever he sat for too long. The occupational therapist suggested ways he could vary his position while on the job and told him how to adjust his seat and work area so as to put less strain on his joints. Another patient, a saleswoman in a boutique, complained that her knees hurt because her job required so much standing. The occupational therapist recommended some strain-relieving postures and shoes that are well padded and offer good support.

You may also be asked about the layout of your house. For example, where is your bedroom in relation to your bathroom? How many steps do you have to take to get there? How is your kitchen arranged? What sort of appliances do you have and where do you store them? The occupational therapist will ask for similar details about the physical layout of your workplace.

The therapist will also be interested in your hobbies and recreational pursuits, since they are a major source of enjoyment for you and their continuation can bring you pleasure and satisfaction.

By the time your history is completed, the occupational therapist will have gathered information about hygiene (bathing, mouth care, use of the toilet), grooming, eating, drinking, dressing, getting in and out of bed, driving, homemaking (cleaning, cooking, and shopping), working, and your sex life.

After taking your history, the therapist will give you a detailed physical examination much like that administered by your physician or physical therapist. The occupational therapist's emphasis, however, is on the way your joint function and range of motion may affect your ability to perform the tasks of daily living. You'll be asked to reach overhead, touch the back of your head or back, reach your mouth or feet, look over your shoulder, or look up to the ceiling. An examination of these motions tells the therapist how well you are able to cook and feed yourself and get dressed. He or she will also look closely for any deformities that could hinder your performance at home or work. These may require assistive devices that can make work and household tasks easier. The occupational therapist will also make a note of whether you need splints, wrist supports, or neck collars.

This entire evaluation procedure may take from one to two hours and may include a follow-up for fitting splints, as necessary.

How to Work with Your Occupational Therapist for Maximum Effectiveness

Occupational therapy is only part of an entire treatment plan that ultimately requires your full participation to make it work. You must take your medications and do the exercises prescribed by your physician and physical therapist; you should also eat properly and get adequate rest. You might analyze your own daily activities and identify possible problem areas that you can share with your occupational therapist. For example, Laura, a forty-three-year-old woman with rheumatoid arthritis, very much enjoyed embroidering. Sometimes, however, the pain in her hands prevented her from doing her needlework, and she was very upset about this. Her occupational therapist directed her to a variety of devices that could help her enjoy her hobby with less wear on her joints: special embroidery frames that can be attached to a table or chair; automatic threading machines; and sewing scissors that require pressure from the palm rather than from painful finger joints. Many times patients are unaware of simple devices that can make their tasks easier. Of course, as patients adopt the principles taught by the therapist, they often find solutions to problems on their own. You may even begin to fashion your own implements for doing things on the job or around the house.

Joint Rest and Protection

While you will receive your own individualized program of joint protection, there are some basic principles that are useful for any activity.

Conserve your energy. Try to plan out your daily activities ahead of time, leaving plenty of time for each task so that you don't have to strain yourself. Divide large jobs into smaller tasks. A compulsive fifty-seven-year-old college professor with ankylosing spondylitis decided to rearrange his extensive book collection. Although he would have preferred getting the job over with all at once, he realized it would be too taxing. He allowed his study to remain in a messy state for a few days and did the job in small increments. Similarly, if you plan to clean your house, don't try to do the job all at once. Do the bathroom one day and the kitchen the next.

It can also help if you organize and rearrange items in your home and workplace so that you don't have to duplicate your efforts. Keep all frequently used items close to your work area. For example, store cooking utensils close to the stove and a set of everyday dishes near the dishwasher.

At work and at home, balance work with rest by taking short rest periods periodically. Try to plan bigger jobs for the time of day you hurt the least. Don't sit in one position for too long. Stretch your muscles out now and then.

Use good body mechanics. Avoid stooping; lift objects with your knees bent and your back straight to avoid straining your back; and stand with good posture. If you normally work at a desk, make sure your work surface is at the proper height: two inches below your elbows. Your chair should have a firm, straight back for good support. You may find that a tilted desk, similar to the ones artists use for drafting, places less strain on your back and neck.

Sit rather than stand when working. At home, you might want to use a high bar stool when you are working at the kitchen counter or ironing. If you must stand at work, be sure to shift your weight often from one leg to the other. If possible, rest one leg on a stool placed in front of you to take the pressure off your lower back. Try to take small, frequent rest breaks throughout the day.

Use larger joints whenever possible. When opening a door, for example, push with your shoulders or hips rather than your hands. Carry a pocketbook on your shoulder rather than in your hands or over your elbow.

When lifting things, use two hands rather than one.

Slide objects instead of lifting them. For example, slide pots on the stove from one burner to another.

Avoid tight gripping and twisting motions of the hands. Use a flat, open hand to do chores rather than your fingers. For example, you can open a jar by pressing on the lid with your open palm and rotating your shoulder, or squeeze a sponge out by pressing on it with your palm. Built-up handles on kitchen and writing implements can reduce strain on finger joints. You can buy them ready-made or build up the existing handles by gluing insulating foam around them.

Use assistive devices for better mechanical advantage. When you are screwing on or unscrewing a lid, use a jar opener that grips the lid while you rotate the jar with your hands. Long-handled tools for cleaning and gardening reduce strain, too. Use a cart with wheels to carry objects from one place to another.

Listen to your pain. Pain is the body's signal that you are doing too much and need to rest.

Specific Tips

Occupational therapy has developed hundreds of ways to make the activities of daily living easier. The following are some of the most important techniques and devices. However, a full list of aids and devices and where to get them is available in the Arthritis Foundation's *Self-Help Manual for Patients with Arthritis,* which you can obtain for a nominal fee. You may wish to write or call the Arthritis Foundation for further information (see resources section).

Personal Hygiene
- Use a raised toilet seat.
- Install a bench in your bath.
- Fit handrails on your tub.
- Use built-up handles on your toothbrush.

- Use built-up faucet handles.
- Use liquid soap to avoid slippage.
- Install a bidet.
- Use an electric shaver or grow a beard.

Dressing
- Wear clothes with front openings or elastic waists.
- Wear clothes with pockets so you can carry several objects and minimize trips around the house or at your workplace.
- Wear slip-on shoes or shoes with elastic shoelaces or Velcro closures.
- Use buttoning aids or zipper pulls. Sew Velcro closures on blouses.

Eating and Cooking
- Slide pots rather than lifting them. Use lightweight cookware.
- Use the same pots or casserole dishes for preparation and serving.
- Use electric appliances—e.g., food processors, blenders, can openers, electric knives.
- Store heavier objects at waist level and lighter objects above. Use a reacher to retrieve items from the cupboard.
- Leave commonly used appliances and items out on the counter.
- Sit on a high bar stool when preparing food.
- Fasten large cloth or yarn loops to drawer handles and refrigerator doors. You can slip your arm into the loop and open the doors using your forearms, without placing strain on your finger joints.
- Use a garbage can with a pedal to open it.

Cleaning
- Use a long-handled mop and an upright vacuum cleaner.
- Let dishes air-dry rather than toweling them.
- To save steps, keep a full set of cleaning supplies in the kitchen and bathroom and on each level of the house.

Driving
- Use extra mirrors to avoid turning your head as much.
- Attach a fabric loop to the inside of the door so that you can close it more easily.
- Drive a car with electric windows, mirrors, and locks and power brakes and steering.

Sleeping
- Use satin sheets or wear pajamas that are slippery so you can slide more easily into a more comfortable position.
- Use a cervical pillow for better neck support.
- Use an electric blanket so you don't need the added weight of heavy covers to stay warm.

Taking Medicine
- Use a large cup that is easier to grip.

Walking
- Use crutches, canes, braces, and special wheelchairs when necessary. However, you don't want to use wheelchairs more than necessary; if you become overly dependent upon them, you may decrease the amount of exercise you do and your range of physical activity. Motorized carts, available in some supermarkets, can help you shop and carry heavy items. These carts require batteries, so they are generally quite heavy and are not practical for everyday use.

Recreation
- Use card shufflers, a stand to hold your book, a golf cart.

Splints

Splints are strap-on devices made of cloth, metal, or plastic. They support and immobilize inflamed joints, reducing painful motions that can worsen deformity. They are available for fingers, hands, wrists, neck, back, knees, and ankles. Wrist splints are the most common. Use them whenever you have a flare-up or on one of your bad days.

Wrist splints and neck collars are available commercially, but custom-made splints of lightweight materials provide the best fit and comfort. Custom splints are generally designed by a physical therapist, an occupational therapist, or a specialist in prosthetics. The designer takes a pliable, heat-sensitive material (orthroplast), cuts it to an appropriate size, and heats it with a hot air gun. The splint is then shaped to promote proper joint alignment and fitted to your joint so that it allows enough motion for comfort. When the fit is perfect, the orthroplast is permanently set with cold water. Velcro straps enable you to take the splint on and off easily.

More elaborate splints for fingers have been devised to correct or prevent deformity and to rest the joints. Splints can be worn day or night.

A special type of splint called a silver ring splint is made of two rings fused together, and is designed for patients whose fingers have swan-neck deformities. The silver ring splint provides a much more functional position for the fingers.

Assistive Devices

Your occupational therapist can also prescribe or create devices to help you with your daily activities. You may be able to purchase some of these devices in pharmacies, but it's best to have a prescription for their purchase to ensure that they are appropriate and that you'll be reimbursed for them by your health insurance provider. You may be able to make some of these devices yourself, using materials widely available in stores.

The following are some of the most common and generally useful assistive devices:

Rocker Knife.
With this curved knife, you can cut meat by simply rocking the blade back and forth. It is much simpler to grip than a conventional knife.

Zipper Hook.
This simple device helps you zipper your clothes. It can be made from a dowel rod and cup hook.

Built-up Handles.
You can enlarge the handles on most utensils simply by wrapping them with pipe insulation material or with a foam rubber hair curler.

Button Hook.
A piece of wire attached to the end of a wooden handle will help you button your clothes, even if you have finger deformities.

Reachers.
Long-handled reachers are very useful for picking things off the floor without bending down or for getting things down from shelves.

Many other devices can be designed for your special needs. Once you figure out which activities you have trouble with, you can work with your occupational therapist to develop imaginative and frequently simple solutions.

Sex and Arthritis

Many people with arthritis continue to have satisfying sexual relations. However, for some, sore and painful joints can interfere with lovemaking. Fatigue may also decrease sexual desire. Sometimes physical changes make people feel self-conscious or less desirable. Your partner may be fearful of hurting you and may avoid sex. You in turn may misinterpret this and feel rejected.

Though many people find it difficult or embarrassing to talk about sex, open communication is the best way to clear up misunderstandings. You should discuss your feelings openly with your partner and when necessary, seek information and advice from members of your health care team. Some people benefit from counseling by sex therapists, who are knowledgeable about issues surrounding chronic disease.

Set aside a time when you can talk to your partner about your feelings without interruptions. You alone know what hurts you as well as what gives you pleasure. Now is a good time to experiment and find different lovemaking positions that will put less stress on affected joints. (The Arthritis Foundation pamphlet *Living and Loving* provides detailed suggestions on more comfortable lovemaking positions.) Some couples say a new frankness and experimentation often draws them even closer to each other.

The following are a few suggestions that you may find helpful.

- Try to pace your daily activities so you don't overtire yourself, and plan sex during the time of day when you feel rested and at your best.
- Take your medication before sexual intercourse so that you can receive the full benefit of its pain-relieving effects.
- Take a warm bath or shower first, to relieve joint stiffness. (Some people even incorporate this into the lovemaking.)
- Try new positions to find those that put the least strain on your joints.

Pain Relief

Painful joints can sometimes make it difficult for you to perform your normal activities. While relief from pain is not exclusively within the province of occupational therapy, it can play an important role in helping you to perform your daily activities. Many medications can effectively relieve the inflammation and pain of arthritis, and these are discussed in chapter 14.

The following is a brief review of temporary pain relief techniques. Some doctors may recommend these techniques, others may not. These methods are used only as a temporary adjunct to the medication and treatment your doctor has prescribed. Their use frequently depends upon the type and severity of your arthritis. You should always consult with your physician, physical therapist, or occupational therapist about the proper use of these techniques.

Heat and Cold Treatments

At one time, rheumatology treatment centered around spas because people believed in the healing power of warm water. In fact, the English city of Bath got its name because it was one of the places where patients with arthritis and other illnesses could come to bathe in hot spring waters. While warmth can make you feel better, however, it shouldn't be confused with long-term therapy.

You can get temporary local pain relief by using hot packs, cold packs, heating pads, electric blankets, and hot wax immersion treatments. Some people find that taking a warm shower or bath prior to exercising helps relax their muscles and ease their stiffness. (Those who have trouble getting in and out of the bathtub may want to consider installing bathrails. If standing in a shower is stressful to your legs and spine, consider sitting on a chair or shower stool.)

Because of many advances in arthritis treatment, physicians place less emphasis on heat and cold therapy. Some doctors have even raised the possibility that such therapy may cause harm by hastening the destructive processes in the joints. Today we are more interested in treatment with drugs and a comprehensive program of physical and occupational therapy than we are in hot wax and heat treatments. However, these temporary adjuncts to therapy can ease morning stiffness and may help you do your prescribed range-of-motion exercises more easily.

Both heat and cold treatments should be used under the guidance of a physical therapist. Heat may not always be appropriate for your condition, and can even aggravate your symptoms. The following are some guidelines:

Heat Treatments
- Don't apply heat to one area for more than twenty to thirty minutes.
- Don't use heat if you have poor circulation, poor sensation, or increased sensitivity to heat; you might inadvertently injure your skin.
- When using heating pads or packs, check your skin every five minutes for signs of burning. Don't place heat directly on the skin; wrap the hot pad in towels. Add extra towels or turn the electric heating pad down if there are signs of burning.
- Keep your skin dry and free from lotions or creams.

Cold Treatments
- Don't apply cold to one area for more than ten to twenty minutes. Remove the pack when the area has numbed.
- Check your skin during and after treatment.
- Don't use a cold pack if you have any sensitivity to cold, decreased circulation, decreased sensation, or any cardiovascular problems.

Paraffin wax baths may sometimes be used to relieve painful fingers or feet. These can be done at home or administered by a physical therapist. Your hand or foot is immersed several times in a mixture of melted wax and mineral oil until a thick coating is formed. You have to hold your fingers or toes perfectly still so the hardened wax doesn't crack. The joints will then be wrapped in waxed paper or plastic wrap and covered with a towel or a piece of cloth to retain the heat. The warmth brings temporary relief and the wax is left on your hands or feet for twenty minutes before being peeled off. Since more effective medications have become available, wax treatments are used less frequently. If you respond well to an NSAID and remittive drugs, I wouldn't make this a routine part of your therapy.

Heat lamps may also be used for heat treatments. This is called diathermy. The bulb used in the lamp is an infrared bulb, not the ultraviolet type found in sunlamps.

Ultrasound is another form of heat that can promote temporary relief. Ultrasonic sound waves can quickly penetrate and warm joints. This method is used more frequently for musculoskeletal injuries than for rheumatoid arthritis or other systemic inflammatory diseases.

Massage

Some people find it soothing to massage stiff or tight muscles in their arms or legs or neck. You can massage yourself or have someone else do it for you. Oils or lotions make your hands glide more easily. While this may bring temporary relief for some, be careful if your joints are painful or inflamed; massage can make the condition worse.

TENS

Transcutaneous electrical nerve stimulation, or TENS, involves the use of an electrical stimulation to the nerves to block pain signals to the brain. This is a last-resort measure used mostly for localized musculoskeletal problems of the spine and back that fail to respond to other treatments. You will be attached by electrodes to a small battery-powered box that emits low-level electrical energy. The electrodes are placed on your skin with a little gel near the painful area. You receive a low-level shock that gives you a tingling sensation. Some people find this brings temporary relief; others do not. A TENS unit is very expensive and is used only for chronic, intractable localized pain. You should not use TENS if you have a pacemaker.

Psychological Techniques

Sometimes the pain of chronic illness causes a vicious cycle. Your health problems may cause you to feel anxious and stressed; stress causes you to tighten the muscles around your joints; the increased muscle tension makes your pain greater.

A certain level of stress in our lives is to be expected and may even have some beneficial effects. Acute stress speeds up your heart rate, increases the tension in your muscles, increases your rate of breathing, and raises your blood pressure. These physiologic changes prepare you for action— they are called the "fight or flight" response. Acute stress may help the athlete win his race and the politician deliver a more dynamic speech. Too much chronic stress, however, can be detrimental to you. It can cause anxiety, depression, insomnia, fatigue, a change in appetite, and chronic muscle tension.

Psychological techniques may help to get you to consciously relax and break the vicious stress-depression-pain cycle. These techniques may be taught by physicians, psychologists, nurses, occupational therapists, and physical therapists. Stress management techniques are also taught in self-help courses offered through the Arthritis Foundation and by various mental health professionals.

You may want to try using one or a variety of the techniques described below. Practice them for a few minutes twice a day during uninterrupted blocks of time. Don't try them just after a meal, because eating may make you sleepy and it may be hard to concentrate. It may be hard for you to relax at first. You may feel guilty about taking the time out for yourself or silly trying these techniques. Relaxation often gets easier with practice, and many people say that they find it very helpful for relieving tension.

These techniques do not replace your medication or your prescribed therapies and should be practiced only under the guidance of your physician.

Deep Breathing

Before you begin to practice this or any other relaxation technique, you need to find a quiet place where you will not be interrupted. You may want to dim the lights. Find a comfortable chair or lie down on a soft quilt. Rest your hands limply on your lap or at your sides. Close your eyes.

Begin by breathing in and out slowly, deeply, and rhythmically. Try inhaling through your nose and exhaling through relaxed lips. Notice the feeling of tension when you inhale and the release of tension as you exhale. Try to clear your mind of everything but your breathing. Watch your breath for a while, and with every breath out, silently repeat a neutral syllable or phrase such as "one," or "I am," or say a soothing word like "peace," "calm," or "relax." If thoughts about your family or your job drift into your mind, don't worry about them. Just let the thoughts drift through and then gently refocus your attention on your breathing. Do this for five minutes at a time at first; then work your way up to fifteen or twenty minutes. You'll be amazed at first at how difficult it is to clear your mind, but you'll improve with practice. At the end of each session, notice how much lighter and less tense your body feels.

Progressive Relaxation

Lie on your back with your legs straight and your arms at your sides. Close your eyes and begin breathing deeply, slowly, and rhythmically. When you feel quite relaxed, begin to systematically tense and relax every muscle in your body, beginning with your feet. Tense your right foot, hold the tension for a few moments, then relax (never tighten muscles to the point of pain). Notice how limp and heavy your relaxed foot feels. Now do the same for your left foot, then for your ankles, calves, knees, thighs, abdomen, buttocks, hands, forearms, upper arms, and shoulders.

Proceed slowly up your body, savoring the feeling of relaxation and release in each muscle. Relax your shoulders and neck. Wrinkle your face and then feel your jaws, eyelids, lips, forehead, and scalp relax. When you are done, take a mental inventory of your body. If any part feels tense, focus on sending a wave of relaxation to that area. End the exercise with more deep breathing and enjoy the sensation of release and freedom from tension.

Creative Imagery

Begin this exercise as you do for progressive relaxation. After several deep, slow rhythmic breaths, watch your breath for a while, and when you feel relaxed, imagine a scene—for example, a beach, a lakeside cottage, a forest glade—that makes you feel safe and happy. Whatever the scene, picture it in vivid detail and experience it with all your senses—sight, touch, and smell. For example, if you are conjuring up a beach, try to feel the warmth of the sun on your skin and the sensation of sand under your feet and between your toes; try to hear the sound of the waves slapping on the shore, the smell of the salt air, and the sound of gulls. Embellish your fantasy scene as much as you like.

Biofeedback

Biofeedback requires instruction. During biofeedback, you will be attached by electrodes to a machine that uses signals or a screen to display your body functions. Using a combination of relaxation and visualization techniques, you will be taught how to achieve voluntary control over such body processes as blood pressure, muscle tension, heart rate, and temperature. Eventually you may be able to control these processes without the machine and reduce the stress you feel. Biofeedback has been used to treat Raynaud's syndrome, enabling some patients to consciously increase blood flow to their fingers. The technique has also been used to treat migraines, high blood pressure, and asthma.

Self-Hypnosis

Self-hypnosis is a form of self-induced deep relaxation that must be learned under the guidance of a physician, psychologist, or mental health counselor. It has been used to help patients cope with the effects of chemotherapy and with migraine headaches, and also as a way to aid in weight reduction and smoking cessation.

Support

Sometimes it helps to know that others feel the same frustrations, sorrows, and joys as you do. Many people say they benefit from joining an arthritis support group. Your local branch of the Arthritis Foundation is a good place to start. They offer a self-help course that includes discussion, exercises, and stress management techniques.

Your family and friends can also be invaluable sources of support, helping you out during days when you feel less well and energetic. Learn how to communicate your needs to others and how to delegate chores and household tasks to other family members. If friends and family offer to help when you're not feeling well, let them do so. You would probably help others out if the situation were reversed, and doing for others makes people feel good.

Your health care team is also an invaluable resource. Talk to them when you are having special problems. Your physician, physical therapist, and occupational therapist are familiar with your history and individual needs. They may be able to suggest solutions that will help you cope better with your everyday activities.

18

Surgery

Paul, a sixty-two-year-old man in excellent health, first came to the Duke clinic ten years ago, when he noticed a pain in his right hip that seemed to come and go. He owned a small hardware store and had to stand on his feet almost all day, but the pain was not bad enough to interfere with his business or with his weekly game of golf and yearly hunting trips. I evaluated Paul and discovered some narrowing of his hip joint, which was encircled by a bony spur. The diagnosis was osteoarthritis. I told Paul to take two 5-grain aspirin four times a day for the pain, as necessary, but didn't think it was necessary for him to limit his activities.

Over the years, Paul's pain grew progressively worse. It became uncomfortable for him to walk. Two years ago he had had to give up hunting and golf, and he was finding it increasingly difficult to work at his hardware store. I prescribed higher, more frequent doses of aspirin. A physical exam showed that Paul had lost considerable motion in his hip joint and X-rays showed the joint space had narrowed even more dramatically than before. At this point, I referred Paul to an orthopedic surgeon, who thought Paul was a good candidate for joint replacement surgery. I sat down with Paul to ask what he thought about undergoing a joint replacement procedure. Paul rejected the idea. His wife was also having health problems, and there would be no one to run his store during the period of hospitalization and recovery the surgery would require.

Over this past year, Paul had been in constant pain and often lay awake at night, unable to sleep. He limped and was no longer able to climb the stairs. None of the NSAIDs helped very much. Occasionally he needed to take codeine. I suggested surgery to him again, and this time he agreed to it. Together we planned the surgery for after the Christmas season, when his hardware store business was a little slower. In the meantime, Paul used a cane to help him get around better.

Paul was able to find someone he trusted to run his business, and he came in for surgery feeling quite comfortable about his decision. The surgery went well, and during his recovery in the hospital over the next few days, he was delighted to be pain-free for the first time in years. He was also surprised that he was able to get up and move around with a walker just days after the operation. By six weeks, he was quite mobile. And after three months, he was walking essentially pain-free, using a cane only occasionally. He is almost ready to go back to work.

Joint surgery is one of the more successful and gratifying tools we have in the treatment of arthritis. Fortunately, most patients do not need joint surgery, and it is viewed largely by physicians as a measure of last resort. Why? Because any surgery carries with it certain risks; and while joint replacement surgery may certainly have dramatic results, a replacement joint is not the same as your own.

Medications, physical therapy, exercise, and rest should all be tried before you consider any type of surgery. If surgery is necessary, your doctor may want to try simpler, more conservative procedures first, in the hopes that they may put off or eliminate the need for joint replacement. A synovectomy (see page 331), for example, can provide a rheumatoid arthritis patient with pain relief for five or more years. Replacement joints have a limited life span, so the longer you can postpone surgery the better. It's also possible that during this interval, a more effective drug may emerge that will enable you to relieve your pain without further surgery.

When surgery is indicated, it has several goals: to relieve pain, improve the functioning of your joints, correct deformities, and prevent further damage to the joint structures. Pain relief is by far the overriding reason for most surgical procedures. While improved joint function is also a goal, the patient who is in a great deal of pain may find it acceptable to sacrifice a certain amount of joint function in exchange for pain relief. In the extreme, there are procedures that fuse painful joints into one position so that they no longer hurt. Such operations are usually done on wrists or ankles (current artificial joint replacements for these structures are not yet as good as they are for hips and knees). Although surgery may correct deformities, doctors don't usually recommend surgery for purely cosmetic reasons. Surgery may occasionally be necessary for repair of conditions of the soft tissue, such as torn ligaments, damaged knee cartilage, or rotator-cuff tears; but a detailed discussion of these surgeries is beyond the scope of this book.

Making the Decision

If you are considering joint surgery, you probably have many questions and concerns. The surgical options available to you depend upon the type of arthritis you have, the joints that are involved, and your overall health and physical condition. With rare exceptions, joint surgery is not usually considered for people with lupus, scleroderma, or gout. Patients with ankylosing spondylitis may occasionally require total joint replacement; however, doctors are sometimes concerned about performing this surgery on AS patients because of problems they have with excess bone growth. Rarely, AS patients may have an operation to straighten the spine.

The most likely candidates for surgery are those with severe and debilitating osteoarthritis and rheumatoid arthritis.

Do you need joint surgery? Since joint surgery is not usually an emergency procedure, you needn't rush into it. You can take ample time to discuss it with your physician and to seek several opinions, if you wish. This is a decision I like to make over time, to make sure it is necessary. Symptoms of many forms of arthritis, including osteoarthritis, can be episodic, becoming less of a problem on their own. So when you're in pain, I want to make sure that the pain will not respond to therapy or remit on its own, and that surgery really is the last alternative. I want to observe you and see what other therapies can do to improve your condition.

One man with osteoarthritis in the base of his thumb told me that the thumb had become so painful at one point that he couldn't even shake hands with business colleagues. His doctor recommended surgery, but the man was reluctant and decided to put it off. In the meantime, the doctor prescribed a pain-relieving medication that worked well. The patient's pain eventually subsided, and he never needed the surgery.

Similarly, I know of a seventy-two-year-old with osteoarthritis who likes to ski and ride a bike. She developed severe hip pain and consulted an orthopedic surgeon because she had read that surgery can correct such problems. Though her hip hurt a lot, the surgeon said that the joint really looked quite good on X-rays. He recommended NSAIDs, and over the next month her pain diminished significantly, and she was able to resume many of her former activities. She never needed the surgery.

In my own practice, when I suggest surgery to a patient, I'll describe the procedure, its benefits, and the possible complications. I like to introduce the subject to patients early on, to see what their feelings are and to allow for the possibility of surgery to sink in. Often I will suggest that my patients speak to others who have undergone the same operation. I also like to bring the orthopedic surgeon in early, as part of our team, since it is the orthopedist who ultimately decides on the best surgical treatment and performs the operation. This initial meeting gives the surgeon a chance to become familiar with the patient in case surgery becomes necessary. After the patient has had the first consultation with the orthopedist, we sit down together and review all information carefully before making a final decision.

If surgery seems imminent, you should discuss the various benefits and risks of surgery at length with your physician. Can you expect that surgery will substantially relieve your pain, correct your deformities, and improve the quality of your life? How long is the anticipated recovery time? What will your physical rehabilitation program involve? What are some of the possible complications of surgery?

The decision concerning surgery is ultimately yours. You are the one who has to decide whether the possible benefits outweigh the risks. And you are the one who has to participate fully in the rehabilitation process in order to get the best results. That decision should be carefully considered and made only when you are ready.

If you have been suffering from significant pain and your doctor recommends surgery, you might decide that you want to go ahead with it immediately. On the other hand, you might feel the pain is still bearable and want to put off deciding. Could such a delay be harmful? If X-rays show there is not much change, your doctor might want to try different medicines and just observe the condition for a while. In many cases, where relief of pain is the goal of therapy, waiting months or even years does not affect the later outcome of surgery.

While it's good to be cautious, I have some patients who obviously need surgery but who refuse it because they are afraid of the procedure. A sixty-five-year-old man with rheumatoid arthritis and serious knee problems was in constant pain. When I introduced the topic of knee surgery, he said he'd like to think about it. He came back several months later, still in pain. Again we talked about surgery, and again he said he'd think about it. A year went by, and he was still in terrible pain. I asked, "What are you afraid of?" and he said, "Don't they cut your leg off?" Although I had described the operation to him in detail, he had somehow gotten the false impression that this surgery was equivalent to an amputation. We talked at length about what goes on during surgery, and he felt much better about it and finally decided to go ahead with it. He did very well and feels gratified by the success of his operation.

Surgery is a very stressful experience, and one sixty-five-year-old woman with rheumatoid arthritis, who also had a very painful knee, was afraid of the problems she would experience during recuperation. She lived alone and worried about who would take care of her. She had tried NSAIDs, remittive drugs, and low-dose steroids. I injected her joint several times with a corticosteroid preparation, but even that failed to provide relief. Finally she couldn't go on anymore and was willing to accept the operation. She was more frightened by what she imagined her life was going to be like after the operation than by the surgical procedure itself. A social worker on our hospital team helped her make arrangements for the recovery period. She had the operation and is doing extremely well.

If you are making a decision about whether to have joint surgery, you might find it helpful to ask yourself the following questions:

Is your pain unacceptable? Constant pain that doesn't respond to NSAIDs, that keeps you awake at night, and that prevents you from working or doing the activities you enjoy is severe enough to require surgery.

Do you require narcotic pain relievers? If you need to take them daily, at full allowable doses to control your pain, you may require surgery.

Have you tried all other avenues to achieve pain relief? This means NSAIDs, physical therapy, rest, exercise, and joint protection measures. For patients with systemic forms of arthritis, this may also mean use of remittive agents or steroid injections in selected joints. For both rheumatoid arthritis and osteoarthritis patients, this would include the use of canes or crutches.

Are your goals realistic? If you have osteoarthritis and your pain is limited to a single joint, then surgery—particularly joint replacement—is likely to bring you considerable improvement. Your bones and other joints are likely to be in good shape, so you can more easily use walkers and crutches during recovery. Correcting the disease in a single problem joint can essentially cure the arthritis, and you may realistically expect surgery to significantly improve your level of activity.

If you have rheumatoid arthritis, however, you're in a somewhat different situation, because the disease is systemic and affects multiple joints. Though surgery may eliminate significant pain in your hip, for example, you may still have to contend with painful knees, elbows, shoulders, and feet. However, I've had patients with RA tell me that even though other joints may still hurt, in general they feel so much better after a joint replacement operation that it was well worth their while. RA patients with hip replacements may be able to sit more comfortably or sleep better, despite the fact that knees and other joints may still hurt.

However, rheumatoid arthritis patients need to be realistic in their expectations of a joint replacement operation. Such surgery will not be as nearly curative for them as it is for people with osteoarthritis who have just one problem joint. In addition, patients with RA frequently have bones weakened by osteoporosis, which complicates certain joint replacement procedures. Since their upper extremities are often involved, especially the hands, people with RA may have trouble using crutches or a walker, making their recovery more difficult. They may also have poorer health overall, which can also influence their recovery.

On the other hand, the lower activity level of patients with rheumatoid arthritis may mean less wear and tear on replacement joints, allowing the joints to last longer. I have certainly had RA patients who have done marvelously well following surgery, though their other joints still hurt. Even though these operations won't cure you, they may restore you to a higher level of health and functioning, and that in itself is very worthwhile.

When a patient with rheumatoid arthritis has multiple joint involvement, the approach to surgery must be carefully planned. If several joints need surgery, you have to decide which joint to treat first. Sometimes it's preferable to operate on the feet first, and then on the hips, so you'll be able to walk more easily. In other cases, your surgeon may decide to do your hands and feet at one time, to limit your exposure to anesthesia and other operative risks and to permit you to have all your rehabilitative therapy during the same hospitalization.

Are you in good physical condition? Older patients are frequently at greater risk for complications during and after any major surgery. Heart, lung, kidney, and blood vessel disease may increase surgical complications. However, age is no bar to surgery. I know some seventy-five-year-olds who are in good shape and are physiologically younger than their age. I'd feel comfortable about recommending surgery to them.

Are you prepared to follow a rehabilitative regimen conscientiously? Recovery from joint surgery may entail months of daily exercises to recover joint function.

Choosing an Orthopedic Surgeon

The orthopedic surgeon, or orthopedist, is a specialist in the problems of bones and joints, of which joint replacement surgery is only one part. He or she is also trained to perform many valuable nonsurgical therapies, including splinting, casting, and certain types of joint injection. In most hospitals, the orthopedist performs arthroscopic procedures that aid in diagnosis and therapy.

Your family physician, general internist, or rheumatologist will probably be able to refer you to a qualified orthopedic surgeon. Not all orthopedists do frequent joint replacement surgeries, so you'll want to inquire whether the specialist you're considering is knowledgeable about current techniques and performs such surgeries on a frequent and regular basis. In orthopedics, as in any specialty, skills are developed through practice.

Your orthopedist must understand your lifestyle and activities, your tolerance for pain, your expectations about surgery, and your work, family, and means of social support. For example, Ralph, a seventy-year-old with advanced osteoarthritis in his left hip, inquired at length about the mechanical aspects of surgery. He was an engineer by profession and had a natural curiosity about the technical functioning of the replacement joint. Having met Ralph several times, the orthopedist understood the things that worried him and took the time to give Ralph full and lengthy explanations about the technical aspects of surgery. Ralph was impressed by the surgeon's grasp of the principles of biomechanics and by his descriptions of the mechanical properties of joint replacements. The resulting rapport built between doctor and patient allayed many of Ralph's initial fears. Ralph had his surgery and is doing very well.

Surgical Procedures

There are a number of different surgical procedures that can be performed to relieve pain in advanced cases of arthritis. Surgery done on major joints requires opening the joint through a large incision (an arthrotomy), usually two or more inches wide, under general anesthesia. Smaller procedures can be performed through an arthroscope, a fiberoptic instrument a little wider than a drinking straw that allows surgeons to look inside a joint. This process, known as arthroscopy, requires several small incisions only a quarter of an inch wide. Arthroscopic surgery is less traumatic, entails less time for hospitalization and recuperation, and may be performed under a local anesthetic (although general anesthesia is sometimes required). Arthroscopy is most frequently used for diagnosing knee and shoulder problems and for surgically repairing sports-related injuries, such as a torn ligament or rotator cuff. This surgery also allows for the removal of fluid and small pieces of bone and cartilage that may be floating around in a joint.

The major types of surgery for arthritis are described below.

Synovectomy

This procedure is performed in the hospital and involves removal of the diseased synovium, or joint lining. A synovectomy is done primarily for patients with rheumatoid arthritis. In RA, the joint lining can become quite inflamed and enlarged, so you have a huge mass of tissue that grows very rapidly. The quickly growing synovial cells can produce substances that destroy cartilage, ligaments, tendons, and bone. The inflammation can often be controlled with medication; however, when there is constant severe pain that is not responsive to remittive agents or joint injections, and the health of the joint appears jeopardized, it may be necessary to remove the joint lining surgically.

Synovectomy can be performed through a surgical incision or an arthroscope, depending on the size of the joint. The joint is opened and tissues and other components are removed, but enough synovial tissue is left to maintain lubrication. It may take several weeks to recover from surgery. Rehabilitation is gradual and includes range-of-motion and strengthening exercises. Scientists are currently exploring ways to use chemicals to shrink the diseased synovium (chemical synovectomy).

Removal of the synovium can relieve your pain, frequently for a few years, and can possibly provide some protection against progressive joint damage. But synovectomy is frequently not a permanent cure. As time passes, the synovium tends to grow back, especially when therapy with remittive agents has not been successful. Physicians sometimes question whether the temporary relief of synovectomy justifies doing a major surgical procedure. However, synovectomies do provide good pain relief and are a more conservative approach than joint replacement. They can buy some time for the patient with rheumatoid arthritis.

Osteotomy

An osteotomy involves cutting the bone around the joint and then resetting the joint into a better position. This procedure is usually recommended in cases of osteoarthritis when the cartilage has worn away unevenly, leaving a joint misaligned and deformed. In corrective surgery of the knee in osteoarthritis, for example, a piece of bone may be removed from one of the leg bones to allow better alignment and more even weight distribution on the joint. The procedure affords good pain relief. It requires hospitalization and the recovery may take several weeks.

Resection

This operation involves the removal of all or part of a damaged bone to relieve pain. A metatarsal resection may be performed on a person with rheumatoid arthritis who suffers from debilitating foot pain (see "Feet" on page 338). Occasionally, this surgery may also be performed on an elbow, to remove part of the painful joint. Also, it is used to remove painful bunions. It may take several weeks to recover from this surgery, but the recovery period can vary.

Arthrodesis (Fusion)

This procedure involves fusing a joint such as an ankle, wrist, knee, or thumb into a fixed position. The bones are surgically repositioned in the best, most functional alignment; new bone growth fuses the joint into a "frozen" position. (Sometimes fusion can be accomplished without surgery, simply by immobilizing a joint.) This is one instance in which motion may be sacrificed for pain relief. Following this operation, you will no longer feel the pain of bone rubbing on bone. Fused joints no longer bend in their usual way, and lose their natural motion; however, they are frequently quite functional, are no longer a source of pain, and allow physical activity within limits. A patient with a fused knee may limp, but at least he is able to walk. This operation may be considered for patients whose bones are not healthy enough for a joint replacement operation; for those who have repeated joint infections that do not allow the insertion of a prosthesis; and for small joints, like the thumb, where joint replacements are done less frequently. Recovery from this procedure can take several months, during which time you may need to wear a special brace.

Arthroplasty

This procedure involves joint reconstruction using both the patient's own tissues and artificial joint components. Most arthroplasties done today involve total replacement of the joint with a prosthesis. Improved surgical techniques, anesthesia, and man-made materials have made hip and knee joint replacement surgeries not only possible but almost commonplace. Several hundred thousand joint replacement operations are done annually in the United States. Hip and knee replacement surgeries are the most common and most successful of these operations. They are over 90 percent effective in relieving pain and in significantly restoring function to the joint.

This is major surgery that requires general anesthesia, a seven- to ten-day hospital stay and a lengthy postoperative rehabilitation period. After hip or knee replacement, you may be able to walk with a cane by six weeks. It may take up to an additional six weeks before you are fully recovered.

Types of Joint Surgery

The type of surgery you may require will depend upon the nature of your arthritis, the joints affected, your age, the strength of your skeletal bone, and your surgeon's judgment concerning the best procedure.

I will briefly review the possible surgical options for each major joint. The hip and knee joints will receive the most emphasis in this discussion because they are the joints most commonly operated on.

Hips

Joint replacement surgery of the hip has become one of the most common operations performed in America, with close to 100,000 such operations done each year. It often brings dramatic relief to patients with osteoarthritis and rheumatoid arthritis who suffer from debilitating hip pain.

Efforts to replace diseased hip joints with artificial joints have gone on since the 1800s, when surgeons used prostheses made of ivory and glass. An all-metal hip prosthesis, anchored to the bone with metal screws, was also used. However, the tremendous stress placed on hip joints—more than three times the weight of one's body—rapidly eroded and loosened such artificial joints.

The modern era of total joint replacement began during the 1960s, with the work of the late Sir John Charnley, a British orthopedic surgeon. After many years of research, he developed a prosthesis made of synthetic, high-density polyethylene that could absorb shock and eliminate the stress of metal rubbing against metal. Rather than being fastened by screws and bolts, his prosthesis was glued into place with methylmethacrylate cement, a dental glue used to hold crowns and tooth inlays in place in a constantly moist environment.

Charnley's original design is the one we basically use today. (See the drawing below.) The worn hip socket (the acetabulum) is replaced by a "cup" made of polyethylene. The head of the thigh bone (the femur) is replaced by a metal ball attached to a stem, which is cemented into the thigh bone.

Total hip replacement operations have been performed in the United States since 1973. At first they were confined to older, more sedentary patients aged sixty and up. Today they are performed on younger, more active patients as well. But younger patients do pose special considerations. Hip joints last approximately ten to fifteen years (sometimes more) with normal wear. A younger person is usually more active; and should the hip wear out, there is a good possibility that he or she might need a second operation. The removal of a cemented joint is a difficult operation. In view of this, a special cementless joint that is easier to remove has been designed. It has a porous metal surface that encourages the patient's own bone to grow around it, anchoring the joint in place. These cementless joints also reduce the chances of infection and mechanical loosening.

Sometimes only the head of the femur needs to be replaced or resurfaced. This procedure, called a cup arthroplasty, is chosen if the patient's hip socket is in good shape and only the head of the femur is damaged. This is a more conservative procedure and may delay the need for a total joint replacement.

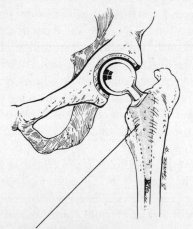

HIP PROSTHESIS

**stem of prosthesis
inside bone of leg**

The major complications of hip replacement surgery are loosening or dislocation of the joint and infection. Loosening occurs at the site where the cement meets metal or bone. You will feel pain and an X-ray will show a characteristic clear space where the loosening has occurred. Dislocation occurs when the ball separates from the socket. You may have a popping sensation and feel the joint slipping. If artificial joints are loosened or dislocated, another operation needs to be done.

Infection also causes persistent pain and sometimes other signs such as fever. Sometimes it can be treated with antibiotics and then suppressed by continuing therapy. However, more severe infections may require removal of the joint. Reinsertion of a prosthesis may be attempted later, after the infection has been brought under control. With today's surgical techniques, the infection rate for artificial hip joints is extremely low (less than 1 percent).

The results of hip surgery are excellent overall. Over 90 percent of patients experience significant relief from pain and an improvement in function. Though patients can be physically active, they are restricted from such vigorous activities as downhill skiing, tennis, and jumping, which could place too much stress on the joint.

Knees

The hip is a relatively stable joint because of its ball-and-socket design and the muscles anchoring it. As such, it is an ideal joint for replacement. Replacements of the knee are technically more complex. Situated between the two longest bones of your body, the knee is exposed and bears all of your body's weight. It is not just a simple hinge, but is required to perform very complicated twisting, gliding, and rotating motions. There are more technical problems involved in replacements of the knee, and the operation is more exacting than hip procedures.

A number of types of surgery other than joint replacement may be useful for the knee, depending on the type and extent of joint damage present. A patient with osteoarthritis, for example, may have an uneven erosion of the cartilage in the knee, so that his or her joint space is uneven and the joint becomes poorly aligned. Instead of replacing the entire joint, the surgeon may want to replace only the inside or outside portion of the joint, building new surfaces. The joint may also be realigned with an osteotomy, in which the bone is cut and then reset into a more functional position. When joint damage is more extensive and the entire knee is involved, a total knee replacement will probably be necessary.

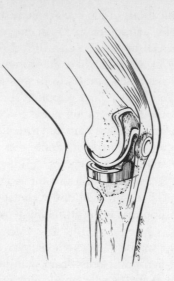

KNEE PROSTHESIS

Most knee prostheses have a bottom part made of high-density polyethylene that sits on top of your shinbone and a top part made from a metal alloy that is attached to the thigh bone. (See the drawing above.) As with hip replacements, loosening and infection are possible complications. The overall results, however, are usually good, and patients can expect pain relief for ten or more years.

In rare cases when your knee joint is infected or the bone is in very bad condition, your surgeon may fuse it. The resulting joint is stiff, but you will still be able to walk and do a fair range of physical activities. Fusion, however, is not usually the treatment of choice.

Hands

Decisions about operating on the hands are made somewhat differently than such decisions about hips and knees. The longer you delay having hand surgery done, the more problems you may have with ruptured tendons and ligaments. Hand deformities are often reversible earlier in the disease, but if the operation is delayed too long, they may become fixed. It is better to treat the hands earlier in the progression of the disease to restore function and prevent further deterioration. Surgery of the hand joints is not viewed as a last resort.

Severe rheumatoid arthritis in the hand is a major reason for surgery.

The rheumatoid process can erode cartilage and bone and weaken the supporting structures that hold ligaments and tendons in place. As the joints are pulled out of alignment, the hands may become deformed and incapable of performing simple functions. The disease process can also rupture tendons and ligaments, disconnecting the joint from its muscle. This leads to further loss of motion. Surgery of the hand aims at halting this disease process.

There are many approaches to hand surgery. A synovectomy, for example, may remove the destructive joint lining and prevent further joint damage, such as rupture of tendons and ligaments. If your tendons have already been pulled out of alignment, surgery can be performed to put them back in place and reestablish proper muscle action. Sometimes, in advanced rheumatoid arthritis, the thumb joint becomes so painful and unstable that it simply gives way when you attempt a grasping motion. In such cases, your surgeon might suggest an arthrodesis procedure, an operation to fuse the thumb into a stable, unbendable position so it will no longer cause you pain.

Artificial finger joints can also be surgically inserted. Since finger joints are so small, they are replaced by small plastic spacers rather than by two-part prostheses. During surgery some of the diseased joint tissue is removed and a small, hinged prosthesis is inserted in its place. Tissue gradually forms around the prosthesis and the finger becomes more functional.

After surgery, your hands will usually have a much improved appearance. However, surgery is undertaken to improve function and relieve pain, not just for cosmetic reasons. Many people are quite satisfied with the amount of hand function joint surgery can give them, although you won't have a complete restoration of function. The disease may progress, and some deformity may return. Loosening of the joints and infection aren't as much of a problem here as they may be for some other man-made joints because the hands are not subjected to as much mechanical stress.

Wrists

Arthrodesis is usually performed for patients with severe rheumatoid arthritis of the wrists. When a surgeon realigns the hand, he or she will frequently fuse the wrist to eliminate the pain that occurs from the movement of damaged joints and to stabilize the wrist. This stability is essential for efficient use of the hands. Synovectomies can also be done on wrists.

Elbows and Shoulders

Shoulders are key joints. While they don't bear weight, they are essential for grooming, eating, and hygiene. Arthritic shoulder joints usually aren't as painful as similarly affected joints used for moving and standing, but they can certainly have functional problems. The development of artificial shoulder joints is less advanced than the development of artificial knees and hips. Normal motions of the shoulder are extremely complex, and artificial shoulder joints don't function or hold up as well as some other man-made joints. There is continued interest in developing a better artificial shoulder joint.

Painful elbows are sometimes treated with a synovectomy, coupled with a partial resection. Prostheses are also available for elbows, but elbow replacements, like shoulder replacements, are not as advanced as hip prostheses.

Feet

Surgery on the joints of the feet is used most successfully to treat the painful deformities of rheumatoid arthritis. Walking is exquisitely painful for some RA patients because the dislocated ends of bones in the deformed foot receive the body's full impact. (In a normal foot, the stresses are absorbed and distributed over the bottom of the foot.) This problem can be surgically corrected with a resection. The joint is removed, making the foot shorter and flatter, and the toes are realigned. Patients are often able to walk comfortably again. If you need hip or knee surgery as well as surgery of your feet, it is best to correct the foot problems first. As I've previously mentioned, this can help speed the rehabilitation process after surgery.

Ankles

We have not yet developed a reliable prosthesis for ankle joints. To relieve pain in the ankle, we sometimes have to fuse it surgically or with a brace. Though the ankle may lose its flexibility, the pain will lessen, since bones no longer rub against each other.

Neck

This is one area where surgery may not be elective. In many cases of advanced rheumatoid arthritis, the vertebrae of the spine may become unstable and slip into one another. The medical term for this is C1–C2 subluxation. This can cause significant neck pain and headaches, which can be persistent. Doctors don't treat this type of pain with surgery, because the operation is difficult and very risky. However, we do perform surgery when the vertebrae impinge on the spinal cord and disturb its function, causing weakness in the arms and legs and loss of bowel and bladder control. This is considered a medical emergency. To protect the spinal cord from permanent injury, the vertebrae must be fixed in place by wiring the bones together, complemented by a bone graft to fuse the bones together. A spinal fusion is not done simply when there is evidence of subluxation. It is only performed when the patient shows symptoms of progressive nerve and muscle problems.

Preparing for Surgery

The following is a checklist of points to consider prior to surgery. Most of the information in this and following sections refers to hip and knee surgery, since these are the most common forms of surgery performed.

Stay in shape. Good muscle strength before surgery will help you to a speedier recovery afterward. Keep practicing your prescribed physical therapy exercises, and if possible, perform some regular exercise such as swimming.

Keep your weight down. Being overweight places additional stress on your already weakened joints and on your heart and lungs during surgery. Strive for your ideal body weight or lose weight as recommended by your physician. This too will aid in a speedier recovery.

Review medications with your physician. Discuss with your doctor whether you should adjust your current medications. You may, for example, be asked to stop taking aspirin because it can prolong bleeding and have a detrimental effect on surgery. Methotrexate may prevent surgical wounds from healing and may have to be stopped.

Make home arrangements ahead of time. Now is the time to prepare for your recovery period after surgery. Ask your doctor if you will need crutches or require any special equipment or chairs for sitting. If you are having surgery on your hands, you may need assistance with the tasks of daily living. Make arrangements ahead of time for nursing or family assistance for when you arrive home.

Review current infections with your doctor. If you have any potential sources of bacterial infection, they should be treated and completely cleared up prior to surgery. Even a minor infection can spread to the site of the operation and cause complications after surgery. You may also need to consult with your dentist, since mouth infections can sometimes be a problem, especially if you have dental decay.

Hospital Admission

Simple procedures on the hand and removals of bunions may be performed on an outpatient basis. However, major joint replacements are extensive procedures that require hospitalization. You may be admitted to the hospital on the day before surgery or on the morning surgery is to take place if you've already had preoperative evaluation and preparation.

You will be told not to eat or drink (even water) from after midnight prior to the day of surgery. This is extremely important, because during anesthesia you could vomit and choke on anything in your stomach.

Make a list of the medications you normally take, including over-the-counter drugs, so that you can inform your physician about them. This information should be recorded on your patient hospital chart. During your hospitalization, the only medications you should receive are those given to you by the hospital staff. Remind the hospital staff about any allergies to drugs (such as penicillin) you may have.

The preoperative evaluation consists of a variety of diagnostic tests, including a chest X-ray, an electrocardiogram, and lung function tests. In addition, your blood will be typed in case a transfusion becomes necessary. Your anesthesiologist and other physicians and medical personnel involved in your care will visit you. The anesthesiologist will tell you what kind of anesthesia he or she is going to administer (general, local, spinal, or epidural), and you may wish to ask questions about how long the anesthesia will last, whether you must stay flat on your back after surgery (spinal), and when you can eat and drink.

You will be shaved and asked to take a shower and shampoo with antiseptic soap. Since infection is by far the major complication of total joint replacement, you will be given an antibiotic. The physical therapist or another staff member may visit you to tell you about the equipment and exercises you will use or perform during your hospital stay.

You will be asked to remove your jewelry (if possible, leave all valuables at home) and dentures. Wedding bands are usually allowed and taped into place. Nail polish should be removed.

You will be given a sedative prior to surgery, and you may be drowsy as you are wheeled to the operating room. Here the anesthesiologist will insert a needle into a vein and begin intravenous fluid replacement; an IV will allow other fluids, and if necessary, blood and drugs, to be administered during surgery. After a short while you will be in a deep sleep. Total joint replacement operations can last up to three to four hours.

Recovery

After the operation, you'll be transferred to the recovery room for monitoring while you wake up from anesthesia. You may feel groggy for a while, but your condition will be closely watched by nurses and doctors who will monitor your heart rate, blood pressure, breathing, and any other reactions you may have to surgery. They'll help you get comfortable and may give you medication for the pain, intravenous fluids, or blood as needed. The nurses will help you cough and breathe deeply to prevent lung complications that slow down recovery.

You may find that a small tube has been placed at the site of the operation to drain off blood. Another tube may have been placed in your bladder to drain away urine. You may be wearing elastic stockings as well, especially after hip surgery, to prevent blood clots from forming in your legs.

Once you are fully awake and stabilized, you will be transferred to your room. Recovery varies, depending on the surgery performed, but generally speaking, a knee or hip procedure requires seven to ten days in the hospital. You should be able to get out of bed and walk around a little after a day or two.

You may not feel very well in the first few days, but after the stress of surgery is over and after the intravenous tubes and drains are removed, you will soon feel more like yourself. Even in the first hours and days, you may notice that your painful joint no longer hurts, a feeling many patients have considered a true miracle. One sixty-two-year-old who'd had extreme, constant hip pain for which he frequently had to take narcotic-type pain relievers said that he noticed the difference as soon as the effects of the anesthesia wore off. For the first time in years, he no longer had pain in his hip. You may not be totally pain-free, however; your surgical incision may hurt, and you may be in an uncomfortable position. You may be placed in a specific position designed to prevent you from moving your joints. For example, if you've had a hip replacement, a special pillow may be placed between your legs to keep them a shoulder-width apart and to prevent your legs from rotating inward; if you've had knee replacement surgery, your knee may be attached to a device called a continuous passive motion machine that will keep your new joint gently exercised.

Your bed will be equipped with a special trapeze to allow you to move on your back or lift yourself up.

Your physical therapist should begin to help you learn to use your new joint as soon as possible. You will learn new exercises to strengthen the muscles around the affected joint and to regain your range of motion. At first you'll walk only a few steps at a time with a walker for support so your new joint doesn't have to bear the body's full weight. You will progress from a walker to crutches and then to a cane. The physical therapist will teach you how to use your new joint to get in and out of bed, walk, sit, go up and down the stairs, get in and out of the shower, and maneuver in and out of cars. You will also learn how to get dressed without bending your hips or knees.

As your recovery progresses and your joint motion is restored, you will be prepared for discharge. Your surgical bandages will be removed and you'll receive final instructions on how to use your new joint and a prescription for pain medications, which you'll probably need for a few days. If you have questions about activities you may or may not perform or about the prescribed exercises, this is the time to review them with your physical therapist. It is also important that all arrangements be made for you prior to your arrival home.

Sutures are generally removed after ten to fourteen days, at which time you may have to make a follow-up visit to the surgeon.

Recuperating at Home

Once home, you will continue to work to regain strength and range of motion in your new joint. In most cases, recovery will be uncomplicated. You should, however, contact your physician should any of the following symptoms occur: pain, swelling, or drainage from the site of operation; fever; chest pain; shortness of breath; or any unexpected new symptom.

Some patients may need to spend time recuperating in an extended care facility, especially if they are older, have more complicated medical problems, or have difficulty getting adequate home care. This will be only a temporary stay, just until your recovery is sufficient to allow independence.

If you've had hip surgery, keep in mind that your safe maximum knee bend during recovery is 90 degrees. After the recovery period, do not overstress or flex your joints too much. The following guidelines can help prevent you from bending too much at the hip and possibly dislocating your hip:

- While sitting, keep your knees below your hips.
- Don't cross your legs while sitting or lying down.
- Avoid bending from the waist.
- Sit with your legs spread three to six inches apart.

To avoid bending, you may want to purchase a raised toilet seat, a bath bench, and special long-handled grippers to help you pick up items from the floor. If you must travel by car, get in and out of it carefully, and sit in the front seat with a pillow underneath you to raise the height of the seat. Enter the car backward, swinging your legs around to face forward. Lift your affected leg using your hands as necessary.

During recovery, follow your orthopedist's instructions on using crutches and a cane to avoid putting your full weight on your joint as it heals. By six weeks you should be using a cane most of the time, and by twelve weeks, your recovery should be essentially complete. Some patients with new joints feel so well that they wish to engage in strenuous physical activity. One sixty-year-old who could just barely hobble before hip surgery is now swimming, cross-country skiing, and hiking again. A professional basketball coach had a hip replacement and is back coaching again. Some exceptional people have even gone out and run marathons with their new hip joints. I would definitely *not* recommend this, but it is an example of how successful the surgery can be. Many of my patients are able to return to work, to drive, to visit friends, and to resume many of their recreational activities.

Remember, replacement joints are not the same as normal joints: they can deteriorate, loosen, or dislodge. Avoid joint overuse and let your physician and your own good sense guide your choice of activities. Continue to eat sensibly and keep your body weight down. Extra pounds on the body impose unnecessary stress on the new joint and may shorten its life span.

Your artificial joint is a foreign body and thus is a site of possible infection. Remind your dentist or doctor that you have a prosthesis before any dental work, minor surgery, or diagnostic procedures that can spread infection (for example, instrumentation of the bladder) are done. You will need to take antibiotics as a preventive measure.

Infection is always a possibility with a prosthetic joint; contact your physician if you have any joint pain—a symptom of infection.

Summary

There are many types of surgery that may help relieve the pain of debilitating arthritis. Most must be approached cautiously, after all other possibilities for treatment have been fully exhausted. Of all the types of surgery, joint replacement has had the most success in improving patients' lives. Patients with artificial joints may be pain-free for the first time in years. They are more independent, and can return to work and to more active and productive lives. Even patients with rheumatoid arthritis—who may still have limited activity because of disease in other joints—are likely to experience improved overall health because of the decrease in pain after the operation. The psychological gains to you and your family can also be significant. Few procedures in medicine can so decisively improve the quality of life as reconstructive joint surgery.

19

Unproven Remedies and Treatments

Mark, a fifty-six-year-old sales manager, developed pains in his hands, feet, elbows, and wrists. His knees were especially affected; the pain grew so severe that he limped constantly. He believed there wasn't much that could be done for arthritis, so instead of seeking conventional medical care, Mark decided to go to Mexico, to a clinic that he'd heard had a cure for arthritis. While in Mexico, he received a number of steroid injections and felt better for a short while. A few months later, after he came back home, his symptoms returned. Mark was very discouraged and came to Duke for a detailed evaluation. X-rays suggested the possibility of gout. We tapped his knee and discovered evidence of gout crystals. The steroid injections Mark received in Mexico were unnecessary and inappropriate for his stage of disease. We placed him on an initial course of therapy with NSAIDs and colchicine, and then on allopurinol. Mark has done well ever since.

Arthritis patients spend billions of dollars a year on untested cures, from wearing copper bracelets and sitting in abandoned uranium mines to eating special foods and taking vitamin supplements. I find this disappointing and sometimes almost tragic. Patients may waste their time and money; but even worse, they may not avail themselves of the many good therapies available for arthritis today. One unfortunate fact of modern medicine is that some patients don't have enough money to obtain the care they need. In this case, patients have enough money but aren't spending it in the right place. Here it's an issue not of adequate finances, but of patient education.

As a physician, I try to keep an open mind when it comes to unproven remedies. I am interested in the possibility that some of these treatments may be of value, and I wait for the studies that will allow them to be appropriately evaluated so I can make an assessment. After all, the history of medicine is filled with treatments that were initially looked upon with suspicion and then were later found to have validity. Before discounting herbal remedies, for example, we should remember that aspirin is a derivative of willow bark and that people used to make a tea of this bark to reduce fever. In the old days, healers used to bleed their patients in the sincere but mistaken belief that too much blood was harmful to one's health. This practice was appropriately stopped when it was found to have no value. Yet a few years ago it became popular to practice plasmapheresis and leukophoresis, more sophisticated procedures that involve the removal of components of patients' blood to cure disease.

The problem is, some unproven remedies can be dangerous, and others, though seemingly harmless, may divert patients away from effective conventional treatment plans. I prefer to use proven standard therapies that have a scientific basis, so I know what these therapies can and cannot do. Certainly it's a tragedy if a patient spends time on unproven remedies and doesn't get the benefit of conventional remedies. The clock is ticking on some diseases. For example, if you wait too long to seek care for rheumatoid arthritis, you may end up with joint deformities. By the time you go to a regular doctor, it may be too late.

Why People Turn to Unproven Remedies

The three biggest groups of patients attracted to unproven claims are those with AIDS, cancer, and advanced arthritis. AIDS and cancer are severe and potentially life-threatening diseases. Arthritis, on the other hand, can involve chronic pain. Patients with these diseases may feel desperate and willing to try almost anything to improve their situation. They may feel hopeless and believe there is nothing to be done to treat their disease. Unfortunately, there are people out there who prey on such fears; these people promise quick and easy cures and prescribe treatments of no value.

What Is an Unproven Remedy?

An unproven remedy is one that has not been satisfactorily put to the scientific test. Some unproven remedies are outright quackery; others fall into a gray area—they may or may not be of any medical benefit. There are four basic categories of what may be called unproven treatments:

New and Experimental Medical Therapies.

By definition, these are unproven remedies; scientists do believe they have some value, even though they have not yet been fully tested.

Unconventional Medical Preferences.

This type of unproven remedy includes therapies that are not necessarily standard practice, but which some health professionals believe may be of some value. Chiropractic falls into this category. While chiropractors are licensed practitioners, and you can get third-party reimbursement for their care, there is some controversy in the medical field about the therapeutic value of this approach. Sometimes individual physicians adopt a style of practice or use drugs that they believe, based on their own experience, to be beneficial for their patients; however, other doctors may prefer not to use these treatments or may believe that they are ineffective or have unacceptable side effects.

Folk Remedies.

These include such things as amulets, vinegar and honey, elderberry wine, or the spraying of lubricant WD-40 on your joints. Patients don't need prescriptions to try such remedies and may just try them on their own without asking a doctor's advice. There's no proof that any of these work.

Quack Medicine.

Finally, some unproven remedies fall into the category of outright quackery. Such treatments have no merit whatsoever and may even be dangerous. Quack practitioners may be a cause for real concern. Though in their hearts many believe they are doing good, they may be practicing unacceptable medicine, such as giving excessively high doses of steroids. Some are outright charlatans whose only motive is profit.

Common Unproven Remedies

Many unproven remedies fall into the category of folk remedies. They are backed by anecdotes and testimonials from patients rather than by scientific studies published in reputable medical journals. Such remedies include special diets and foods and a variety of natural herbs and products. If my patient wants to try a folk remedy, I won't encourage it, though I may have to tolerate it and let him do what he wants. One of my patients, for example, said he read in some magazine that elderberry wine was good for rheumatoid arthritis and asked what I thought. I didn't think there was anything wrong with moderate consumption of elderberry wine, though I doubted it would help his swollen joints. I said that if he wanted to give it a try, it was really up to him. Another patient asked me if avoiding red meat would improve his arthritis. My response to this, as to dietary changes in general, is that I'm not in the position to say whether this could help or not. I have no evidence that abstaining from red meat will provide any benefits or that eating it will do you any harm. Since this patient was overweight and his diet included lots of fatty cuts of red meat, I certainly didn't mind his giving the diet a try, as it might do him some good, but not necessarily for the arthritis. In most instances, avoidance of specific foods is not an approach that I can recommend with any enthusiasm, given our current understanding of arthritis.

Similarly, I can't tell you with certainty whether herbal remedies can be of any help. It's conceivable that there may be some medical benefits from certain herbs. Many of today's medicines were originally derived from plants. Belladonna, which relaxes spasms, is derived from the leaves, roots, and flowers of the deadly nightshade. Colchicine, used to treat gout, also comes from a plant; so does digitalis, a drug that stimulates the heart. A popular Chinese herbal folk remedy for arthritis is currently being studied seriously by scientists. Since some herbs can have medicinal effects, they should be taken as cautiously as you would take any drug, and I recommend you discuss them with your doctor; however, don't be surprised if your physician disapproves of such therapy.

Some patients ask about elimination diets. As I discussed in chapter 16, there may be a small percentage of people whose arthritis is influenced by foods in their diet. Some people are highly sensitive to certain foods, and others are concerned about the effects of additives and antibiotics in our food supply.

The only way to know for certain whether a particular food is making your arthritis worse is to eliminate possible food sources one by one to see if the arthritis improves and then to reinstate foods in the same manner, to see if the arthritis returns. This is a long and difficult process, and because of the natural fluctuations of the disease, it is sometimes hard to find a direct relationship. Is it worthwhile to have everyone go on an elimination diet? Given the very small number of people this would help, and the lengthy and difficult process of an elimination trial, I don't think so. However, if an individual believes a particular food is having an adverse effect on him, I will work with him to test his theory.

What about devices like copper bracelets? I doubt very much that a copper bracelet can do anything to improve your arthritis. In fact I'm surprised this folk remedy has stuck around for so long. As a physician, I'm interested in why certain unproven remedies persist. Does such a remedy represent a collective delusion, or could there be something there that doctors have missed? Could it be possible, for instance, that copper is absorbed from the bracelet? We give patients with rheumatoid arthritis shots of gold, also a heavy metal; and we know that penicillamine, also used to treat rheumatoid arthritis, binds with and removes metals from the blood. Could there be a tie here? I suppose it is within the realm of possibility; however, such a relationship has not been proven.

Another unproven remedy you may have heard about is DMSO (dimethyl sulfoxide), an industrial solvent that when rubbed on the skin has a local analgesic activity. Currently, DMSO has been approved for the treatment of interstitial cystitis, a rare bladder disease. Does it work for some forms of arthritis? I don't think so, but I really don't know. To date, scientific studies have shown no such benefits. Nor have benefits been shown for such other unproven remedies as snake or bee venom, which carry a danger of severe allergic reaction; vitamin therapies; or topical applications of the lubricant WD-40.

The Placebo Effect

Sometimes patients feel temporarily better after trying an unproven remedy. This may be pure coincidence. Arthritis frequently comes and goes in an unpredictable fashion, and you may attribute a naturally occurring remission to an unproven remedy. But you may also sense improvement because practitioners of these "cures" offer the reinforcement and psychological support that can make you feel good.

When scientists do a controlled, double-blind study, they divide participants into two groups. One group receives the substance being tested.

The other group receives a sugar pill, or placebo, that looks just like the active drug. *Double-blind* means that neither the scientists interpreting the results nor the study participants know who is getting the active drug and who is getting the placebo. Scientists have observed that as many as 30 percent of people in any placebo group may experience an improvement in their condition. Patients' emotions and expectations seem to influence their symptoms independent of the substance taken. This is known as the placebo effect. There is very likely a physiologic basis to the placebo effect, relating to the production of chemical substances that influence brain function and perception of pain.

Unproven remedies appear to provide a very powerful placebo effect, at least temporarily. A placebo effect can play a positive role in conventional therapy, but it can also be exploited by quack practitioners. A support group, for example, may offer a placebo effect. But that's okay, because participating in the group supports and reinforces the other good therapies you may be receiving. On the other hand, quack therapies are not okay, even if they do offer a placebo effect, because they deflect you from seeking good treatment and expose you to potentially dangerous substances.

We used to see evidence of what may have been the placebo effect at work years ago when we put rheumatoid arthritis patients in the hospital for bed rest. Such patients were removed from the stresses of their everyday lives, they were fed and cared for by a supportive staff, and they felt a lot better. The same thing happens when a patient goes to an exotic clinic that promises a quick cure. He may pay a lot of money and travel a great distance to be treated at the clinic, and he may feel supported and encouraged once he gets there. This, too, can have a very powerful placebo effect.

Aside from banking on the placebo effect, quack healers commonly practice in warm and exotic locales, such as Mexico and the Bahamas. Such practitioners rarely set up clinics in cold and unappealing areas. So the patient travels with great anticipation to a warm, attractive setting, and that in itself may make him feel better.

One of my rheumatoid arthritis patients, Roger, had invested so much time, energy, and money in traveling to a clinic in the Bahamas that he hated to admit defeat. However, he returned to America feeling just as bad, if not worse. I put him on a course of gold treatment. Within a few weeks, Roger was responding quite well. His first response was "See, the treatment in the Bahamas is finally working."

While quacks profit from the harmless placebo effect, they also commonly give patients steroids. In the short run, steroids can make someone feel good, and you could probably send anyone to the Bahamas and administer steroids and induce a feeling of well-being. However, steroids are very powerful drugs that, depending on your condition, may or may not be beneficial for you. You may feel temporarily better, but you subject yourself to the risk of side effects and potential harm, and such treatments may deprive you of more appropriate long-term therapy.

Part of being a good doctor means giving that same sense of support and encouragement that an exotic clinic can provide, not in order to manipulate a desperate patient, but in order to facilitate good therapies. When a patient trusts you and knows that you are looking out for his or her best interests and will use effective, well-proven treatments, the resulting rapport can have very beneficial results.

For example, Gary, a fifty-nine-year-old with active, severe rheumatoid arthritis that was not responding to gold and penicillamine, volunteered to participate in a collaborative study at Duke on methotrexate, a drug then being studied for treatment of RA. (Methotrexate has since been approved for this use.) Although he didn't know it at the time, Gary was placed in the active drug group and received methotrexate for several months. The drug did not appear to help him at all. Several months following the study, Gary was still feeling poorly. I was having good results using methotrexate with other patients and decided to try him on the drug once more. Within a few weeks, Gary got dramatically better. Just out of curiosity, I asked him why he thought the methotrexate hadn't worked for him previously. Gary said that while he was in the study, he had been plagued by constant worry: "When I didn't feel any better, I got worried that I was on the inactive drug, or else that I was on the active drug and that it wasn't working. It was my last hope, and I was scared. Now you've recommended it to me. I've always trusted you. You're a good doctor, and now I can see it's working and that it's a good drug."

Unproven Remedies and Your Doctor

It is not always easy to distinguish between the different types of unproven remedies, to determine which are quackery and which are merely unproven. Sometimes there is a fine line between the two. For example, some people believe that sitting in an abandoned uranium mine can help to cure arthritis. Physicians would consider such unsupervised treatment, without careful monitoring or study, an unproven remedy; and if such a treatment was advocated in an unscrupulous way, we'd consider it quackery. On the other hand, treating rheumatoid arthritis with radiation therapy in well-defined doses was actually considered in a scientific trial in the 1980s. There is a certain irony here.

Gold treatment emerged as a therapy in the 1930s, but it wasn't until the 1960s that it was considered an acceptable, proven treatment for RA. Sulfasalazine was originally developed to treat RA in the 1940s, but not until the past few years has it been acknowledged as a valuable therapy. Methotrexate, too, was first tried for RA twenty or thirty years ago, yet has only recently been approved as an effective RA drug.

So at one time many currently respected treatments were viewed as unproven remedies. Past studies may have used inadequate methods, too few patients, or the wrong patients. The benefits of the drugs being tested were not immediately recognized or clear-cut, and scientists were suspicious of their side effects. Subsequently, these same drugs have been retested under scientifically vigorous standards and have emerged as part of our standard medical arsenal.

Sometimes, to advance the field, physicians have to try unconventional new therapies. This is very different from quack cures. A reputable physician will carefully identify a patient whose illness may justify experimental therapy, ask for his or her informed consent, and always make sure the patient understands the possible benefits and risks. Reputable physicians are also willing to report their results in scientific journals. Unorthodox healers don't operate under these strictures or safeguards.

Almost every physician at one time or another has performed what was in essence an experiment on individual patients with drug treatments that have not been tested scientifically. This usually happens when they've exhausted all conventional therapies. For example, I may first try to treat a patient with polymyositis by giving him steroids along with Imuran or methotrexate. If my patient gets no relief from these conventional approaches, I have to ask myself, "Is there something else out there I might try that has some scientific rationale?" I might reason that polymyositis is an immune-mediated disease and that cyclosporine is a good immunosuppressive drug, so I might be willing to give this drug a try for this patient. Although this is an unproven treatment and no studies have been published on it, as a doctor I have an obligation to explore possible options that may help improve my patient's condition.

As a doctor I must be completely honest about unproven therapies. In such cases, I'll explain to my patients that the therapy is unproven in the strict sense of the word and that I'd like to try it because other available therapies don't seem to be working. Though based on a strong scientific hunch, this is essentially an experiment. If my patient improves after undergoing this unproven treatment, I would try to prove that the treatment, and not the placebo effect, caused the good result by verifying it in a scientific trial with other patients. If the results were reproducible, I'd let other medical professionals know about it. I may publish it as a case study or as a commentary in a medical journal so that other doctors may hear of my experience.

If your doctor suggests trying an unproven treatment, gather as much information about it as you can and discuss the possible risks and benefits with him or her in depth so you'll have a better idea of whether it makes sense for you to participate. Being an active patient who takes control of your health care choices will help you obtain the best results.

How to Evaluate Unproven Remedies

Different doctors approach therapies differently, and one doctor's regimen may be deemed unconventional by another. How do you, as a patient, sort it all out? First, I think you should see a qualified rheumatologist who has been recommended by another doctor you know and trust. The Arthritis Foundation is another good source of referral. If you've received a word-of-mouth recommendation from a friend or acquaintance, make sure the doctor is reputable. Check him or her out with your local Arthritis Foundation or call the local county medical society for a listing of the physician's credentials.

Second, you should become educated about your disease on your own. Reading this book is a good start, and you'll find helpful literature published by the Arthritis Foundation. If you find a discrepancy between the therapy you are receiving and what the literature says, discuss this with your physician; and if necessary, get a second opinion.

The following are possible signals to you that you may be involved in a disreputable program:

- The cure being touted does not appear anywhere in the medical literature.
- The cure is backed solely by patient testimonials and endorsements rather than by scientifically rigorous studies.
- The doctor doesn't take insurance and wants cash up front.

- The staff running the program allege that the medical community is "conspiring against them" to suppress their treatment methods.
- The treatment is being offered in an exotic, distant location, usually in a tropical climate.
- The program offers a secret, undisclosed cure.
- You're unable to verify the doctor's credentials.
- The program promises unrealistic "overnight" cures.

The Doctor-Patient Relationship

Sometimes a patient comes to my office and requests an unproven therapy that I honestly don't think is of any merit. I don't want to encourage my patients to waste their time and money or to delay getting the good treatments that are currently available to them. When I express my reservations, we may have a potentially contentious situation.

One patient kept asking me for a prescription for a drug unproven for arthritis. I had to tell him that I didn't think the drug would work and that I didn't want to get involved in this particular experimental treatment. I did direct him to a clinic where the drug was being tested and told him that he could seek treatment there if he wished. He told me that he couldn't afford to travel to the clinic because he'd already spent thousands of dollars traveling to different cities to meet with people who had already tried the cure. Some time after our conversation, published results of a scientific trial showed the drug to be of no value in treating arthritis. The patient's response was, "They probably didn't do the experiment right, anyway."

So with some patients, I feel like we are both in a no-win situation. On the other hand, I really am willing to be open-minded and flexible about treatments that seem medically reasonable. I encourage my patients to at least bring me some literature on the therapy they want to try so that we can sit down and review it together. If I think there's some merit in the approach, I may work along with the patient. If the therapy seems counterproductive, I feel it's my responsibility to warn my patients so that they don't waste their money or harm their health.

Occasionally I get angry patients who say, "Why are you keeping this therapy from me?" My response is, "Why haven't the people espousing these therapies shared them with the medical community? Why haven't they published articles about these therapies in reputable journals accepted by medical professionals?" I am not trying to keep the therapy from my patients; rather, the methods of those who are promoting those therapies keep them from the medical community.

What we really need is education, especially of patients and their families. There are many good therapies available for arthritis, and there is no need to feel desperate and seek out unorthodox cures. We physicians must also educate one another, because this is a field where there are so many changes and new developments in therapy that it's sometimes difficult to keep up with the latest approaches. Sometimes doctors aren't completely up-to-date on what's available. They may not be as encouraging of therapies as they might be and may unintentionally develop a mind-set that there's nothing to be done for a particular type of arthritis. One of the things we can do as academic physicians is to write and lecture and bring physicians into medical centers to correct this information gap.

Patients should recognize that arthritis is treatable and some forms are even curable with medication. For every disease, we have reasonable, reliable approaches. Research on new drugs continues, and in the years ahead there are certain to be more breakthroughs in this field.

I realize that patients and their families may sometimes have difficulty dealing with chronic pain and illness, and I try to understand their concerns and behavior and be sensitive to their needs. I try to convey to them the sense that there are many things that can be done to help them. Desperation makes people susceptible to quacks and drives them away from good, proven therapies that can really help.

PART FOUR

What's in the Future?

20

The Genetic Connection

At birth, we receive roughly 100,000 genes, one set from each of our parents. These genes determine all of our inherited traits, from gender and eye color to facial appearance and body build—in short, the entire blueprint of life. Genes are composed of a substance called DNA (deoxyribonucleic acid), the material of heredity for all living things. Encoded in DNA's long, thin intertwining strands are complex sequences of instructions that direct the growth and development of all the cells in your body. DNA tells the cells to manufacture enzymes and other proteins at exactly the right time and in precisely the right amounts so that your body functions smoothly.

Your immune system, like other important body functions, is under genetic control. As a result of this hereditary influence, the immune system of one individual differs from that of another in ways that may be important to health and disease. We now have good evidence that individuals vary in their genetic susceptibility to arthritis. Just as a person's hair and eye color may differ from someone else's, so may his susceptibility to arthritis.

Although we do not yet understand the exact nature of this genetic connection, researchers have a tremendous interest in its exploration. We hope that the pieces of the genetic puzzle will one day come together so that we can use our knowledge to prevent or treat arthritis. For now, the issue of the genetics of arthritis remains a complex and fascinating subject being probed in research laboratories.

Genetic Research: A Brief Overview

Much of what we know about the genetics of immunity and of individual susceptibility to arthritis springs from research done in an entirely different field—organ transplantation. An important set of genes that control the immune response was found serendipitously while scientists were trying to discover why donor organs were rejected by unrelated individuals.

In the early 1950s, when the first kidney transplants were performed, many of the operations were unsuccessful. Although donor blood type matched that of recipient, the immune system of the recipient still rejected the transplanted organ. The most successful transplant operations were those in which both donor and recipient were one of a set of identical twins or in which organ recipients had received powerful drugs to suppress their immune systems and prevent rejection.

Scientists sought to discover why organ transplants are rejected when donors and recipients are unrelated. The process of organ rejection is regulated by the immune system and very much resembles the inflammatory process. The body treats the transplanted organ as foreign and uses the same strategies that it would use to fight off a foreign antigen.

This process of organ rejection was not a surprise to physicians involved in transplant surgery. Studies from organ grafts in animals, especially mice, indicated that tissue from unrelated animals would be rejected in much the same manner as if the animals were fighting an infection.

Most of these animal experiments involved strains of mice that were inbred over many generations, so that like identical twins, they were all genetically the same. It was observed that mice from one group, which we'll call strain A, could accept skin grafts from other strain A mice; but A-strain skin grafts were promptly rejected by mice in B-strain groups, and vice versa. Since A and B strains differ genetically, it appeared that the acceptance or rejection of skin grafts was under genetic control.

Scientists performed further breeding experiments to try to identify the genes involved in organ rejection. They discovered that in all species a single set of genes was responsible for the prompt and powerful rejection of foreign tissues. This gene set was called the major histocompatibility complex, or MHC (*histo* = tissue; *compatibility* = acceptance; *complex* = many closely linked genes). A similar set of genes was found in humans. This set of genes was called the human leukocyte antigen, or HLA. HLA was so named because this system was first discovered on leukocytes, or white blood cells; however, we know that these antigens are distributed on *all* of the body's cells. There are many different forms of each gene in the MHC complex. In humans there are at least six MHC genes labeled as A, B, C, DQ, DP, and DR. Each gene in turn can take as many as thirty different forms (scientists label each possible gene variant with a letter-number tag; for example, A9, B27, DR3, etc.).

Later experiments with mice revealed that the MHC appears to determine whether a mouse responds to a particular antigen and the magnitude of that response. So while this gene system had originally been recognized in the context of organ transplantation, its true role seemed to involve the body's ability to distinguish self from non-self. Similar studies in humans now indicate that our immune responses are also controlled by MHC.

Arthritis and Genetics

Since some forms of arthritis appear to involve an immune response to something in the environment, scientists reasoned that genetics might help explain why some people seem more susceptible to disease than others. Using the tools for tissue typing—the technique used to determine MHC types—developed for transplantation, scientists began to test patients to see if there was an association between certain MHC markers and any forms of arthritis. In 1973, ankylosing spondylitis was the first type of arthritis in which scientists found such an association. Over 90 percent of patients with AS have the genetic marker HLA-B27. In the general population, only 8 percent of whites normally have this marker. Scientists subsequently found an association between Reiter's syndrome and HLA-B27; lupus and HLA-DR2 and HLA-DR3; and rheumatoid arthritis and HLA-DR4.

It appears that your MHC type may have a great deal to do with the way you react to *some* antigens in the environment (although your response to many other environmental antigens may be perfectly normal). So if you have a predisposition for inflammatory arthritis, you may respond to certain antigens by producing excessive amounts, or certain kinds, of antibodies. This could eventually lead to inflammatory arthritis. Someone else with a different MHC type, when faced with the same antigen, would not have this type of reaction. Similarly, if you have a genetic predisposition for arthritis but are never exposed to the antigen, you won't develop the disease.

Relative Risk

The question is, if you have a particular MHC marker, how much more likely are you to develop arthritis than someone who does not have this marker? The risk varies, depending upon the disease. The association between ankylosing spondylitis and the HLA-B27 marker is probably the strongest. If you have HLA-B27, your chances of getting ankylosing spondylitis are anywhere from ten to fifty times greater than if you don't have this marker. If you have the markers associated with rheumatoid arthritis and lupus, your chances of getting these diseases are anywhere from two to five times higher than for someone without those tissue types.

These numbers say only how much more *likely* you are to get the disease. They do not tell you what your absolute risk of getting the disease is. In other words, if the disease is rare and occurs in only a very small percentage of the population, and you are ten times more likely to contract the disease, your absolute risk of ever getting this form of arthritis is still very low. If your risk of having a certain disease is five times higher than the general population, for example, and the disease affects 1 of every 10,000 people, your absolute risk for the disease is 1 in 2,000. So in reality the risk of many of these diseases is really quite low, and many people with these genetic markers never get arthritis.

If arthritis is triggered by an antigen, as hypothesized, the likelihood of your developing arthritis may also depend on the chances of your being exposed to the antigen that triggers the disease. Since scientists do not really know what triggers inflammatory arthritis, or the rate of exposures to such triggers, the likelihood for acquiring this disease is hard to evaluate.

The pattern and severity of disease, even in people who have the same risk, may also differ from person to person and even within the same family. A father may have severe ankylosing spondylitis, eventually developing a bamboo spine, while his son may have only mild back pain that never gives him much trouble. So if you are at genetic risk for the disease, you can't assume you will get the disease as severely as someone else in your family.

Most forms of inflammatory arthritis, while influenced by genetic background, do not usually appear in more than one family member. Rheumatoid arthritis and lupus, for example, most commonly affect a single family member. Perhaps there are other genes that interact with the MHC and alter the expression of disease in different individuals. It's also possible that one person in the family has frequent, repeated exposure to something in his environment that acts as a trigger, while the other family members do not receive such exposure. In addition, a person's immune system may be altered by stress, diet, gender, or age.

Up until now, I've been discussing mainly inflammatory forms of arthritis. But what about osteoarthritis, which is primarily a degenerative disease? Does this too have a genetic connection? So far we have not established genetic markers for osteoarthritis. To do so is more difficult because of the frequency of OA in the general population (over 50 percent of us eventually show signs of OA). Since OA occurs so commonly, it's not surprising to find that several members of a family may have it. My feeling is that OA has more to do with such traits as joint alignment, cartilage composition, physique, and obesity, all of which may be under genetic control. However, OA is unlikely to involve the same genes as those associated with inflammatory arthritis. For example, people in the same family have a tendency to walk alike or have a similar stature, and I wouldn't be surprised if that contributes to OA. Metabolic factors may also be involved.

Tissue Typing

Although we have the ability to detect MHC antigens for several forms of arthritis, we don't do such tests routinely. That's because we don't need to know your tissue type in order to make an adequate diagnosis. Rheumatologists can make very fine diagnoses from medical histories, physical exams, X-rays, and laboratory tests.

Moreover, tissue typing is not usually useful even in those cases where we are uncertain about the diagnosis. That's because the MHC type can tell you no more than the likelihood that someone may acquire the disease; it is not diagnostic in and of itself.

In arthritis, as in the case of many diseases with a genetic component, tissue typing may eventually enable us to adopt a preventive approach to treatment. Again, genetic testing at our current level of sophistication would be of no help in this instance. The relative risks of acquiring arthritis are low, and even if you do develop the disease, tissue typing cannot tell us how severe your symptoms will be.

MHC typing tests don't yet have a well-established role in predicting arthritis. While studies of large populations have shown an association between arthritis and certain HLA types, doctors don't commonly see several members of the same family with arthritis. In fact, I am caring for a fifty-five-year-old identical twin who has deforming RA, and his identical twin brother is perfectly fine. So even in identical twins, heredity may not tell the entire story. In addition, HLA markers linked to certain forms of arthritis may be modified by a number of other genes; for example, it appears from animal studies that as many as six genes may influence whether an experimental animal gets lupus. If this holds true for humans as well, having a particular HLA marker is not by itself an indication of whether you will or will not develop arthritis.

I don't think that tissue typing for genetic counseling is necessary or that the recognition of the role of heredity in arthritis should influence a couple's decision to have children. Although some forms of arthritis can run in families, the only thing that can be inherited is a susceptibility to arthritis, not the disease itself. In most instances, only a small proportion of genetically susceptible individuals ever acquire the disease.

Research Prospects

Research is one area in which genetic analysis is of enormous value. We've been able to identify genes that cause many diseases. Once you can identify the gene involved, you can attempt to figure out the mechanism of disease and begin to design better ways to treat it. Recently, scientists have learned how to identify the gene for cystic fibrosis; as a result, we have new clues as to what causes this disease and have begun to think about new therapies. As we continue to learn more about the role of heredity in human disease, we also hope eventually to understand why some people with certain genetic markers appear more susceptible to inflammatory arthritis. In the near future, we hope to have an even more precise knowledge about the causes of arthritis and would like to be able to take steps to cure or prevent it.

21

New Research

Rheumatology is among the most dynamic fields in all of medicine. Over the past fifty years we have learned how to classify, diagnose, and effectively manage many forms of arthritis. Chronic gout, for example, once a serious disease, can now be well controlled by medication. The survival rates for lupus patients have risen dramatically. Arthritis associated with rheumatic fever has virtually been eradicated in the United States. Artificial joint replacements now offer patients with some crippling forms of arthritis a second lease on life.

New and promising leads and emerging technologies offer hope for further advances. Researchers in immunology, genetics, and microbiology are trying to determine what triggers inflammatory arthritis and why some individuals seem more susceptible to these diseases than others. Other researchers are studying cartilage and bone metabolism to find out what goes wrong in degenerative joint disease. Discoveries in these areas should help us to intervene in disease processes and should produce even more effective treatments.

Changes in the field are occurring rapidly, an encouraging note both for medical professionals and for you as a patient. While the following presents much-simplified versions of some complex areas of research, it should give you an overview of the major areas currently under investigation.

Genetics

Genetics has become a major focus in the study of many diseases. We now recognize that genetic factors are involved in such conditions as Alzheimer's disease, heart disease, diabetes, and hypertension. Arthritis also appears to be under genetic influence, and there is much research at present focusing on the types of genes that could predispose an individual to some forms of arthritis.

Many investigators feel that arthritis is triggered when a genetically susceptible individual is exposed to certain infections in the environment. Indeed, we already have good evidence that some forms of arthritis are associated with infections. The arthritis resulting from rheumatic fever, for example, is caused by a streptococcal infection; Lyme arthritis is caused by the spirochete bacterium, which is spread by deer ticks. We do not yet know if infectious agents cause rheumatoid arthritis or lupus; however, we are studying the possibility.

As researchers look for possible triggers, they ask themselves two basic questions about the contribution of genetics to some forms of arthritis: (1) Is inflammatory arthritis a response to some rare type of organism that we have not yet identified? (2) Is inflammatory arthritis an abnormal response to an infection that most healthy people would fight off more easily? The latter hypothesis currently seems the more likely of the two. People with arthritis, who otherwise appear healthy, may have an exaggerated response to specific infections and, as a result, develop joint problems.

We are currently testing these theories using several major research approaches.

Genetic Mapping

This approach allows us to identify genes that may cause an individual to be susceptible to arthritis. Scientists study people with certain forms of arthritis to see if they have genetic markers in common that would distinguish them from other, healthy people. The markers are identified by studying specific parts of different chromosomes. When we find such a marker, we focus on the portion of the chromosome where that gene lies, and then on the gene itself, to determine what it encodes. Once we have identified the gene, we can try to determine its function and then develop therapy based on this function. This is a very difficult study, especially for a disease that is likely influenced by multiple genes or sets of genes. However, genetic mapping has recently been used successfully to identify the genes responsible for such diseases as cystic fibrosis and muscular dystrophy.

Spontaneous Disease Models

Arthritis does not appear to be unique to humans. Many animals spontaneously develop similar diseases. Mice and dogs, for example, may develop a form of arthritis that resembles rheumatoid arthritis and lupus. Chickens can develop a disease like scleroderma. However, in all these species only some strains of animal develop these diseases; this confirms the suspicion that arthritis is under a genetic influence, and allows us to identify the genes associated with disease in susceptible animal strains. Scientists study animals that develop arthritis and then test whether the genes involved are similar to those in humans. This may be a faster approach than genetic mapping.

Induced Disease Models

Induced disease models follow principles similar to spontaneous disease models. Rather than waiting for disease to arise spontaneously, however, scientists cause the disease to occur. For example, if you inject a rat with collagen, you can induce a type of arthritis that has features in common with rheumatoid arthritis. Rats injected with organisms similar to those that cause tuberculosis can also develop an induced form of arthritis. Again, not all strains of animals develop induced disease, which allows scientists to identify the genes responsible for disease susceptibility.

Transgenic Technology

One of the most important new research techniques, transgenic technology is being used in the study of many diseases, including arthritis, cancer, and heart disease. Using this method, scientists take human genes associated with a susceptibility to arthritis and create a new strain of animal; the human gene is expressed by injecting the purified human genes into the embryos of rats and mice and allowing a new strain of "transgenic" animal to develop. This allows us to take a gene that's been identified as a possible contributor to arthritis and test it in animals in a way that we can't with humans. For example, injection into rats of the HLA-B27 gene for ankylosing spondylitis leads to a disease with a remarkable similarity to Reiter's syndrome. In this way we create a new strain of animal that bears this susceptibility gene in a prominent way and that can pass the gene on to its offspring. We can now investigate how high levels of expression of this gene actually cause disease.

Our goal is to identify common genes that may predispose some people to arthritis. In some forms of arthritis, the major histocompatibility complex (MHC) plays a role (see chapter 20); but there are probably other genes that may also influence the development of arthritis. We do not have a clue as yet to the nature of such genes and the types of changes they cause. All may not be directly related to immune function. For example, one of the findings that has emerged from animal studies is that our response to stress may be under genetic control. Some rats seem to react to stressful stimuli by producing higher than normal levels of cortisol, an anti-inflammatory substance. This may influence the animal's immune system, and consequently, whether or not that animal develops arthritis.

It is very difficult to identify genes that may cause arthritis in people. So scientists first try to identify possible target genes on the basis of animal studies and then investigate whether humans have a similar gene. From laboratory work with mice, we've learned that there are several distinct ways of getting lupus. Different mice get the disease in different ways, and different genes appear to be responsible in different mice. These studies have shown us that lupus is more heterogeneous than we previously thought. In other words, two people may get lupus, but different genes may cause it in each one.

Animal studies also allow us to scrutinize the possible relationships between genes and triggering agents in ways that are not possible with human studies. For example, we can take rats expressing the B27 gene and see if they will develop a more severe disease if infected with bacteria known to be associated with reactive arthritis.

Through such animal research we eventually hope to pinpoint the infectious agents responsible for many forms of arthritis. When we are able to do this, we may be able to prevent and more effectively treat these diseases.

Another current area of research, one in which I myself am involved, is the study of a phenomenon called molecular mimicry. This research is based on the fact that something foreign—a part of a bacteria or virus—can closely resemble human substances. It is believed that when some foreign substances resembling the body's molecules invade the body, they appear to confuse the immune system, which starts to manufacture antibodies against its own healthy substances. We are searching for bacteria, viruses, or fungi that mimic normal substances in the body and that may be a trigger for arthritis. If we can find such substances and the bacteria or viruses that produce them, we may be able to prevent or eradicate the infection before it leads to arthritis.

We have already identified genetic markers associated with ankylosing spondylitis, Reiter's syndrome, lupus, and rheumatoid arthritis. Scientists are working to identify other genes that may influence whether or not an individual with these markers will actually develop arthritis. We are also trying to identify genes associated with other forms of arthritis such as osteoarthritis. Perhaps one day we will be able to map out all of the interacting sets of genes responsible for the different forms of arthritis. Then we'll be able to identify what predisposes susceptible individuals to disease and perhaps take early preventive measures.

The Immune System

Scientists continue to devote much effort to trying to understand the normal actions of the immune system and the specific roles various immune cells play in helping us fight disease. At Duke, we are trying to answer such questions as: How do problems of immune regulation predispose a person to arthritis? What types of specific immune disturbances are capable of provoking arthritis? Can we manipulate these disturbances in a therapeutic way to prevent arthritis? What is the role of viruses and other infectious agents in causing disturbances in the immune system? The development of our knowledge about the specialized cells that regulate the immune system has exploded within the past few years. Among the substances we've discovered are hormone-like proteins called interleukins, which modify the function of immune cells. These molecules are produced by white blood cells, and we are only beginning to understand how interleukins act under normal circumstances and how their functions alter with disease. We hope eventually to be able to manipulate specialized immune cell regulators such as interleukins and administer them by injection the way we now administer human hormones to control various diseases. Once we fully understand the role of interleukins, we may also be able to design drugs that mimic their actions or alter their levels in the body.

Another area of interest is the study of a series of proteins called adhesion molecules that are found on the surface of white blood cells. These molecules make the cells sticky and allow them to migrate across blood vessels and attach at sites of inflammation. Adhesion molecules are thought to play an important role in maintaining inflammation and are found in high concentrations in inflamed synovium. We are trying to develop agents that will block the function of adhesion molecules so that inflammatory cells don't settle in the joints, causing pain and possible joint injury.

The Brain

We have known for a long time that the nervous system has an impact on many diseases, including rheumatoid arthritis and lupus. It has become increasingly clear that many substances in the brain affect immune cell function and vice versa. This opens up whole new avenues for therapy. As I mentioned earlier, animal studies indicate that an individual's response to stress is under genetic control and can affect the natural production of cortisol, a steroid that can reduce inflammation. We are studying ways to manipulate brain function, using both psychological techniques and medications, to see how brain substances can affect the immune system.

Viruses

By studying the viruses associated with AIDS, scientists now know that certain viruses can have profound effects on the immune system and can lead to diseases that resemble inflammatory arthritis. In certain animal species, slow-acting viruses called lentiviruses can also lead to a disease that resembles inflammatory arthritis. Scientists are investigating these and other viruses that may act as environmental triggers in people genetically susceptible to arthritis.

Cartilage

Many of the approaches we've discussed so far have to do with inflammatory forms of arthritis. Research is also being conducted into the degenerative diseases of joint and bone. The study of the properties of cartilage, for example, may hold the key to new approaches to the prevention and treatment of osteoarthritis.

Some people mistakenly think that osteoarthritis is a bone disease, because the term *osteo* means bone. OA actually involves the erosion of cartilage, the substance that normally protects the ends of the bones. In the normal joint, cartilage is constantly breaking down and being replaced. This process may be disturbed in some people with OA.

Cartilage has extraordinary mechanical properties that results from its complex structure. Scientists are studying the structure of cartilage and are trying to identify the cells involved in normal cartilage metabolism. They are trying to understand why cartilage metabolism appears to become unbalanced in osteoarthritis, resulting in more cartilage breakdown than repair. When these processes are better understood, whole new treatment therapies may be developed.

Research is also needed to define the relationship between the long-term impact of exercise and osteoarthritis. Some people worry that strenuous exercise will lead to later joint problems, but that hasn't really been proven. With the recent exercise boom, however, we'll have a good opportunity to study the long-term effects of exercise on OA. We'll begin to learn which types of exercise may be potentially harmful and which may be beneficial. As we study the long-term effects of exercise on this generation, we'll have a better idea of the consequences of activity and can establish sensible recommendations.

Bone Metabolism

Osteoporosis, when it appears alone or when it is associated with some forms of arthritis, is another focus of ongoing research. Patients with osteoporosis experience an excessive loss of bone, which puts them at risk for fractures and breaks. Scientists are trying to find out why people with osteoporosis seem to lose bone at an increased rate. We are studying the normal activities of cells responsible for bone growth and breakdown so that we may one day be able to modify bone metabolism.

Osteoporosis can sometimes be a side effect of steroid therapy; we're also trying to come up with better ways to use steroid drugs so that we may prevent this complication.

This bone disease affects mainly women and can take many years to develop. One emphasis in research is on preventive measures. We already have a sense about the things we can do to avoid osteoporosis. Sufficient calcium intake and weight-bearing exercise early in life appears to promote denser, healthier bones; this seems to provide a margin of safety for the later years, when bone loss accelerates, especially in women after menopause. Women today seem to be consciously exercising more; such activities are probably going to help prevent this disease. More studies will be directed toward establishing the precise role of diet and exercise in osteoporosis.

Osteoarthritis and osteoporosis are primarily diseases of older people;

they will undoubtedly receive more attention in the years to come as the population in this country continues to age.

Replacement Joints

We've certainly made dramatic strides in the field of joint replacement surgery, but more work needs to be done. As we operate on younger and younger patients, we will need to develop new kinds of artificial joints that will last longer and that are easier to replace.

Treatments

Scientists are constantly learning about new substances produced by various white blood cells to regulate the inflammatory process. With each new substance we identify, we have a potential new target for therapy—drugs that either increase its action or decrease its action.

In addition, computer modeling techniques now allow us to see the structure of inflammatory substances and their receptors in three dimensions. This technology enables us to learn how to block the actions of such substances and helps us design new drugs more quickly and precisely.

Animal models, which I discussed earlier, allow us to test new drugs safely. One of the most exciting advances has been the breeding of the SCID (severe combined immunodeficiency) mouse, which allows us to re-create a human immune system in a mouse. With the development of the SCID mouse, we can test the effects of various new drug agents on human cells without any danger to human life.

While we have many effective drug treatments for arthritis, we are seeking ways to use these drugs more safely and measures to prevent side effects. Scientists are also researching new treatments that will enable us to manipulate the immune system; these include the administration of interleukins and modifiers of immune cell function and removal of problem-causing cell types.

Diagnostic Tools

Currently, it can take many years to see the effects a particular treatment may have on the progress of your arthritis. Researchers are looking for simpler, more reliable, faster techniques to measure disease activity and determine whether a therapy is working. We hope to develop a blood test that can measure cartilage breakdown products and help diagnose osteoarthritis in its early stages. We are also looking at different ways to measure immune cell function so that we can measure the disease activity of lupus and rheumatoid arthritis. New advances in X-ray technology include magnetic resonance imaging (MRI), for example, which allows us to see erosions that don't show up on regular X-rays and may help us detect some forms of arthritis at earlier stages.

Educational Measures

Medical treatments are just one area of arthritis research. As practitioners, doctors also recognize how important it is to educate patients about their disease and to encourage their participation in self-care measures. Organizations such as the National Institutes of Health and the Arthritis Foundation seek to disseminate information about arthritis to medical consumers and help people cope with the daily emotional and physical challenges of chronic disease. Psychological techniques for coping with pain continue to be an exciting new field of exploration as an adjunct to drug therapies.

Future Prospects

Rheumatology is a vibrant, dynamic field that continues to change at a swift pace. The things we are learning about genetics and the immune system bring us closer than ever to an understanding of what causes arthritis. That means we are getting closer to new and better avenues for prevention and treatment. Our increased knowledge about the immune system is helpful not only to people with arthritis, but to those with other immune-related conditions, including cancer; endocrine diseases such as diabetes; AIDS; and neurological diseases such as multiple sclerosis. Conversely, research in all these related fields is bound to expand our knowledge about arthritis. I am quite optimistic that in the next several decades we will unlock many important doors in the field of rheumatology.

Epilogue:

A Good Life in Spite of Arthritis

I recently had the opportunity to attend the meeting of an arthritis support group: a group of patients had gathered to hear a nurse talk about living with arthritis. The nurse told the group that adjustment to any disease may at first be difficult, because it may mean a change in your lifestyle and in your usual activities. Everyone goes through this adaptation process somewhat differently, within his or her own time frame, but most people ultimately make a good adjustment.

Your first reaction upon learning that you have any disease is usually denial, she said. You may think, "Oh, no, not me. This can't be happening." Then slowly the realization will dawn on you that you have a condition that may require you to change how you live day to day. Understandably, you may feel angry or upset. You may want to know "Why me?" Finally you will probably come to understand and accept what you can and cannot do.

"Sometimes," said the nurse, "you have to admit to yourself, 'I'm annoyed, I don't feel so good, I hurt today.' At least say it to yourself, if not to others. And then you begin to sense that it's something you can deal with."

It helps to focus on the things you *can* do. You can take an active role in helping yourself to live well despite your condition. You can see to it that you learn as much as possible about your disease, get a thorough evaluation by a qualified physician, and avail yourself of the full medical care that's currently out there. You can look to friends or relatives for support, but ultimately you have to care for yourself, follow your treatment schedule, do your exercises, and take your medications.

Later, several of the participants in the support group talked about how they had adjusted to arthritis. One thirty-four-year-old woman with rheumatoid arthritis said that it took her several years to accept her disease, but that she's learned to "put it in its place." While not ignoring her arthritis, she doesn't let it take over. The mother of two young children, she's taken a part-time job as an administrative assistant at an advertising agency.

Another woman in her fifties with rheumatoid arthritis said that it took her a long time to realize that when she is mentally and physically active, she feels better. "I stopped focusing on my illness and decided to go out in the community and do some volunteer work at a day care center. And I feel much better for it."

The way you handle your arthritis probably depends as much on your personality as your condition. In my own practice, I see people handle their arthritis in various ways. Some focus all their attention on their disease, while others try to deny it entirely and may even abuse their bodies and disregard medical advice. Others find a happier medium: they pay attention to their illness and take good care of themselves, but try not to let it become the center of their lives.

You too have to find the delicate balance between denial and acceptance. Denial is an understandable reaction to disease, but it can make you delay seeking appropriate treatment. You should focus enough on your arthritis so that you get input from a medical team consisting of physicians, occupational therapists, physical therapists, and other health professionals who can help you reorganize your life, find a way around your limitations, and get the right medication.

On the other hand, it's disconcerting to see people focus so much on their illness that they close themselves off from life and deny its pleasures. You wouldn't sit idly by if someone you loved allowed himself to be consumed by an illness he could live with, so don't let it happen to you. I've had patients who let their illness dominate their relationships. Put your illness in its place and continue to go to work and enjoy yourself and lead as perfectly normal a life as possible. I have patients at Duke who have serious disease yet are actively working in a diverse number of fields—they're teachers, farmers, nurses, roofers, mechanics, lawyers, and doctors. Their work is very important to these people, for both financial and emotional reasons, and most manage very well to continue on the job, as well as to stay active in hobbies and family life.

It seems to me there is a relationship between your understanding of your arthritis and how well you manage it. If you educate yourself about your disease, you're more likely to weather its ups and downs and to understand the importance of taking your medication and its possible side effects. You're likely to put your problems into perspective, to interpret your symptoms better, and to understand when and when not to worry. So to a certain extent, the more you know, the better your response to your illness is likely to be.

Part of what you know about your condition will come from your own experience with your illness, from reading, and from talking to other people who share your condition. But one of the major sources of information is your doctor. I've emphasized throughout this book how important the doctor-patient relationship can be in arthritis treatment. In my own experience, I find that patients do better and feel better when their doctor takes time to sit down with them, listen to them, and provide them with information and reassurance. Most physicians have your interest at heart, care about you, and want to help you as much as they can.

Frequently the doctor-patient relationship is a very satisfying one; however, it isn't necessarily an easy one, because when you visit your doctor it's usually when you're unhappy or under stress. This imbalance of circumstances makes it an imperfect marriage. Doctors are often very busy people who see many patients and are under time limitations. They too are under stress, and they're not perfect, either. You have to trust your doctor's good intentions and expertise and work together to build a good relationship.

If there's a message I'd like to leave you with, it's that there is much to be done for you by physicians, nurses, occupational therapists, physical therapists, arthritis organizations, and supportive employers, family, and friends. There are many excellent therapies available based on state-of-the-art techniques. With proper medical evaluation, most forms of arthritis can be well managed. Even those conditions thought only a short time ago to be untreatable now have a good prognosis. And researchers are actively unraveling clues that promise new avenues for treatment and prevention.

Scientific knowledge about arthritis has rapidly expanded in recent decades; and if our recent progress is any yardstick, chances are excellent that advances in our understanding and treatment of arthritis will continue. This doesn't mean that that knowledge will be translated into therapy tomorrow, but there's great interest in research and many distinguished scientists are involved in the field. Several recent Nobel prizes have been awarded to scientists whose research has direct relevance to arthritis. New breakthroughs in the future seem inevitable. This is an area where you as a patient or relative of a patient might want to be involved. Medical research needs support and financing, especially during these times of spending restrictions. You may want to write to your representatives in Congress to express your support of this research or contribute to organizations such as the Arthritis Foundation that are active in promoting research.

Another area where we've made progress is in our understanding of disease prevention. While we don't know how to prevent all forms of arthritis, we can to some extent lessen the chances of developing certain conditions by changing our patterns of eating and exercise. We are beginning to appreciate the benefits of exercise not only as a cardiovascular conditioner, but also as a way of keeping our bones strong. Exercise and reasonable eating habits can also help you to avoid becoming overweight, possibly slowing down or preventing the wear and tear that can lead to osteoarthritis in your later years. It's important to develop a healthful lifestyle not because you're sick, but so that you don't *get* sick. If you start some of these habits when you're young, you'll lead a happier and better life, and that's really the bottom line.

Many of my patients tell me there's more in their lives than their disease. They've learned to go beyond their arthritis. I hope that you too will gain satisfaction from working with your doctor and doing all that you can to help yourself to a good life in spite of arthritis.

Frequently Asked Questions About Arthritis

Questions About Causes . . .

Does aging cause arthritis?
In general, people are more likely to get arthritis with advancing age, and it's likely that certain forms of the disease, particularly osteoarthritis, result from age-related changes to cartilage and the musculoskeletal system. Not every person who develops degenerative arthritis will have significant symptoms, however, and some forms of arthritis can occur at any age.

My mother had arthritis; will I get it too?
There is some evidence that a susceptibility to some forms of arthritis may be inherited. However, only a small percentage of genetically susceptible people will actually develop arthritis. This suggests that other factors, such as environment, also play a role in the disease.

Can children have arthritis?
Children can develop various forms of arthritis, collectively referred to as juvenile rheumatoid arthritis (JRA). Most children with JRA outgrow their disease by adulthood; a few do not. Treatment is similar to that for adults, except that some of the NSAIDs are not approved for children and corticosteroids are to be avoided, if possible, because they stunt physical growth.

Is arthritis caused by an infection?
Some forms of arthritis develop as a result of infections. These include rheumatic fever, Lyme disease, reactive arthritis, and arthritis that

appears after a viral illness. Extensive research has been conducted to try to pinpoint an infectious agent that might cause rheumatoid arthritis. So far no such agent has been found.

Can stress cause arthritis?
Though stress by itself does not appear to cause arthritis, there is some evidence that it may be one of the factors that contributes to its development and that it may worsen the perception of pain in arthritis sufferers. Learning to relax is therefore helpful for most patients.

Can jogging cause arthritis?
There is no evidence that moderate jogging, in the absence of injury, contributes to arthritis. However, a sports-related injury such as a torn cartilage, ripped tendon, or fracture can lead to long-term musculoskeletal damage, especially if you continue to use the affected joint excessively and don't heed the warning signs.

Are tendonitis and bursitis forms of arthritis?
In common usage, the term *arthritis* is used to describe many different musculoskeletal problems throughout the body. The strict medical definition of arthritis, however, is "inflammation of the joints." According to this definition, tendonitis and bursitis are not considered to be forms of arthritis. Tendonitis is an inflammation of a tendon, frequently caused by excessive or abnormal use. Bursitis is an inflammation of a bursa, the small sac that cushions the tendons and muscles. Treatment of both involves the use of nonsteroidal anti-inflammatory drugs, rest, local application of heat, and sometimes injection of corticosteroids. While these conditions may go away, they can recur, especially if the predisposing activity is not modified.

I was told I had bursitis. Now the doctor says I have a frozen shoulder. What is that?
A frozen shoulder is a condition characterized by a loss of shoulder movement. It frequently follows an inflammation or injury that prevents you from moving your shoulder for a prolonged period of time. Bursitis, if it is painful and prevents shoulder motion, may lead to this condition. The medical term for frozen shoulder is adhesive capsulitis; the word *adhesive* refers to the small scars or adhesions that form, making movement difficult and painful. A frozen shoulder is treated with physical therapy, with NSAIDs, and sometimes with local injections of corticosteroids.

What is Lyme disease?
Lyme disease is an infectious form of arthritis transmitted by a tick that infests deer. It is named after the town of Lyme, Connecticut, where this disease was first observed. The first symptom is a characteristic skin rash followed by joint pain and fever. Lyme disease generally responds to antibiotics and usually disappears after a number of weeks or months.

Questions About Remedies and Daily Living . . .

Will moving to a warm climate improve my arthritis?
Many people say their arthritis feels better when the weather is warm or dry, though there are patients who find that excessive heat or cold worsens their symptoms. We don't know why certain climatic conditions make some people feel better, but we don't feel that the weather itself causes arthritis. It is unlikely that moving to a warm climate will alter the course of your disease, although it may make you feel more comfortable.

Can avoidance of certain foods influence arthritis?
Physicians believe in the value of a healthy, well-balanced diet for everyone, but there is no scientific evidence that any specific diet will help cure arthritis. Excess weight can add stress to joints, however, so maintaining a body weight as close to ideal as possible is recommended. A diet low in saturated fat and cholesterol should help you do this.

I have heard that fish oils are good for arthritis. Should I increase my intake?
Evidence suggests that fish oils may reduce atherosclerosis (hardening of the arteries) and may also benefit people with arthritis, but at present there are no long-term studies confirming the benefits of fish-oil supplements. Increasing the amount of fish in the diet appears to make good sense nutritionally.

Will nutritional supplements help my arthritis?
A well-balanced diet that provides adequate vitamins and minerals is essential for everyone's good health and is especially important for those with chronic disease. If you have such a diet, you probably don't need to take nutritional supplements. There are some conditions, such as iron-deficiency anemia, that do call for supplementation. Be sure to consult your doctor before taking any nutritional supplements.

Is exercise good for arthritis?
Range-of-motion exercises, prescribed by your physician or physical therapist, should be done regularly, to help keep your joints mobile. Other types of regular exercise, such as walking or bicycling, are useful for everyone, even for people with arthritis, providing that they can tolerate it within the limits of their disease. You should discuss with your doctor the type of activities that are best for you and exercise within sensible limits.

Can wearing copper bracelets help arthritis?
There is no evidence that copper bracelets are helpful in arthritis (they are considered to be unproven remedies), but wearing them seems harmless. While these bracelets don't appear to have any benefits, it's interesting to note that some of the drugs used to treat arthritis contain metal. Gold is a metal and penicillamine may be activated by the copper present in the body.

Will heat applications provide pain relief?
Heat applications, such as heating pads, can produce temporary relief of local pain. Some RA patients find that a warm shower in the morning helps to ease morning stiffness. An electric blanket may also provide warmth and has the benefit of being lightweight. However, heat applications are sometimes inappropriate, especially when joints are inflamed. Consult your doctor before using heat.

Should I use Ben Gay for arthritis pain?
Ben Gay (and related preparations that go by a variety of brand names) is a cream or gel containing methyl salicylate (a relative of aspirin) and oil of wintergreen (menthol). It produces local warmth and can temporarily alleviate pain. It can be useful for minor muscle pains but is not part of the long-term therapy of arthritis.

Does DMSO work for arthritis?
DMSO, a chemical solvent that some people apply to their skin to alleviate joint pain, is not an approved treatment for any form of arthritis and can be classified as an unproven remedy.

If I have arthritis, can I drink alcohol?
Alcohol can interact with many medications, causing undesirable side effects; for example, alcohol can cause gastric irritation and bleeding, which can exacerbate some of the side effects of NSAIDs. Alcohol is also

a contributing factor to gout. Physicians are concerned about problems associated with excessive alcohol intake and are recommending that all patients restrict its use.

Should I bandage an arthritic joint with an Ace bandage?
Such bandages are useful to restrict motion when you sprain an ankle or another joint, but doctors do not usually recommend their use in arthritis. If such immobilization is helpful, you need a splint made by a professional.

I have been told I have arthritis in my neck and notice that some people wear special collars. Can they be helpful?
Neck collars can relieve neck pain for people with arthritis by limiting motion. Do not buy a collar without getting professional advice.

Questions About Drugs . . .

What is an OTC drug?
OTC is short for "over the counter" and refers to drugs that may be purchased without prescription.

What is a generic drug?
When a drug is first developed, it is patented and the manufacturer has the exclusive right to sell it. Such proprietary (meaning belonging to somebody) drugs are usually expensive because the costs of the research leading to their discovery and development have to be recouped. After a number of years, the patent runs out and other drug companies can manufacture the same drug, sometimes at lower costs. It is then referred to as a generic drug. To get FDA approval, a generic drug must be proven to be equivalent to the proprietary drug in efficacy and metabolism; it is usually cheaper.

What is arthritis-strength aspirin?
Arthritis-strength aspirin contains more aspirin per tablet than the standard dose (about one and a half times the amount). When used as the label recommends, however, it is unlikely to provide adequate anti-inflammatory levels in the blood to alleviate the symptoms of arthritis.

Should I use Tylenol instead of aspirin? I've heard it's safer.
Tylenol (acetaminophen) is a different medication from aspirin. It does

not irritate your stomach the way aspirin may. Tylenol relieves pain but not inflammation and is not useful when an anti-inflammatory drug is required.

Aspirin helps my arthritis, but it irritates my stomach. Is there anything I can do?
There are various aspirin preparations—some buffered, others coated—that reduce stomach problems. In addition, it's best to take aspirin with your meals. Sometimes taking an antacid with aspirin helps.

I've read that steroids may have harmful side effects, but I've also heard that they can be helpful. Should I take them?
Steroids are powerful drugs that can be of significant benefit in the treatment of arthritis when used at low doses or for short periods of time. Sometimes steroids are used for longer periods and at higher doses to treat serious inflammatory diseases such as lupus or polymyositis. In such cases, it is felt that the benefits of suppressing inflammation outweigh the risks of potentially serious side effects. Discuss the risks and benefits with your doctor.

My doctor prescribed methotrexate for my arthritis. Isn't this a drug used to treat cancer?
Methotrexate has been used to treat psoriasis and cancer. It has recently been approved for treatment of rheumatoid arthritis as well and is marketed under the name Rheumatrex. Methotrexate is used increasingly by many physicians for severe, progressive rheumatoid arthritis that fails to respond to NSAIDs.

Can antibiotics be used to treat arthritis?
A number of doctors have advocated the treatment of many different kinds of arthritis with antibiotics. We have no definite proof that antibiotics are of benefit in the treatment of rheumatoid arthritis, despite our interest in the possibility that infection may cause the disease. Other forms of arthritis, such as Lyme disease, clearly respond well to antibiotics.

The drugs used to treat arthritis are expensive. Any suggestions?
The personal cost of drugs to patients depends on the nature of their health care coverage. Some plans include the cost of prescription medicine, although you may have to meet a deductible. You can also obtain savings if you are a member of an organization such as the American Association of Retired Persons, which has a mail-in pharmacy service.

Questions About Symptoms . . .

I have been told that I have rheumatoid arthritis. How long can I expect my symptoms to last?
This is hard to predict. In some patients, the disease goes away within a year, while others have it indefinitely. Rheumatoid arthritis may wax and wane over time, and you may have flares, when you may feel worse, and periods of remission, when you feel better. The severity of the disease also varies from patient to patient.

I frequently feel tired. What can I do?
Fatigue is a symptom of most forms of inflammatory arthritis. Additional rest is part of the treatment. When working, whether at home or on the job, try to divide your work load into a series of smaller tasks and to balance periods of work and rest. Your aim should be to rest *before* you feel overly fatigued.

I have bony swellings on my knuckles and fingers. Will they eventually go away?
These are called Heberden's or Bouchard's nodes, and they are a sign of osteoarthritis. Although usually painless, they may become inflamed and tender. An NSAID such as aspirin will usually relieve the pain. The nodes usually become less swollen and tender, but they do not go away. Development of nodes is hereditary.

Is there something I can wear to keep my fingers from drifting?
Yes. Resting splints designed for you by a physical therapist can be useful. Splints can be worn at night or during the day.

How can I remain informed about new developments in arthritis care?
Every two months the Arthritis Foundation publishes a magazine entitled *Arthritis Today*. For information, write or call your local arthritis chapter or the national office listed in the Helpful Resources section of this book.

Helpful Resources

The Arthritis Foundation

The Arthritis Foundation is the leading national organization devoted to promoting research and education on all forms of arthritis. The Foundation provides patients with information and support through local arthritis self-help workshops, patient support groups, lending libraries, lectures, and literature. The Arthritis Foundation publishes self-help materials and distributes an excellent series of patient brochures on various topics relating to arthritis. Local chapters work to raise funds for training of physicians and scientists and investigation into the causes, treatment, and prevention of all forms of arthritis.

To avail yourself of services available in your area, contact your local Arthritis Foundation, or write or call:

THE ARTHRITIS FOUNDATION
1314 Spring Street
Atlanta, GA 30309
(404) 872-7100

Other Organizations

There are a number of other national organizations that provide educational literature on arthritis. You may wish to write to them for additional information.

Ankylosing Spondylitis
ANKYLOSING SPONDYLITIS ASSOCIATION
511 North La Cienega
Suite 216
Los Angeles, CA 90048
1-800-777-8189

Juvenile Arthritis
AMERICAN JUVENILE ARTHRITIS ASSOCIATION
1314 Spring Street
Atlanta, GA 30309
(404) 872-7100

Lupus
THE AMERICAN LUPUS SOCIETY
23751 Madison Street
Torrance, CA 90505
(213) 373-1335

L.E. SUPPORT CLUB (LUPUS ERYTHEMATOSUS)
8039 Nova Court
North Charleston, SC 29418
(803) 764-1769

LUPUS FOUNDATION OF AMERICA
1717 Massachusetts Avenue N.W., Suite 203
Washington, DC 20036
(202) 328-4550

LUPUS NETWORK
230 Ranch Drive
Bridgeport, CT 06606
(203) 372-5795

NATIONAL LUPUS ERYTHEMATOSUS FOUNDATION
5430 Van Nuys Boulevard, Suite 206
Van Nuys, CA 91401
(818) 885-8787

Scleroderma
SCLERODERMA ASSOCIATION
P.O. Box 910
Lynnfield, MA 01940
(508) 535-6600

SCLERODERMA FEDERATION
1725 York Avenue #29F
New York, NY 10128
(212) 427-7040

SCLERODERMA INTERNATIONAL FOUNDATION
704 Gardner Center Road
New Castle, PA 16101
(412) 652-3109

SCLERODERMA RESEARCH FOUNDATION
Box 200
Columbus, NJ 08022
(609) 261-2200

UNITED SCLERODERMA FOUNDATION
P.O. Box 350
Watsonville, CA 95077
(408) 728-2202

Sjögren's Syndrome
SJÖGREN'S SYNDROME FOUNDATION
29 Gateway Drive
Great Neck, NY 11021
(516) 487-2243

Glossary

ALLOPURINOL: A drug used to prevent gout attacks by blocking uric acid formation.

ANA: *See* antinuclear antibody.

ANALGESIC: A class of drugs that primarily relieves pain. Acetaminophen (Tylenol) is a good example.

ANKYLOSING SPONDYLITIS: A type of arthritis that primarily affects the spine and sacroiliac joints. Tendons and ligaments may become inflamed where they attach to the bone. Advanced forms may result in formation of bony bridges, causing the spine to become rigid.

ANTIBODY: A type of blood protein made by the body in response to a foreign substance (antigen); its purpose is to bind to that antigen and eliminate it from the body.

ANTI-DNA: Antibodies to DNA often produced by people with lupus. A useful diagnostic marker for lupus. Levels of anti-DNA generally rise and fall with disease activity, making this a good monitoring tool for lupus as well.

ANTIGEN: Any substance that the body regards as foreign or potentially dangerous and that results in production of an antibody.

ANTINUCLEAR ANTIBODY (ANA): Antibodies to the cell nucleus found in people with many connective tissue diseases, including lupus, rheumatoid arthritis, scleroderma, and polymyositis. Their presence is considered a marker of the disease.

ANTI-SM: Antibodies to Sm, a substance found in the cell's nucleus. Almost exclusively seen in lupus patients and therefore useful in diagnosis.

ARTERITIS: An inflammation of the walls of the arteries.

ARTHRITIS: A disease often involving inflammation of the joints. In common usage, any of many conditions causing pain and inflammation in tendons, ligaments, joints, and muscles.

ARTHRODESIS: A surgical procedure that fuses joint bones together into a "fixed" position, usually performed for pain relief.

ARTHROPLASTY: A surgical procedure involving joint reconstruction using the patient's own tissues as well as artificial joint components. Most arthroplasties involve total joint replacement with a man-made prosthesis.

ARTHROSCOPY: Examination of the inside of a joint through a slender fiberoptic instrument (an endoscope) inserted through a small incision. Arthroscopy is used commonly in diagnosing and treating sports-related injuries or for minor surgical repairs, such as removal of small pieces of torn or loose cartilage.

AUTOIMMUNE DISEASE: A disease caused by a malfunctioning of the immune system in which the body appears to attack its own tissues.

BIOPSY: Removal of a small piece of living tissue for microscopic examination.

BOUCHARD'S NODES: Bony enlargements in the middle joints of the fingers that may occur in patients with osteoarthritis.

BURSA: A fibrous sac that acts as a small cushion between muscles and bones. It is lined with a membrane that releases fluid and permits muscles, tendons, and bones to slide over each other.

BURSITIS: Inflammation of a bursa.

CARTILAGE: A resilient material that cushions the ends of the bones so they don't rub against each other.

CHEMISTRIES: Blood tests that measure the concentrations of various chemicals in the plasma.

COLCHICINE: A drug used to treat gout and prevent future attacks.

COLLAGEN: The principal component of cartilage and other connective tissue.

COMPLEMENT: A complex set of proteins that helps the body fight foreign substances and that becomes activated when antibodies bind to antigens. Depressed levels may indicate the presence of immune complexes and can be used to help determine disease activity in lupus.

COMPLETE BLOOD COUNT: A diagnostic test that measures blood components, including white blood cells, red blood cells, and platelets.

CONNECTIVE TISSUE: Tissue found throughout the body that supports and connects other tissues and body organs.

CONTRACTURE: A joint deformity caused by loss of joint motion and shortening of the surrounding tissues. May be prevented by daily stretching exercises. Also called a flexion contracture.

CORTICOSTEROIDS: Potent and effective drugs related to the hormone cortisol that quickly reduce swelling and inflammation.

CPK TEST (CREATIVE PHOSPHOKINASE TEST): A blood test to determine muscle damage. When muscles are damaged, CPK, an enzyme found mainly in muscles, leaks into the bloodstream, causing CPK levels to rise.

CPPD DISEASE: A form of arthritis induced by crystals of a salt called calcium pyrophosphate dihydrate (CPPD) that are deposited in the joints. Pseudogout is one form of CPPD disease.

CREATININE TEST: A diagnostic test that measures the presence of creatinine, a normal waste product, in the blood. Excess levels may indicate possible kidney problems.

CREST SYNDROME: A milder form of scleroderma, generally more contained.

CYTOTOXIC DRUG: A drug that kills dividing cells.

DERMATOMYOSITIS: A disease involving muscle weakness and inflammation, accompanied by a rash. *See also* polymyositis.

ELECTROMYOGRAM (EMG): A test that measures electrical activity of the muscle. It helps to distinguish between muscle weakness caused by nerve damage and that caused by muscle fiber damage.

ENTHESIS: An attachment structure; the place where tendons and ligaments are anchored to the bone.

EROSION: A wearing away of areas of bone or cartilage caused by synovitis, most usually in rheumatoid arthritis. A sign of joint damage that may predispose to deformity.

ERYTHROCYTE SEDIMENTATION RATE (ESR): A diagnostic test that measures the rate at which red blood cells fall to the bottom of a tube. Red blood cells settle more quickly in the presence of inflammation. Also known as the sed rate.

FASCIA: Bands or sheets of connective tissue that surround muscles.

FIBROMYALGIA: *See* fibrositis.

FIBROSITIS: A disease involving pain in muscles or joints with no clinical signs of inflammation. Linked to stress and certain compulsive, hard-driving personality types.

FLEXION CONTRACTURE: *See* contracture.

FLUORESCENT ANTINUCLEAR ANTIBODY (FANA): A diagnostic test to measure antinuclear antibodies in the cell nucleus, revealed microscopically by the addition of a fluorescent dye.

FUNGAL ARTHRITIS: A rare and slowly progressing arthritis caused by fungi, a type of microorganism found in plants and soil, among other places.

FUSION (OF BONES): *See* arthrodesis.

GIANT CELL ARTERITIS: An inflammatory condition involving the arteries that sometimes accompanies polymyalgia rheumatica.

GONOCOCCAL ARTHRITIS: A common form of infectious arthritis, caused by the same bacteria that cause gonorrhea.

GOUT: A form of arthritis caused by deposits of monosodium urate crystals in the joint. Gout usually strikes a single joint with a sudden, violent onset.

HEBERDEN'S NODE: A knobby enlargement of the joint of the finger nearest to the fingertip in patients with osteoarthritis.

HUMAN LEUKOCYTE ANTIGENS (HLA): Also known as histocompatibility antigens, these genetic markers may be associated with a predisposition to certain forms of arthritis. HLA-B27 is associated with an increased risk for developing ankylosing spondylitis and Reiter's syndrome. HLA-DR4 is associated with rheumatoid arthritis.

HYPERURICEMIA: Excess levels of uric acid in the blood, sometimes associated with gout but also with other conditions such as kidney dysfunction or use of diuretics. Not diagnostic of gout.

IMMUNOSUPPRESSIVE DRUGS: Potent drugs that decrease immune responses. Some are cytotoxic—that is, they kill dividing cells. Immunosuppressive drugs include Imuran and Cytoxan. Some doctors place methotrexate within this group, too. Can be used in treatment of rheumatoid arthritis, but more commonly for more severe inflammatory problems such as lupus and vasculitis.

INFLAMMATION: A reaction to injury or infection resulting in redness, heat, swelling, pain, and loss of function in the affected area.

JOINT: The structure in the body where two bones come together. Allows varying kinds and degrees of motion.

JOINT ASPIRATION: Removal of joint fluid.

JOINT CAPSULE: A fibrous capsule encasing joint contents, including the ends of the bones and cartilage. Also called the synovial sac.

JUVENILE RHEUMATOID ARTHRITIS (JRA): A term used to describe several types of arthritis that can occur in childhood. Also called juvenile arthritis.

LE TEST: A diagnostic test for lupus erythematosus that measures the presence of an antibody to the cell nucleus. This test has been supplanted by antinuclear antibody testing, which is easier to perform.

LIGAMENTS: Thick, cord-like fibers that are anchored to bones to keep them in correct alignment.

LYME DISEASE: A joint infection caused by bacteria transmitted by a tick that infests a variety of animals, including deer, mice, and domestic animals such as dogs.

MAJOR HISTOCOMPATIBILITY COMPLEX (MHC): A closely linked set of genes, called HLA in man, recognized initially in its role in determining organ transplant acceptance. Now recognized as the set of genes that regulates the immune system. MHC appears to be involved in some forms of inflammatory arthritis. See human leukocyte antigens.

MUSCLES: Elastic tissues with contractile properties that support the joint and allow all bodily movement.

NODULE: An accumulation of inflammatory tissue under the skin commonly seen in rheumatoid arthritis. Their presence may denote a more serious disease pattern.

NONGONOCOCCAL INFECTIOUS ARTHRITIS: A form of arthritis caused by bacteria other than gonococci that spread through the bloodstream to the joints.

NONSTEROIDAL ANTI-INFLAMMATORY DRUGS (NSAIDS): A class of drugs that includes aspirin and is useful in reducing pain and inflammation for virtually all types of arthritis.

OCCUPATIONAL THERAPIST: A licensed practitioner who helps to evaluate the impact of arthritis on daily activities at home and on the job. Occupational therapists can help devise ways of performing tasks that put less stress on joints and can design and prescribe splints and assistive devices.

OPHTHALMOLOGIST: A physician who specializes in eye disease.

ORTHOPEDIC SURGEON: A physician who specializes in surgery of the musculoskeletal system, its joints, and related structures.

OSSIFICATION: The transformation of tissues into bone-like substances. In ankylosing spondylitis, ossification may cause the spine to become rigid.

OSTEOARTHRITIS: A degenerative arthritis caused by a change in the nature of the cartilage, possibly from wear and tear to a joint over time. Movement of an affected joint may be stiff and painful.

OSTEOPHYTES: In osteoarthritis, small bony growths that form at the ends of bone at joints where the cartilage has degenerated.

OSTEOPOROSIS: A condition resulting in the thinning of bones and an increased susceptibility to fractures.

OSTEOTOMY: A surgical procedure during which bone is surgically removed to allow realignment in a better position.

PAUCIARTICULAR DISEASE: An arthritis that involves only a few joints, most commonly referring to a form of juvenile arthritis that affects four or fewer joints.

PHYSIATRIST: A physician certified in rehabilitative medicine.

PHYSICAL THERAPIST: A licensed professional involved in the physical aspects of medical illness and a specialist in the use of exercise to treat physical conditions. The physical therapist can also prescribe splints, canes, and special shoes.

POLYARTICULAR DISEASE: Any type of arthritis that affects more than five joints. The term is sometimes used to delineate a form of juvenile arthritis that is most similar to adult rheumatoid arthritis.

POLYMYALGIA RHEUMATICA (PMR): An inflammatory condition that involves severe muscle pain and stiffness in the neck, shoulders, and hips. Not usually associated with obvious signs of joint inflammation. Responds promptly to corticosteroids. Sometimes accompanied by a more serious blood vessel involvement (*see* giant cell arteritis).

POLYMYOSITIS: A disease of muscle weakness resulting from an inflammation of the muscle tissues. Sometimes accompanied by a rash (*see* dermatomyositis).

PROSTAGLANDINS: Chemicals in the body that appear to play a key role in inflammation.

PSEUDOGOUT: A crystal-induced arthritis clinically similar to gout. *See* CPPD disease.

PSORIATIC ARTHRITIS: A form of arthritis that accompanies the skin condition psoriasis.

RANGE OF MOTION: A quantifiable range of normal movement for each joint, used to measure the severity of arthritis and the presence of contractures. Term also applied to a type of exercise.

RAYNAUD'S PHENOMENON: An extreme sensitivity to the cold and to emotional upsets that may cause a narrowing of the blood vessels of the fingers and a burning, tingling, and numbness.

REACTIVE ARTHRITIS: A form of arthritis that arises as a reaction to certain types of infections. Reiter's disease is an example.

REITER'S SYNDROME: An inflammation of joints that often follows severe intestinal or genital/urinary tract infections, although it may occur with no evidence of previous infection. Also called a reactive arthritis because the joint inflammation appears to be a reaction to an infection elsewhere in the body.

REMITTIVE DRUGS: A group of drugs used primarily to treat rheumatoid arthritis when other, less potent drugs fail. Also called second-line, slow-acting, or disease-modifying drugs. Included in this group are gold, penicillamine, Plaquenil, and methotrexate.

RESECTION: The surgical removal of all or part of a damaged bone to relieve pain.

RHEUMATIC FEVER: A systemic illness that usually follows a streptococcal infection and which, if untreated, may result in a migratory type of arthritis.

RHEUMATISM: An imprecise term sometimes used to describe conditions that cause pain and swelling in joints and surrounding supportive tissues, ligaments, and muscles.

RHEUMATOID FACTOR (RF): An antibody found in large amounts in the blood of people with rheumatoid arthritis. Its presence in the blood is a useful diagnostic tool.

RHEUMATOLOGIST: A physician who specializes in the diagnosis and treatment of arthritis.

SALICYLISM: A condition associated with excessive doses of salicylate-containing drugs. Symptoms include tinnitus (ringing in the ears), hearing loss, mental confusion, excitability, and abnormal breathing.

SCLERODACTYLY: In scleroderma, a thickening of the skin of the fingers.

SCLERODERMA: A relatively rare systemic form of arthritis in which the body produces too much collagen. Excess collagen may be deposited in the skin, joints, and other body organs.

SED RATE: *See* erythrocyte sedimentation rate (ESR).

SPURS: Bony growths seen in people with osteoarthritis.

STEROID DRUGS: *See* corticosteroids.

STILL'S DISEASE: A form of juvenile arthritis that often involves high fevers, rash, and enlargement of the spleen and lymph nodes.

SYNDESMOPHYTE: In ankylosing spondylitis, a bony bridge that forms between vertebrae of the spine.

SYNOVECTOMY: Surgical removal of diseased synovium or joint lining.

SYNOVIAL FLUID: A viscous, clear fluid produced by the synovial membrane that acts as a lubricant for the joints.

SYNOVIAL MEMBRANE: The lining of the inside of a joint.

SYNOVIAL SAC: *See* joint capsule.

SYNOVITIS: An inflammation of the joint lining.

TELANGIECTASIAS: In scleroderma, fine networks of dilated blood vessels visible below the skin.

TENDONS: Strong bands of tissue that connect muscle to bone.

TISSUE TYPING: A technique used to identify major histocompatibility types, a set of genetic markers whose identification aids in organ transplantation. Sometimes useful in arthritis because of the association of certain tissue types with various forms of arthritis. *See* human leukocyte antigens *and* major histocompatibility complex.

TOPHI: Lumps under the skin from an accumulation of monosodium urate crystals, associated with gout.

TRIGGER POINTS: Certain places on muscles that appear exceptionally tender to touch in people with fibrositis. Also known as tender points.

URIC ACID: A waste product normally present in the blood, resulting from the breakdown of purines. Excessive amounts can lead to crystal formation in the joints and gout.

URICOSURIC DRUGS: Drugs used to treat gout by increasing the excretion of uric acid in the urine.

URINALYSIS: A diagnostic test to measure the presence of red and white blood cells and/or protein in the urine.

VASCULITIS: Inflammation of blood vessels that causes tissue damage. Can be a component of other conditions or occur by itself.

VIRAL ARTHRITIS: A self-limited arthritis that disappears when the viral infection is cured.

Index

ABOUT THE AUTHORS

David S. Pisetsky, M.D., Ph.D., is Professor of Medicine and Assistant Professor of Immunology at Duke University Medical Center in Durham, North Carolina. He is also Chief of Rheumatology and Associate Chief of Staff for Education at the Durham Veterans Administration Hospital. Dr. Pisetsky graduated from Harvard College magna cum laude, and attended the Albert Einstein College of Medicine in the Bronx, where he earned his Ph.D. in molecular biology and his M.D. He served his internship and residency at the Yale–New Haven Hospital, and received further training in immunology as a clinical associate in the Immunology Branch of the National Cancer Institute in Bethesda, Maryland. He was certified in internal medicine in 1976 and joined the faculty at Duke University in 1978.

Among the many professional organizations with which he is affiliated are the American Association of Immunology, the American Federation of Clinical Research, the American Society of Clinical Investigation, and the American College of Rheumatology. He is also active in the Arthritis Foundation and serves on editorial boards for journals in the fields of immunology and rheumatology.

Dr. Pisetsky conducts research in arthritis and immunology and has published his findings in over a hundred articles and chapters in leading medical journals.

He lives in Durham, North Carolina, with his wife, Dr. Ingrid Buhler Pisetsky, a psychiatrist, and their two children, Michael and Emily.

Susan Flamholtz Trien is a writer who specializes in the health field. She has written extensively for national magazines and is author of two previous consumer health books for Ballantine/Fawcett: *The Menopause Handbook* and *Parent's Book of Breastfeeding*. Ms. Trien lives in Rochester, New York, with her husband, David, and their two children, Stacey and Adam.